## Your *Clinics* subscription just got better!

You can now access the full text of this *Clinics* title online at no additional cost! Activate your online subscription today and receive...

- Full text of all issues from 2002 to the present
- Photographs, tables, illustrations, and references
- Comprehensive search capabilities
- Links to MEDLINE and Elsevier journals

**Activate Your Online Access Today!**

Plus, you can also sign up for E-alerts of upcoming issues or articles that interest you, and take advantage of exclusive access to bonus features!

## To activate your individual online subscription:

1. Visit our website at **www.TheClinics.com**.
2. Click on "Register" at the top of the page, and follow the instructions.
3. To activate your account, you will need your subscriber account number, which you can find on your mailing label (note: the number of digits in your subscriber account number varies from six to ten digits). See the sample below where the subscriber account number has been circled.

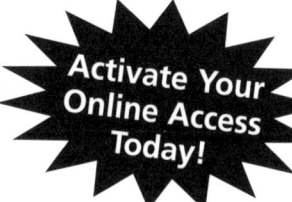

This is your subscriber account number

```
************************************3-DIGIT 001
FEB00  J0167  C7  (123456-89)  10/00  Q: 1

J.H. DOE, MD
531 MAIN ST
CENTER CITY, NY 10001-001
```

4. That's it! Your online access to the most trusted source for clinical reviews is now available.

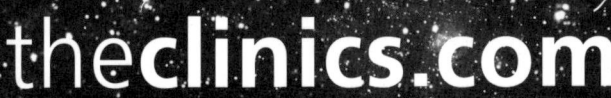
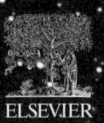

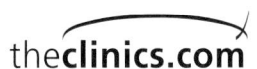

# INFECTIOUS DISEASE CLINICS OF NORTH AMERICA

Travel and Tropical Medicine

GUEST EDITORS
Frank J. Bia, MD, MPH
David R. Hill, MD, DTM&H

CONSULTING EDITOR
Robert C. Moellering, Jr, MD

March 2005 • Volume 19 • Number 1

**SAUNDERS**
An Imprint of Elsevier, Inc.
PHILADELPHIA   LONDON   TORONTO   MONTREAL   SYDNEY   TOKYO

**W.B. SAUNDERS COMPANY**
*A Division of Elsevier Inc.*

The Curtis Center • Independence Square West • Philadelphia, Pennsylvania 19106

http://www.theclinics.com

INFECTIOUS DISEASE CLINICS  Volume 19, Number 1
OF NORTH AMERICA  ISSN 0891–5520
March 2005  ISBN 1-4160-2667-3
Editor: Carin Davis

Copyright © 2005 by Elsevier Inc. All rights reserved. No part of this publication may be reproduced or transmitted in any form or by any means, electronic or mechanical, including photocopy, recording, or any information retrieval system, without written permission from the Publisher.

Single photocopies of single articles may be made for personal use as allowed by national copyright laws. Permission of the publisher and payment of a fee is required for all other photocopying, including multiple or systematic copying, copying for advertising or promotional purposes, resale, and all forms of document delivery. Special rates are available for educational institutions that wish to make photocopies for non-profit educational classroom use. Permissions may be sought directly from Elsevier Inc. Rights & Permissions Department, PO Box 800, Oxford OX5 1DX, UK; phone: (+44) 1865 843830, fax: (+44) 1865 853333, e-mail: permissions@elsevier.co.uk. You may also contact Rights & Permissions directly through Elsevier's home page (http://www.elsevier.com), selecting first 'Customer Support', then 'General Information', then 'Permissions Query Form'. In the USA, users may clear permissions and make payments through the Copyright Clearance Center, Inc., 222 Rosewood Drive, Danvers, MA 01923, USA; phone: (978) 750-8400, fax: (978) 750-4744, and in the UK through the Copyright Licensing Agency Rapid Clearance Service (CLARCS), 90 Tottenham Court Road, London WIP 0LP, UK; phone: (+44) 171 436 5931; fax: (+44) 171 436 3986. Other countries may have a local reprographic rights agency for payments.

The ideas and opinions expressed in *Infectious Disease Clinics of North America* do not necessarily reflect those of the Publisher. The Publisher does not assume any responsibility for any injury and/or damage to persons or property arising out of or related to any use of the material contained in this periodical. The reader is advised to check the appropriate medical literature and the product information currently provided by the manufacturer of each drug to be administered to verify the dosage, the method and duration of administration, or contraindications. It is the responsibility of the treating physician or other health care professional, relying on independent experience and knowledge of the patient, to determine drug dosages and the best treatment for the patient. Mention of any product in this issue should not be construed as endorsement by the contributors, editors, or the Publisher of the product or manufacturers' claims.

*Infectious Disease Clinics of North America* (ISSN 0891–5520) is published in March, June, September, and December (For Post Office use only: volume 19 issue 1 of 4) by W.B. Saunders Company. Corporate and editorial offices: The Curtis Center, Independence Square West, Philadelphia, PA 19106-3399. Accounting and circulation offices: 6277 Sea Harbor Drive, Orlando, FL 32887-4800. Periodicals postage paid at Orlando, FL 32862, and additional mailing offices. Subscription prices are $165.00 per year for US individuals, $272.00 per year for US institutions, $83.00 per year for US students, $196.00 per year for Canadian individuals, $328.00 per year for Canadian institutions, $215.00 per year for international individuals, $328.00 per year for international institutions, and $108.00 per year for Canadian and foreign students. To receive student rate, orders must be accompanied by name of affiliated institution, date of term, and the *signature* of program/residency coordinator on institution letterhead. Orders will be billed at individual rate until proof of status is received. Foreign air speed delivery is included in all *Clinics* subscription prices. All prices are subject to change without notice. POSTMASTER: Send address changes to *Infectious Disease Clinics of North America*, W.B. Saunders Company, Periodicals Fulfillment, Orlando, FL 32887-4800. **Customer Service: 1-800-654-2452 (US). From outside of the US, call 1-407-345-4000. E-mail: hhspcs@wbsaunders.com**

*Infectious Disease Clinics of North America* is also published in Spanish by Editorial Inter-Médica, Junin 917, 1$^{er}$ A 1113, Buenos Aires, Argentina.

Reprints. For copies of 100 or more, of articles in this publication, please contact the Commercial Reprints Department, Elsevier Inc., 360 Park Avenue South, New York, New York 10010-1710. Tel. (212) 633-3813 Fax: (212) 462-1935 email: reprints@elsevier.com

*Infectious Disease Clinics of North America* is covered in *Index Medicus, Current Contents/Clinical Medicine, Science Citation Alert, SCISEARCH, and Research Alert.*

Printed in the United States of America.

TRAVEL AND TROPICAL MEDICINE

## CONSULTING EDITOR

**ROBERT C. MOELLERING, Jr, MD,** Herrman L. Blumgart Professor of Medical Research, Harvard Medical School; and Physician-in-Chief and Chairman, Department of Medicine, Beth Israel Deaconess Medical Center, Boston, Massachusetts

## GUEST EDITORS

**FRANK J. BIA, MD, MPH,** Professor of Medicine and Laboratory Medicine and Co-Director, International Health Program, Department of Medicine, Yale School of Medicine, New Haven, Connecticut

**DAVID R. HILL, MD, DTM&H,** Director, National Travel Health Network and Centre; Honorary Professor, London School of Hygiene and Tropical Medicine, London, England

## CONTRIBUTORS

**ALBERTO M. ACOSTA, MD, PhD,** Medical Director, Traveler's Medical Service of New York; Clinical Assistant Professor of Medicine, Weill Medical College of Cornell University; Assistant Attending Physician, The New York-Presbyterian Hospital, New York, New York

**REBECCA WOLFE ACOSTA, RN, MPH,** Executive Director, Traveler's Medical Service of New York, New York, New York

**SONIA Y. ANGELL, MD, MPH, DTM&H,** Director, Cardiovascular Disease Prevention and Control, New York City Department of Health and Mental Hygiene, New York, New York

**RON H. BEHRENS, MB, ChB, MD, FRCP,** Consultant in Tropical and Travel Medicine, Travel Clinic, Hospital for Tropical Diseases, London School of Hygiene and Tropical Medicine, London, United Kingdom

**FRANK J. BIA, MD, MPH,** Professor of Medicine and Laboratory Medicine and Co-Director, International Health Program, Department of Medicine, Yale School of Medicine, New Haven, Connecticut

**MICHAEL V. CALLAHAN, MD, MSPH, DTM&H,** Director, Biodefense and Mass Casualty Care, Center for Integration of Medicine and Innovative Technologies, Division of Infectious Diseases, Massachusetts General Hospital, Cambridge, Massachusetts

**MARTIN S. CETRON, MD,** Division of Global Migration and Quarantine, National Center for Infectious Diseases, Centers for Disease Control and Prevention; Department of Medicine, Emory University School of Medicine, Atlanta, Georgia

**LIN H. CHEN, MD, FACP,** Assistant Clinical Professor of Medicine, Harvard Medical School; Director of the Travel Medicine Center, Division of Infectious Diseases, Mount Auburn Hospital, Cambridge, Massachusetts

**PETER L. CHIODINI, MBBS, PhD, MRCS, FRCP, FRCPath,** Consultant Parasitologist, Department of Clinical Parasitology, The Hospital for Tropical Diseases; Honorary Professor, The London School of Hygiene & Tropical Medicine, London, United Kingdom

**RACHEL S. BARWICK EIDEX, PhD,** Division of Global Migration and Quarantine, National Center for Infectious Diseases, Centers for Disease Control and Prevention, Atlanta, Georgia

**HERMANN FELDMEIER, MD, PhD,** Professor of Tropical Medicine, Institute of Infection Medicine, Department of Microbiology, Charité-University Medicine Berlin, Berlin, Germany

**PHILIP R. FISCHER, MD,** Professor, Department of Pediatric and Adolescent Medicine, Mayo Clinic College of Medicine, Rochester, Minnesota

**DAVIDSON H. HAMER, MD, FACP,** Assistant Professor of International Health, Center for International Health and Development, Boston University School of Public Health, Boston; Adjunct Associate Professor of Nutrition, Gerald J. and Dorothy R. Friedman School of Nutrition Science and Policy, Tufts University, Massachusetts

**GUNDEL HARMS, MD, MPH, PhD,** Senior Lecturer in Tropical Medicine, Institute of Tropical Medicine, Charité-University Medicine Berlin, Berlin, Germany

**DAVID R. HILL, MD, DTM&H,** Director, National Travel Health Network and Centre; Honorary Professor, London School of Hygiene and Tropical Medicine, London, United Kingdom

**TOMAS JELINEK, MD, DTMP,** Berlin Institute of Tropical Medicine, Berlin Germany

**JAY S. KEYSTONE, MD, MSc (CTM), FRCPC,** Professor of Medicine, University of Toronto; Staff Physician, Center for Travel and Tropical Medicine, Toronto General Hospital, Toronto, Ontario, Canada

**PHYLLIS E. KOZARSKY, MD,** Division of Global Migration and Quarantine, National Center for Infectious Diseases, Centers for Disease Control and Prevention; Department of Medicine, Emory University School of Medicine, Atlanta, Georgia

**ALAN J. MAGILL, MD, FACP,** Science Director, Walter Reed Army Institute of Research, Silver Spring; Associate Professor of Medicine and Preventive Medicine and Biometrics, Uniformed Services University of the Health Sciences, Bethesda, Maryland

**LEONARD C. MARCUS, VMD, MD,** Consultant in Tropical Medicine, Parasitology and Travelers' Health, Travelers' Health & Immunization Services; Clinical Professor, Department of Environmental and Population Health, Tufts University School of Veterinary Medicine, North Grafton; Adjunct Associate Professor, Department of Medicine, University of Massachusetts School of Medicine, Worcester, Massachusetts

**ANTHONY A. MARFIN, MD, MPH,** Division of Vector-Borne Infectious Diseases, National Center for Infectious Diseases, Centers for Disease Control and Prevention, Fort Collins, Colorado

**JEANNE M. MARRAZZO, MD, MPH,** Associate Professor of Medicine, Division of Allergy and Infectious Diseases, University of Washington; Medical Director, Seattle STD/HIV Prevention Training Center, Seattle, Washington

**MARIA D. MILENO, MD,** Director, Travel Medicine Service, Miriam Hospital; Associate Professor, Brown Medical School, Providence, Rhode Island

**NIKOLAI MÜHLBERGER, DVM, MPH,** Berlin Institute of Tropical Medicine, Berlin, Germany

**GEOFFREY PASVOL, MA, MB, ChB, D Phil, FRCP, FRCPE,** Professor, Department of Infection and Tropical Medicine, Imperial College; Director, Wellcome Centre for Clinical Tropical Medicine, Imperial College, London, United Kingdom

**RICHARD J. POLLACK, PhD,** Instructor in Tropical Public Health, Laboratory of Public Health Entomology, Department of Immunology and Infectious Diseases, Harvard School of Public Health, Boston, Massachusetts

**DAVID R. SHLIM, MD,** Medical Director, Jackson Hole Travel and Tropical Medicine, Kelly, Wyoming

**MUHAMMAD R. SOHAIL, MD,** Fellow, Division of Infectious Disease, Department of Medicine, Mayo Clinic College of Medicine, Rochester, Minnesota

**KATHRYN N. SUH, MD, FRCPC,** Division of Infectious Diseases, Children's Hospital of Eastern Ontario; Assistant Professor of Paediatrics, University of Ottawa, Ottawa, Ontario, Canada

TRAVEL AND TROPICAL MEDICINE

# CONTENTS

**Dedication**
Alberto M. Acosta and Rebecca Wolfe Acosta — xiii

**Preface: Coming of Age in Travel Medicine and Tropical Diseases: A Need for Continued Advocacy and Mentorship**
David R. Hill and Frank J. Bia — xv

**Surveillance of Imported Diseases as a Window to Travel Health Risks** — 1
Tomas Jelinek and Nikolai Mühlberger

> Surveillance of imported infectious diseases can provide valuable information for potentially exposed travelers and for affected populations in endemic countries. Reliable data quality, fast data management, and immediate communication of reports to all involved partners are crucial. Clinical networks are in an excellent position to achieve this. TropNetEurop, the largest network worldwide for surveillance of imported infectious diseases, is presented as an example. This network collects information on malaria, dengue fever, and schistosomiasis. Regular summary reports benefit all network members and their clinical practice. Screening tools used by the network enable timely and efficient detection of sentinel events even from small report numbers.

**Challenging Scenarios in a Travel Clinic: Advising the Complex Traveler** — 15
Kathryn N. Suh and Maria D. Mileno

> As international and adventure travel continue to increase in popularity, so too does the spectrum of travelers. Extremes of age, pregnancy, disability, and underlying medical conditions no longer present formidable barriers to rewarding travel. These factors may influence the choice or administration of prophylactic medications and immunizations, however, and can significantly alter both

the risk of acquiring travel-related illnesses and their severity. With adequate planning and appropriate pretravel counseling provided by a qualified travel medicine expert, most travelers can still enjoy healthy and rewarding travel experiences.

## Risk Assessment and Disease Prevention in Travelers Visiting Friends and Relatives 49
Sonia Y. Angell and Ron H. Behrens

Travelers to developing regions for the purposes of visiting friends or relatives are at known increased risk for a number of travel-related illnesses, especially when compared with those traveling for other purposes. This article reviews the unique contributors to their infectious disease risks and provides recommendations for the prevention of selected high-risk illnesses. These include some diseases against which vaccination is routinely recommended during childhood, including also varicella and hepatitis A and B, as well as typhoid fever, malaria, and tuberculosis.

## Health Risks to Air Travelers 67
Muhammad R. Sohail and Philip R. Fischer

There are infrequent yet potentially important risks for air travelers. Good hand washing during flights and avoidance of close contact with sick patients decreases the risk of infection. Pretravel screening can help determine the need of supplemental oxygen. Acute medical conditions might prompt delays in travel until recovery is established. Nonpharmacologic methods are usually adequate to prevent complicated deep vein thromboses. Safety seats can be considered for infants. By implementing these interventions, adverse effects of air travel can largely be avoided.

## On the Medical Edge: Preparation of Expatriates, Refugee and Disaster Relief Workers, and Peace Corps Volunteers 85
Michael V. Callahan and  Davidson H. Hamer

Travelers to medically remote areas require special pretravel evaluation and environmentally specific education. Using a case-based format, this article provides information on approaches to the predeployment medical, dental, and psychologic preparation of long-term travelers and expeditions to extreme environments.

## Sexual Tourism: Implications for Travelers and the Destination Culture 103
Jeanne M. Marrazzo

The destination culture affords travelers ample opportunity for sex while away from home. The seemingly endless advance of the HIV pandemic, a resurgence of syphilis in most industrialized countries, continued high endemic rates of chlamydial infection and genital herpes, and steadily evolving antimicrobial resistance in *Neisseria gonorrhoeae* worldwide all contribute to a high likelihood that travelers who engage in unprotected sex will encounter a sexually transmitted infection. Medical encounters before and after travel provide an excellent opportunity to review the traveler's risk, screen appropriately for sexually transmitted infection and indications for relevant immunizations, discuss risk-reduction measures, and diagnose and treat any evident infection.

## The Impact of HIV Infection on Tropical Diseases 121
Gundel Harms and Hermann Feldmeier

HIV and tropical infections affect each other mutually. HIV infection may alter the natural history of tropical infectious diseases, impede rapid diagnosis, or reduce the efficacy of antiparasitic treatment. Tropical infections may facilitate the transmission of HIV and accelerate progression from asymptomatic HIV infection to AIDS. This article reviews data on known interactions for malaria, leishmaniasis, human African trypanosomiasis, Chagas' disease, schistosomiasis, onchocerciasis, lymphatic filariasis, and intestinal helminthiases.

## Update in Traveler's Diarrhea 137
David R. Shlim

Despite 50 years of research, the rates of traveler's diarrhea (TD) have not diminished in travelers. Restaurant hygiene has emerged as one of the main risk factors for TD. Antibiotic prophylaxis can prevent up to 90% of infections, but is not routinely recommended. Empiric treatment of TD has been the best approach to dealing with this problem, but its usefulness is being undermined by growing antibiotic resistance in many parts of the world.

## Yellow Fever and Japanese Encephalitis Vaccines: Indications and Complications 151
Anthony A. Marfin, Rachel S. Barwick Eidex, Phyllis E. Kozarsky, and Martin S. Cetron

Appropriate administration of yellow fever or Japanese encephalitis vaccines to travelers requires an assessment of the traveler's risk for infection with these vector-borne flaviviruses during their travels and the presence of risk factors for adverse events following immunization. Japanese encephalitis and yellow fever vaccines have been more frequently associated with serious adverse events following immunization since the early 1980s and the late 1990s, respectively. This article describes the adverse events, the magnitude of their risk, and associated risk factors.

## A Travel Medicine Guide to Arthropods of Medical Importance 169
Richard J. Pollack and Leonard C. Marcus

Travelers in North America and abroad can suffer arthropod-induced injuries and infestations, and be at risk of vector-borne disease. This article describes clinically relevant aspects of the biology, ecology, and epidemiology of the main kinds of arthropods that directly injure people or transmit infections. Guidance is offered to clinicians so they might better educate and advise travelers how to protect themselves, and evaluate and manage complaints by travelers on their return.

## New Strategies for the Prevention of Malaria In Travelers 185
Lin H. Chen and Jay S. Keystone

Malaria incidence in travelers has increased dramatically in the past two decades, and resistance to recommended drugs has become established if not widespread. New strategies to assess the incidence, risk, and prevention of travelers' malaria have evolved. Recent developments in prevention of malaria in travelers include sentinel surveillance of malaria in travelers, seroprevalence studies of travelers' malaria, molecular techniques to evaluate drug resistance, the combination drug atovaquone-proguanil, the addition of primaquine as a primary prophylaxis, the evaluation of the new antimalarial tafenoquine, the use of standby emergency treatment, and rapid diagnostic tests for malaria.

## Management of Severe Malaria: Interventions and Controversies 211
Geoffrey Pasvol

All cases of falciparum malaria in travelers are potentially severe and life threatening, especially when managed inappropriately. Prevention is the cornerstone of good malarial control. In cases of malaria in travelers, however, a major reason for progression to severe disease is missed or delayed diagnosis. Once diagnosed, the parenteral administration of adequate safe doses of an appropriate antimalarial in the setting of the highest possible level of clinical care is the priority. All other modalities of management, although important, remain secondary.

## Cutaneous Leishmaniasis in the Returning Traveler 241
Alan J. Magill

Infection with protozoan parasites of the genus *Leishmania* leads to a wide variety of clinical disease syndromes called leishmaniasis, or more appropriately the leishmaniases. The three major clinical syndromes are cutaneous leishmaniasis, mucosal leishmaniasis, and visceral leishmaniasis. All three of these syndromes have been documented in returning travelers. This article focuses on cutaneous leishmaniasis with some comment on mucosal leishmaniasis.

## New Diagnostics in Parasitology 267
Peter L. Chiodini

This article considers new diagnostics in the context of a diagnostic clinical parasitology laboratory receiving samples from an infectious and tropical disease service. Mention of a particular product does not imply endorsement. Laboratory directors should assess the suitability of individual diagnostic kits for the practice that they manage and should be aware that competing products may be available.

### *Online extra*

Full text of article, Chiodini PL. New diagnostics in parasitology. Infect Dis Clin N Am 2005;19:267-270, is available at www.id.theclinics.com, doi:10.1016/j.idc.2004.11.002.

## Index 271

## FORTHCOMING ISSUES

June 2005
### Sexually Transmitted Infections
Jonathan Zenilman, MD, *Guest Editor*

September 2005
### Pediatric Infectious Diseases
Jeffrey Blumer, MD, PhD, and
Philip Toltzis, MD, *Guest Editors*

December 2005
### Musculoskeletal Infections
John James Ross, MD, *Guest Editor*

## RECENT ISSUES

December 2004
### Lower Respiratory Tract Infections
Thomas M. File, Jr, MD, *Guest Editor*

September 2004
### Antibacterial Therapy and Newer Agents
Donald Kaye, MD, *Guest Editor*

June 2004
### Historical Aspects of Infectious Diseases, Part II
Burke A. Cunha, MD, *Guest Editor*

---

**The Clinics are now available online!**

Access your subscription at:
www.theclinics.com

Dedication

# Martin S. Wolfe, MD, FACP

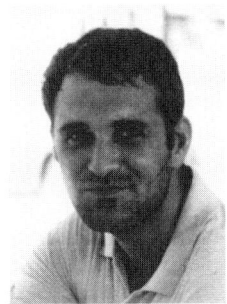
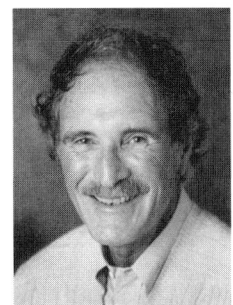

Marty Wolfe, MD in Ghana, 1963     Martin S. Wolfe, MD, FACP

Martin S. Wolfe, MD, FACP has seen more tropical and travel medicine in his four decade career than most. He is not only highly regarded for his clinical expertise, but also for his enthusiasm and love of the field of clinical tropical medicine with its colorful history and characters. A native of Scranton, Pennsylvania, Marty attended the Cornell University Medical College where he met and was inspired by Benjamin H. Kean, MD who encouraged him to: "... go out and do some field work. Get your hands dirty." He did just that. After completing internship, Marty spent two years in Ghana as a US Public Health Service Officer attached to the NIH West Africa Research Laboratory studying schistosomiasis. He returned to Cornell to complete his internal medicine residency and subsequently attended the London School of Hygiene and Tropical Medicine as a Rockefeller Foundation Fellow where he received a Diploma in Clinical Medicine of the Tropics. Marty then spent two years in Lahore Pakistan at the University of Maryland International Center for Medical Research Training (ICMRT) identifying the distribution of Bancroftian filariasis in what is now Bangladesh. He returned to the US and began a 31-year career in the Office of Medical Services in the US Department of State where he dealt with thousands of State Department personnel who presented with a great diversity of tropical and travel-related diseases. On a historical note, Marty served as the personal physician to Henry Kissinger, the US Secretary of State, during the years of "shuttle diplomacy" in the Middle

East and Africa. In a parallel path, Marty developed an independent consultative practice in tropical medicine, a private diagnostic parasitology laboratory, and in the 1970s established one of the first travel clinics in the US where today thousands of travelers are seen each year.

Marty's intellectual curiosity, keen insight, and unparalleled clinical experience produced over 135 articles and chapters on a wide variety of subjects in tropical and travel medicine. He has served on various editorial boards, was a member of the Armed Forces Epidemiology Board, and a member of the board of the Gorgas Institute of Tropical Medicine. Marty was elected a Fellow of the American College of Physicians and of the Infectious Diseases Society of America.

The lecture hall has been a place where Marty has shared his zeal for tropical medicine by passing on knowledge and lore to young students. He has taught the parasitology course at the Georgetown School of Medicine for more than 35 years and serves as Clinical Professor of Medicine at both the George Washington University and the Georgetown School of Medicine. His enthusiasm, humor, and fascinating clinical cases are fondly remembered by generations of students, many of whom were stimulated to pursue careers in tropical and travel medicine.

For over 40 years Marty has been a member of the American Society of Tropical Medicine and Hygiene (ASTMH). He has been a Council Member, served on numerous committees, and was a major catalyst in establishing the American Committee on Clinical Tropical Medicine and Traveler's Health (a.k.a. the Clinical Group) serving as its first president. Marty has guided and mentored countless scientists and clinicians, including many of the leading members of the Clinical Group, with his vast clinical experience, intellectual rigor, and affable personality. For his teaching and mentorship in tropical medicine he received the Ben Kean Award from the ASTMH in 1998.

His many contributions have helped to establish tropical and travel medicine as distinct fields of clinical practice. As Marty becomes respectfully and fondly known as one of the "grandfathers" of the field, he continues to make contributions by practicing, teaching, and writing. Dedicating this latest volume of *Infectious Disease Clinics of North America* to a clinician who has seen, taught, and cared so much about clinical tropical and travel medicine and those who practice it could not be more fitting.

Alberto M. Acosta, MD, PhD
*Traveler's Medical Service of New York*
*Weill Medical College of Cornell University*
*The New York-Presbyterian Hospital*
*New York, NY*

Rebecca Wolfe Acosta, RN, MPH
*Traveler's Medical Service of New York*
*New York, NY*

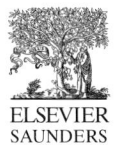

# Preface

# Coming of Age in Travel Medicine and Tropical Diseases: A Need for Continued Advocacy and Mentorship

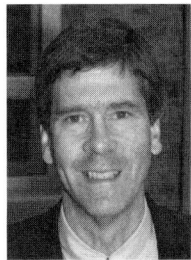 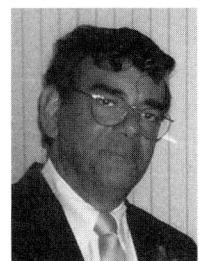

David R. Hill, MD, DTM&H    Frank J. Bia, MD, MPH
*Guest Editors*

Travel medicine has come of age. In the United States, it found its start 25 years ago in a small group of like-minded individuals who gathered informally at the meetings of the American Society of Tropical Medicine and Hygiene (ASTM&H; www.astmh.org) and discussed interesting clinical cases in travel medicine and tropical disease. There is now a large, active group that is leading the way in clinical care, education, training, and certification of knowledge in the fields of travel and tropical medicine: the American Committee on Clinical Tropical Medicine and Travelers' Health (www.astmh.org/subgroup/acctmth.asp). Many of the authors featured in this issue of the *Infectious Disease Clinics of North America* were instrumental in providing the early leadership and continue to do so.

Simultaneously, there was a movement on the international front to create a global body devoted to travel medicine: the International Society of Travel Medicine (ISTM; www.istm.org). Founded in 1992, again with leadership from many of the authors in this issue, the ISTM now has a global membership of nearly 2000 health professionals who span all disciplines and levels of training. The authors in this issue reflect the international membership and perspective in travel medicine.

Why has this happened? There appear to be several reasons for the growth and establishment of travel medicine. First, travel has increased dramatically: in 2003, there were 694 million visits across international borders [1]. A total of $514 billion was spent during these trips, indicating the huge investment made in travel. This level of travel continues despite the threat of terrorism, the reality of war and conflict, and the emergence of new diseases such as severe acute respiratory syndrome, Ebola virus, and avian influenza.

Second, the type of trips and travelers has become more challenging and has required a level of expertise in giving advice to travelers that may not be available in general practice settings. People of all ages who have varied medical conditions visit all corners of the globe. The destinations of travelers who have attended a travel medicine service in Connecticut compared with all global travelers are illustrated in Fig. 1. Travelers who have HIV infection or chronic medical conditions and women who are pregnant necessitate a provider who is knowledgeable and experienced in preparing these types of patients to undertake international travel. The complex itineraries demand knowledge of disease epidemiology and changing patterns of resistance for organisms such as *Plasmodium falciparum* and *Salmonella enterica* serotype Typhi, and how to use new vaccines and chemoprophylactics in prevention.

The third reason has been the maturing of science in travel medicine. The literature has moved from descriptive to formal studies of disease risk, vaccine efficacy, and prevention methods. The field has moved from reliance upon the opinion of experts to a growing evidence base. Clinical practice of travel medicine requires that the practitioner follow the literature and apply this evidence to everyday practice. Established journals such as *Clinical Infectious Diseases* and *The American Journal of Tropical Medicine and Hygiene* have increased their coverage of both travel medicine and clinical tropical diseases. New journals have appeared; they include the *Journal of Travel Medicine* and *Travel Medicine and Infectious Diseases* and reflect the increasing literature of science in these areas.

This growth of travel medicine has been paralleled by needed clinical expertise in the United States in tropical medicine [2]. Although it is not expected that those who practice travel medicine are also experts in tropical medicine, they do need to be competent in recognizing, evaluating, and perhaps triaging such key syndromes in returned travelers as fever, diarrhea, rash, and respiratory complaints [3,4]. As a reflection of the healthy nature of these fields, there has been development of courses in travel and tropical medicine and two examinations that certify knowledge: one is administered by the ASTM&H and covers tropical and travel medicine; the other is given by the ISTM and covers travel medicine alone.

With the coming of age for travel medicine, it is now appropriate that a standard be developed [5]. It is not sufficient to dabble in travel medicine by only giving 'shots' and not also providing detailed advice about personal safety and responsible behavior, insect avoidance, environmental illness, travelers' diarrhea management, malaria prevention, and access to medical care overseas. A committee of the Infectious Diseases Society of America

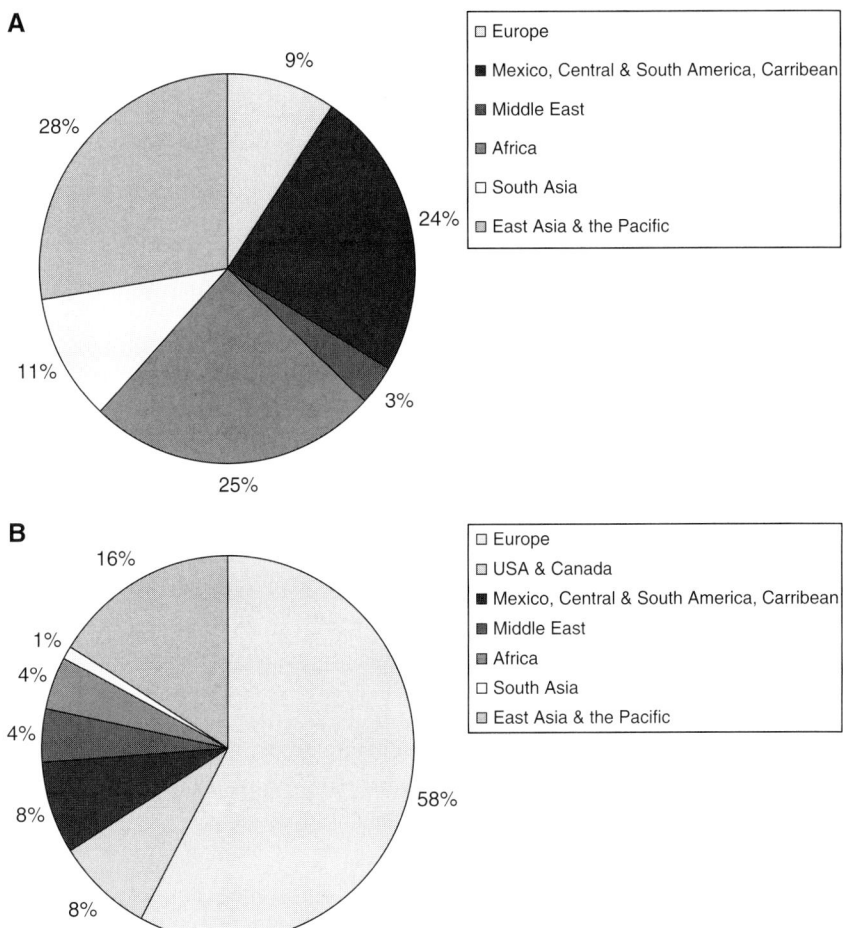

Fig. 1. Destinations of international travelers. (*A*) Destinations of travelers who received pretravel care at the University of Connecticut International Traveler's Medical Service from 1984 to 2002 (n = 14,701). Ninety-one percent of destinations were to developing regions in Latin America, the Middle East, Africa, and Asia. (*B*) Arrivals for all world travelers for the year 2003 (n = 694 million). Thirty-four percent of visits were to developing regions in Latin America, the Middle East, Africa, and Asia. (*Data from* World Tourism Organization. International tourism receipts. World Tourism Barometer 2004;2:2–3.)

guidelines panel has come together to define guidelines for care in travel medicine [6]. This follows a similar Canadian initiative [7], and efforts in other countries to develop standards [8,9]. Boxes 1 and 2 outline the areas in which the guidelines committee feels expertise is needed to practice in the field.

This maturing of travel medicine can only be sustained if there is a steady flow of new clinicians who are entering the field. Travel medicine has

> **Box 1. Provider qualifications for travel medicine**
>
> *Requisite knowledge of broad subject areas*
> - The geography of major disease entities, including travel-associated infectious diseases and their epidemiology, transmission, and prevention.
> - The use and complications of travel-related drugs and vaccines: storage and handling, indications for usage, contraindications, pharmacology, immunology, drug interactions, and adverse events.
> - The noninfectious medical and environmental travel risks, including their prevention and management.
> - The ability to recognize major disease patterns and syndromes in returned travelers (eg, fever, diarrhea, rash, and respiratory illnesses).
> - The ability to access travel medicine resources (eg, texts, articles, Internet sites).
>
> *Requisite experience and continuing education*
> - Several months working experience in a travel clinic with at least 15 pretravel consultations per week.
> - Continuing education: short or long courses in travel medicine and active membership in a specialty society dealing with travel and tropical medicine, and subscription to appropriate journals. Organizations include the American Society of Tropical Medicine and Hygiene and the International Society of Travel Medicine.
>
> ---
> See also the body of knowledge defined by the ISTM [3].

attracted a diverse group of health care providers, and not only clinicians with an interest in clinical tropical medicine, parasitology, or vector-borne diseases, but also internists, emergency medicine specialists, occupational medicine professionals, and nurses from all disciplines [10]. It is fortunate that both the ISTM and ASTM&H have attempted to keep pace with the increasing need for education through provision of formal courses and experiences in travel and tropical medicine. However, as internists with subspecialty board certification in infectious diseases, we could not let the opportunity to preface this issue of the *Infectious Disease Clinics of North America* go by without posing a question and a challenge to our infectious disease colleagues: Who will be the advocates for travel and tropical medicine in our medical schools and residency programs, and who will be the role models for careers focused on these disciplines? We believe that it

> **Box 2. Services provided in a travel medicine practice**
>
> Assessment of the health of travelers and their underlying medical conditions, allergies, and immunization histories. Information should be maintained in permanent, accessible records.
>
> Assessment of the health risk of travel, including evaluation of itineraries, duration of travel, reasons for travel, and planned activities.
>
> Preventive advice, which should be available in verbal and written form. The following subject areas are of greatest concern:
> - Vaccinations and vaccine-preventable illness
> - Travelers' diarrhea prevention and self-treatment
> - Malaria prevention and insect avoidance measures
> - Vector-borne and water-borne illnesses
> - Personal safety, security issues, appropriate behavior
> - Sexual health and sexually transmitted diseases, including HIV prevention
> - Environmental illness, including altitude, heat, cold, diving, motion sickness, and jet lag
> - Animal bites and their treatment; rabies avoidance
> - Problems specific to long-term travelers, expatriates, and business travelers
> - Travelers with special needs (eg, pregnant women, individuals who have diabetes, immunocompromised individuals, individuals who have had a transplantation)
> - Travel medical kits with information on travel health maintenance, medical evacuation insurance, and access to medical care overseas.
> - Posttravel assessment for returning travelers

will be infectious disease clinicians who will increasingly be needed to advocate for classroom and residency training time and to be the role models and personal mentors for our students.

In the late 1960s, many of us who now treat infectious diseases were drawn to the study of tropical disease by experienced and often charismatic mentors. In the case of one of us (F.J.B.), it was Dr. Benjamin Kean at Cornell University Medical College. In the years following World War II and the Vietnam conflict, one of the driving forces that kept this discipline alive in the medical school curriculum was the perceived need for tropical medicine expertise that followed those national experiences abroad. Although times are different, and the generation who taught us is now retiring or has left the field, the need for expertise remains equally great for several reasons.

The first reason has been noted and includes the incredible growth of travel in a continually shrinking world. Any clinician who sees patients in a travel medicine context is aware of the vast diversity of travelers and the reasons for their trips. The second reason has been an AIDS pandemic that affects large parts of the world where HIV has a complex interaction with an environment of multiple tropical pathogens. Those of us at the level of medical student education have also seen a more subtle yet rapid change: the current generation of students has a far different perception of the world than the one in which we grew up professionally. It is a world contracted by the Internet and by rapid transit times between continents. Students have an appreciation of medicine as a universal language—one that can influence the course of individual disease and public health almost anywhere and at any time. If nineteenth- and twentieth-century missionary activity or global warfare underscored the importance of understanding complex tropical diseases, the need for understanding is now also driven by a global sense of citizenship, social justice, and responsibility.

The demand for understanding those diseases that affect persons in developing regions and including them in the curriculum is coupled with an intense interest in actually working in such a context. Some medical educators consider 1- or 2-month rotations in Africa, Asia, or Latin America to be just "safari medicine" unless there is a long-term commitment on the part of the student or resident. This attitude simply misses the point. Would one say the same about a 6-week rotation in a cardiac intensive care unit? Does this 6-week experience merely serve to make the resident a "cardiac dilettante"? For another of us (D.R.H.), a month-long medical service trip to Guatemala in 1968 led to a profound change in world view and to a commitment to a career in infectious disease, travel, and tropical medicine. The young trainees who seek such experiences are very much in need of advocates within the medical school and residency curriculum committees on which we who are established in our careers may serve. That being the case, we must set the standard in our professional schools for what is taught in the classroom and on the wards, and what constitutes a valid clinical experience abroad. We must retain and elevate the crucial roles of mentors and role models for this current generation of students and residents.

This issue of the *Infectious Disease Clinics of North America* covers many of the essential topics in travel medicine that reflect the type of consultative advice—both complex and straightforward—sought by those who seek out members of our subspecialty. In addition, we have added some of the crucial topics in tropical disease that we feel are important for persons practicing in the specialty to understand (eg, management of severe malaria). We have asked our colleagues to approach the subjects from a perspective that provides classic case examples as well as their new insights, while still delivering the key messages for those who practice. We believe they have accomplished this most successfully, and we sincerely thank them for their efforts.

David R. Hill, MD, DTM&H
*National Travel Health Network and Centre, and*
*London School of Hygiene and Tropical Medicine*
*Mortimer Market Centre, Capper Street*
*London WC1E 6AU, UK*

*E-mail address:* david.hill@uclh.org

Frank J. Bia, MD, MPH
*Departments of Medicine and Laboratory Medicine*
*Yale School of Medicine*
*CB 608c 333 Cedar Street*
*New Haven, CT 06520-8030, USA*

*E-mail address:* frank.bia@yale.edu

## References

[1] World Tourism Organization. International tourism receipts. World Tourism Barometer 2004;2:2–3. Available at: www.world-tourism.org/facts/barometer/WTOBarom04_2 excerpt_en.pdf. Accessed September 15, 2004.
[2] Barry M, Maguire JH, Weller PF. The American Society of Tropical Medicine and Hygiene initiative to stimulate educational programs to enhance medical expertise in tropical diseases. Am J Trop Med Hyg 1999;61:681–8.
[3] Kozarsky PE, Keystone JS. Body of knowledge for the practice of travel medicine. J Travel Med 2002;9:112–5.
[4] D'Acremont V, Ambresin AE, Burnand B, et al. Practice guidelines for evaluation of fever in returning travelers and migrants. J Travel Med 2003;10(Suppl 2):S25–52.
[5] Spira A. Setting the standard. J Travel Med 2003;10:1–3.
[6] Hill DR, Pearson RD, Ericsson CD, et al. Guidelines for the practice of travel medicine. Clin Infect Dis, in press.
[7] Committee to Advise on Tropical Medicine and Travel (CATMAT). Guidelines for the practice of travel medicine. An Advisory Committee Statement (ACS). Can Commun Dis Rep 1999;25:1–6.
[8] Leggat PA, Ross MH, Dürrheim DN, et al. Linking yellow fever vaccination centre registration and training in travel medicine. Travel Medicine and Infectious Diseases 2003; 1:17–8.
[9] Beeching NJ, Hill DR. NaTHNaC—the National Travel Health Network and Centre (England). Travel Medicine and Infectious Diseases 2003;1:123–5.
[10] Hill DR, Behrens RH. A survey of travel clinics throughout the world. J Travel Med 1996; 3:46–51.

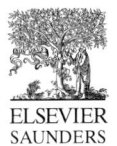

# Surveillance of Imported Diseases as a Window to Travel Health Risks

Tomas Jelinek, MD, DTMP*,
Nikolai Mühlberger, DVM, MPH

*Berlin Institute of Tropical Medicine, Spandauer Damm 130, Berlin 14050, Germany*

From being treated as a mere hobby of interested practitioners, travel medicine has developed into a serious medical discipline. Counseling in this field can draw on a growing wealth of evidence. Studies on various travel health risks have multiplied in the last years: while PubMed lists only 447 entries for "travel medicine" in the years 1980 to 1989, 961 are listed for 1990 to 1999, and already 796 for the short time from 2000 to May 2004 [1]. It was recognized very early that local disease information from travel destinations was not sufficient for assessing travel-associated health risks. Travelers behave differently than inhabitants of traveled regions and tend to have other health risks. An increasing series of studies aiming directly at the various populations of travelers are being performed and are yielding information that has already changed travel medicine practice profoundly. Instead of assessing health risks by deducting from information gained from other populations, health professionals can now draw on results from studies that are directly concerned with the traveler. They are assisted increasingly by networks that collect and provide updated information. In the United Kingdom, the National Travel Health Network and Centre has been specifically created by the government to promote clinical standards in travel medicine with the goal of "protecting the health of the British traveler" [2].

Although surveillance of infectious diseases has a long history, surveillance of imported diseases in travelers has started comparatively recently. Most systems are based on national notification schemes that are diagnosis-oriented. These conventional surveillance programs largely depend on public health departments and laboratories. Direct patient contact by the person doing the reporting is an exception. National systems of infectious diseases

---

* Corresponding author.
 *E-mail address:* tomas.jelinek@charite.de (T. Jelinek).

surveillance generally focus on complete coverage, attempting to obtain all relevant data. The potential advantage of this approach is that no cases are overlooked. In reality, however, compliance with notification regulations is very limited. Estimated coverage rates at or below 50% are normal rather than the exception. The lack of motivation among those requested by law to report is one of the major stumbling points for traditional surveillance systems.

In addition to systems aiming at complete coverage, an increasing number of national and international sentinel networks are being established. The use of sentinel sites has the disadvantage that complete coverage cannot be achieved. A prudent selection of members, however, can ensure that a sentinel network produces representative information. In general, sentinel networks consist of voluntary members who are more focused on surveillance. Information flow is often faster than in systems that are aiming at complete coverage. Examples for this are multinational networks like FluNet, the World Health Organization global influenza network [3], and the European Legionellosis Surveillance Scheme [4].

Increased awareness of emerging infectious diseases has fostered the creation of syndrome-based surveillance networks. They work almost exclusively in sentinel settings. Unlike traditional notification systems, their aim is not to collect information on predefined diagnosis. This type of network rather tries to collect open, possibly even nonstandardized information, to detect new outbreaks and emerging pathogens within a short time. Possibly the most ambitious project of this type is the US Department of Defense Global Emerging Infections system [5]. Clinical sentinel networks represent another broadening of conventional surveillance programs. The clear advantage of these systems is that the persons reporting the requested data have seen the patients themselves and can relay first-hand information. Several provider-based sentinel networks have been implemented during the last years, in particular in the United States as part of a national response plan against emerging infectious diseases [6,7]. The first sentinel surveillance effort focusing explicitly on travelers was Geosentinel, by design a global network that attempts to capture emerging infectious diseases [7].

The lack of surveillance data for imported infectious diseases in Europe prompted the foundation of the European Network on Imported Infectious Disease Surveillance (TropNetEurop), which focuses on the surveillance of imported diseases in travelers [8]. This is a clinician-based sentinel network. The network is designed effectively to detect emerging infections of potential regional, national, or global impact at their point of entry into the domestic population. Sentinel surveillance reporting is performed by participating sites using a standardized and computerized reporting system. Immediate transmission of anonymous patient and laboratory data to the central database ensures timely detection of sentinel events. Membership is voluntary and self-selected by participating centers and monitored by the steering committee of the network. Although the organization of the network does not guarantee a representative data collection for Europe, most major referral centers of the continent are represented. Within a very short time, it has grown to 45 members in 16 countries that represent most of the centers of excellence for imported infections on the continent. Network members overlook approximately 57,000 patients annually, making it the largest infectious disease sentinel network worldwide. Although focusing on diagnosis-based reporting, TropNetEurop is strongly encouraging reporting of unexpected events and syndromes. The network has been very successful in detecting outbreaks of emerging diseases in the past and has proved its value as an additional surveillance tool [9].

**Systematic observations**

At least for large referral centers, reporting of all patients seen by a sentinel site is clearly an overwhelming task if not supported by financial compensations. TropNetEurop settled on regular reporting of only three disease entities: (1) malaria, (2) dengue fever, and (3) schistosomiasis. Concentration on this very limited amount of reports eased the effort for all member sites while still keeping a steady flow of reports that provide valuable information in monthly bulletins that are mailed to all members and, in abbreviated form, to other interested health professionals outside the network [8].

*Malaria reporting*

Results from the collection of malaria reports showed that, depending on the regional impact of immigrants (persons born outside of Europe) versus the amount of travel in the local European population, data from national sources in Europe can be heavily skewed toward one or the other group [10]. Judging from the data provided by national systems of disease notification, TropNetEurop covers approximately 10% of all malaria patients seen in Europe [10,11]. Review of the reported data on falciparum malaria showed that West Africa contributed by far the most malaria patients to TropNetEurop sites: 68.2% of all immigrants and 58.8% of Europeans were infected there [10]. Relatively fewer immigrants and more tourists were infected in East and Southern Africa. Reports of the World Tourism Organization show that only 0.6% to 2.4% of European travelers to potentially malarious areas chose West Africa as a destination [12,13]. This suggests a comparatively high relative risk of acquiring falciparum malaria in West Africa. In comparison, the World Health Organization reports that 16% to 21% of travelers visited South East Asia. Because only very few cases of malaria were reported from this area, the relative risk seems to be very low. These findings are comparable with previous investigations from other nonendemic countries [14–16]. Only a minority of patients with falciparum malaria took drugs or drug combinations appropriate for drug-resistant malaria at the respective destination [17]. Probably a high percentage of the malaria cases could have been avoided by an appropriate malaria prophylaxis regimen. This information can be used directly for travel counseling.

The course of illness tended to be milder in immigrants as compared with Europeans, although available data are not sufficient to show significant differences (Table 1). A large number of patients of the former group were semi-immune inhabitants of malarious areas, whereas European patients were all nonimmune. It is notable, however, that 3.7% of immigrants developed complications during their clinical course. Although this percentage is lower than in European patients (6.3%), some immigrants were critically ill when presenting at the reporting centers. Immigrants who plan to visit their home country after several years may have only a limited perception of travel risks and necessary prophylactic measures. This is a group that is underrepresented in travel clinics and should be actively sought.

It is also TropNetEurop's impression that business travelers have a higher-than-average risk for complications in falciparum malaria. Judging from the reports to TropNetEurop, they tend to seek pretravel counseling less frequently; to follow advice less reliably; and, if symptomatic, to seek medical help later than other travelers.

In analysis of falciparum malaria in travelers, it was conclusively shown that increasing age is a risk factor for severe falciparum malaria in nonimmune patients [18]. Altogether, 1181 nonimmune patients with falciparum malaria met the study's inclusion criteria. Results from adjusted analyses, controlling for potential confounding, yielded that the risk of dying from falciparum malaria (odds ratio [OR] 1.85, 95% confidence interval [CI] 1.30–2.62), experiencing cerebral malaria (OR 1.66, 95% CI 1.31–2.12) or severe disease in general (OR 1.32, 95% CI 1.14–1.53), and to be hospitalized (OR

Table 1
Signs and symptoms in Europeans and immigrants with falciparum malaria

| Symptom | Immigrants (N = 790) (%) | Europeans (N = 869) (%) |
| --- | --- | --- |
| Fever | 603 (76.3) | 704 (81) |
| Headache | 388 (49.1) | 432 (49.7) |
| Fatigue | 189 (23.9) | 302 (34.8) |
| Myalgia, arthralgia | 136 (17.2) | 202 (23.2) |
| Diarrhea | 77 (9.7) | 121 (13.9) |
| Vomiting | 96 (12.2) | 104 (11.9) |
| Respiratory complaints | 21 (2.7) | 30 (3.5) |
| Neurologic complaints | 10 (1.3) | 22 (2.5) |
| Skin affections | 10 (1.3) | 11 (1.3) |
| Otitis | 56 (7.1) | 8 (0.9) |
| Other | 157 (19.9) | 153 (17.6) |
| None | 49 (6.2) | 0 |

Multiple entries possible.

*Data from* Jelinek T, Schulte C, Behrens R, et al. Clinical and epidemiological characteristics among travellers and immigrants with imported falciparum malaria in Europe: sentinel surveillance data from TropNetEurop. Clin Infect Dis 2002;34:572–6.

1.21, 95% CI 1.06–1.39) increased significantly per decade of life (Table 2). Comparing elderly (60 years and older) with younger patients showed that case fatality was almost six times higher among elderly patients (OR 5.74, 95% CI 1.78–18.47). Cerebral complications occurred three times more often (OR 3.29, 95% CI 1.20–9.01). Antimalarial chemoprophylaxis was significantly associated with lower case fatality (OR 0.17, 95% CI 0.04–0.74) and less frequent cerebral complications (OR 0.44, 95% CI 0.20–0.96). The study provided evidence that falciparum malaria is more serious in older patients, and demonstrated that clinical surveillance networks are capable providing quality data for investigating rare events or diseases.

## Dengue fever

Analysis of the data on dengue fever showed that most patients were Europeans who traveled for tourist reasons [19]. Asia contributed the most dengue patients to TropNetEurop sites: 23.3% visited South East Asia, 22.9% the Indian subcontinent, and 6.5% Indonesia. Numbers were slightly lower for the Americas, which contributed a total of 38.2% of all patients. One patient was reported from Hawaii in 2000, heralding the later outbreak of dengue fever on Maui [20]. Reports of the World Tourism Organization show that 16% to 21% of European travelers traveled to South East Asia and only 6% to 8% to India [12,13]. This suggests a high relative risk of acquiring dengue fever in the latter region, whereas numbers from South East Asia seem to reflect the high number of tourists to that area. The low number of infections that were acquired in Africa is consistent with all previous epidemiologic data [21–29]. Dengue importation into Europe shows a seasonal pattern. This is likely to reflect the travel habits of European tourists rather than true variations in disease activity.

Table 2
Age-specific frequency of outcomes of severe falciparum malaria

| Age group (y) | Number of patients | Fatal cases % | Cerebral complications % | Other complications % | Hospital admissions* % |
| --- | --- | --- | --- | --- | --- |
| 10–19 | 50 | 0 | 0 | 4 | 70 |
| 20–29 | 290 | 0.7 | 1 | 5.2 | 79 |
| 30–39 | 369 | 0.5 | 1.9 | 5.4 | 79.7 |
| 40–49 | 225 | 2.2 | 6.2 | 7.6 | 81.8 |
| 50–59 | 169 | 2.4 | 4.7 | 9.5 | 85.2 |
| 60–69 | 56 | 3.6 | 5.4 | 3.6 | 73.2 |
| 70–79 | 20 | 10 | 10 | 20 | 95 |
| 80–89 | 2 | 0 | 0 | 0 | 100 |
| Total | 1181 | 1.4 | 3.1 | 6.4 | 80.3 |

* Missing values in 39 cases.

*Data from* Mühlberger N, Jelinek T, Behrens R, et al. Age as a risk factor for severe manifestations of falciparum malaria in non-immune patients: observations from TropNetEurop and SIMPID surveillance data. Clin Infect Dis 2003;36:990–5.

From the beginning of reporting in TropNetEurop, there has been an increase in the total number of dengue observations per year. This may reflect increased awareness of the disease and its signs by the clinicians who are involved in TropNetEurop. Changes in the pattern of imported activity of dengue were considerable: the proportion of patients from South East Asia increased from 29% in 1999 to 66.1% in 2002 and decreased again to 47.8% in early 2004. A similar tendency was observed in reports from India (14.5% in 1999 to 21.1% in 2001 and 8.4% in 2002), whereas reports from the Americas decreased. This may reflect changes in travel patterns but reports from the World Tourism Organization do not indicate major shifts in travel activities of Europeans away from the Americas toward Asia [12,13]. More likely, these numbers reflect the activity of dengue in the regions that are visited by European travelers. An increase of reports in returnees from an endemic area can serve as an early indicator for increased disease activity. Symptoms commonly associated with dengue, like fever, myalgia, arthralgia, and exanthema, can be helpful for diagnosis when present, but missing typical symptoms does not exclude infection (Table 3). Most dengue patients in this group were symptomatic and they complained of fever and headache. Other symptoms included myalgias; fatigue; skin problems (exanthema); and diarrhea.

## Risk estimates

Estimating risk based on sentinel surveillance in travelers is hampered by the lack of true denominator data. It is very difficult, if not impossible, to obtain reliable estimates regarding the travel activities of the population

Table 3
Signs and symptoms in 294 Europeans and immigrants with dengue fever

| Symptom | N | % |
| --- | --- | --- |
| Fever | 236 | 80.3 |
| Headache | 158 | 53.7 |
| Fatigue | 115 | 39.1 |
| Myalgia, arthralgia | 113 | 38.4 |
| Exanthema | 79 | 26.9 |
| Diarrhea | 54 | 18.4 |
| Vomiting | 22 | 7.5 |
| Respiratory complaints | 17 | 5.8 |
| Neurologic complaints | 7 | 2.4 |
| Psychologic complaints | 5 | 1.7 |
| Otitis | 22 | 7.5 |
| Genitourinary | 3 | 1 |
| Other | 30 | 10.2 |
| None | 21 | 7.1 |

Multiple entries possible.

*Data from* Jelinek T, Mühlberger N, Harms G, et al. Imported dengue fever in Europe: sentinel surveillance data from TropNetEurop. Clin Infect Dis 2002;35:1047–52.

contributing to the patient data. This problem is increased by the contribution of asylum seekers and refugees coming into the area where surveillance is being established. A large number of patients with a particular infectious disease returning from a destination may only reflect increased travel to the destination and not an increased risk for the infection.

Clinical sentinel units are able to recognize disease importation from countries where the disease usually does not occur or is highly unlikely. Their ability to detect increased risks of infection in endemic countries, however, is very limited. This is because importation of tropical diseases is not a frequent event and the number of potential countries of infection is large, so that even large clinical units usually observe too few cases of disease importation from single countries to be able to discern a true change in risk. For example, if a unit on monthly average observes one case of malaria importation from an endemic country even a doubling of infections from that country does not raise suspicion, because small numbers are subject to large chance variation. Detection of unlikely notification increases from single endemic countries requires a minimum number of cases, which for tropical diseases is only feasible by combining surveillance data from several sentinel units.

As a network of clinical sites that are also responsible for pretravel counseling, TropNetEurop has a strong interest in promptly detecting increased risks of infection in tourist countries. Pooled TropNetEurop surveillance data are screened for unexpected notification increases in monthly intervals. Because data from imported disease surveillance lack a true denominator, unexpected notification increases may be caused by increased transmission rates; changes in travel or migration patterns; or altered notification behavior (eg, triggered by outbreak rumors). Unexpected increases are certainly no proof for increased risks of infection in tourist countries, but rather should be understood as warning signals to focus attention on significant observations and trigger further investigation. Because further investigations are time consuming, a priori exclusion of nonsignificant signals saves recourses and improves vigilance. Especially when disease importation from several dozen potential countries of infection is monitored, attention needs to be focused, to prevent the relevant findings being obscured by the large amount of information.

To screen TropNetEurop data for unexpected notification increases, a software tool was developed for comparing the number of recent cases with the number of cases from previous reference periods. Poisson probabilities, expressing the likelihood of detecting as many or more cases over a recent time period compared with the expected number of cases from past surveillance, are calculated for each country and presented in tables and maps. On the maps, levels of significance are indicated by different coloration. To account for the multiple-testing situation, observations are considered unexpected, representing a possible increase in risk, if the Poisson probability is less than 0.001.

An example of the described screening approach is given in Fig. 1. Displayed are screening results from spring 2002 that triggered the detection of a dengue fever outbreak among tourists in Thailand. Altogether, 37.5% of the dengue infections observed within the recent 6 months were imported from Thailand. Compared with the same period the previous year when the country accounted for only 11.1% of the cases, the recent observation was unlikely, and may have heralded a true increase in risk. Further signals were received from the Ivory Coast and some Central American and Caribbean countries. Those signals were caused by single observations, however, which were unexpected because the countries had not contributed cases to the database in the previous reference period.

## Detection of sentinel events

TropNetEurop has demonstrated on several occasions that sensitive detection of sentinel events in travelers can lead to outbreak detection.

### Falciparum malaria in the Dominican Republic

One example is falciparum malaria in the Dominican Republic [30]. Similar to most countries in the Caribbean, large parts of the Dominican Republic are considered as low-risk areas for falciparum malaria [31]. In general, only border regions with Haiti and provinces in the northwest of the country have been associated with endemicity. This pattern was reversed a few years ago: starting with an index patient in June 1999, 12 additional European patients presented with falciparum malaria acquired in the Dominican Republic during the period from November 1999 until February 2000. The patients were identified and reported within TropNetEurop. As a reflection of the nationalities traveling currently to the Dominican Republic on package tours, all but two Spanish and one Austrian patient were German nationals. All patients had traveled to Punta Cana, a town that is situated at the Eastern tip of the Dominican Republic, or to nearby beach resorts. This area had not been implicated as being malarious and in accordance with almost all European recommendations at that time, none of the patients took malaria chemoprophylaxis. Similarly, mosquito exposure prevention was not practiced. Within 1 to 2 weeks after return from their journey, patients presented with fever at their general practitioner's or at the emergency departments, and were admitted after diagnosis of falciparum malaria was established. Drug treatment proved successful in all patients and the clinical course was uneventful.

The clustering of cases during a comparatively short time seemed to indicate a change in the epidemiology of malaria and might herald further outbreaks among tourists during subsequent travel seasons. According to information from the Malaria Department in the Dominican Republic, there had been an increase in malaria in 1999 following hurricane George:

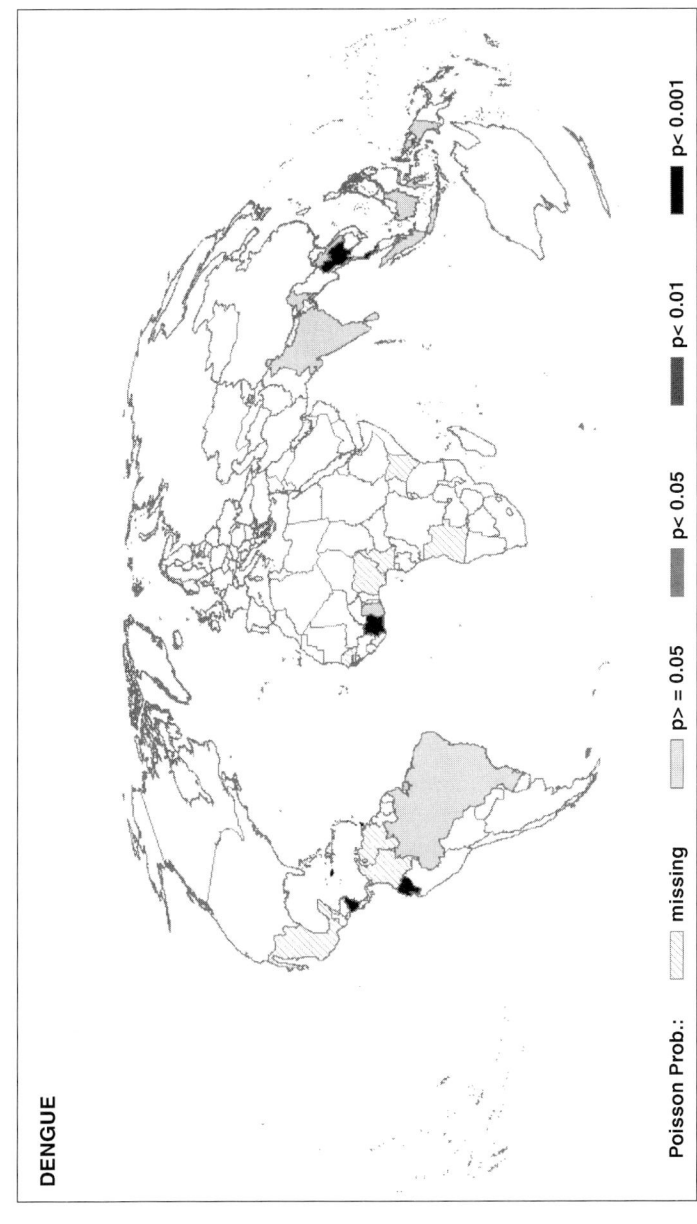

Fig. 1. Result map from TropNetEurop screening for unexpected increases of dengue fever notifications in Spring 2002. The probabilities express the likelihood of detecting as many or more cases over the previous 6 months, given case expectations from the same period 1 year previously. Dark areas indicate unexpected observations, and a possible increase in risk for dengue. "Missing" indicates that cases were observed in the past reference, but not in the recent observation period.

3003 cases up to November 20, 1999, which was an increase over the 2000 cases for the whole of 1998. In the east of the country, an outbreak of falciparum malaria among the local population was noted and traced back to building activities on behalf of the tourist industry. Here, Haitian builders were brought in and some of them imported *Plasmodium falciparum* strains. With anopheline vectors present and abundant breeding sites in that area, transmission of falciparum malaria was technically easy [32]. No reports were received from infections among tourists from other nations, especially the United States, Canada, and the United Kingdom. This may reflect a different use of malaria chemoprophylaxis or mosquito exposure prophylaxis for travel to the Dominican Republic. The discussion of the index case among the member sites of TropNetEurop triggered increased awareness within the network and led to reporting of other patients within days after presentation that might otherwise have gone unnoticed because they presented at different hospitals all over Europe.

*African trypanosomiasis from Tanzania*

Another example is African trypanosomiasis from Tanzania [33]. African trypanosomiasis (sleeping sickness) is a severe protozoan infection (*Trypanosoma brucei*), usually spread from infected animals and humans to man by the tsetse fly. Although the World Health Organization is reporting an increase in its incidence in Africa, it has remained a rare, but well-documented cause of fever in travelers returning from endemic areas. Prompt, appropriate therapy has resulted in favorable outcomes for many patients in Europe. Game parks in Tanzania have long been considered to be low-risk areas for African trypanosomiasis [34]. During February 2001, however, two index patients, followed by an additional six European and one South African patient, presented with trypanosomiasis [35]. The patients were identified and reported within TropNetEurop. All patients had in common travel to the Tarangire and Serengeti National Parks. This area has been implicated as being endemic for African trypanosomiasis. Case incidence among Tanzanian and foreign nationals had been exceedingly low, however, in the last decades.

During their journey or briefly after their return, patients presented with fever at general practitioners or emergency departments. Diagnosis was established by thin and thick blood film. Although specific medication was difficult to obtain, drug treatment proved successful in all but one patient, even though three patients presented with multiorgan failure. The temporal clustering of imported cases suggested a change in the local epidemiology and could have heralded future cases in tourists during the travel season. Reaction of the Tanzanian authorities on being informed involved strengthening of the installation of insecticide-impregnated targets in Serengeti around roads, lodges, staff quarters, and campsites. The effects of this initial program showing a dramatic decline of tsetse flies in the

Serengeti during the second half of 2001. Drugs for treatment of African trypanosomiasis were extremely difficult to obtain, and in some of the European patients treatment with suramin was only possible after informal help from member sites of the network.

*Falciparum malaria in illegal Chinese immigrants*

Falciparum malaria in illegal Chinese immigrants presents a third example [36]. Between November 2002 and March 2003, 17 cases of malaria among illegal Chinese immigrants were observed in seven hospitals of Central and Northern Italy (15 cases of *P falciparum*, one case of *P malariae*, and one mixed infection *P falciparum–P malariae*). One patient died. Before 2000, *P falciparum* malaria had not been reported in Chinese immigrants, despite many thousands living in Italy and other parts of Europe [10]. Although malaria is still endemic in parts of China, mostly at low-level of transmission [37], the major species is the benign form of *P vivax*. *P falciparum* transmission is confined to provinces bordering Lao PDR and Vietnam. All patients reported a stay varying from some days to several months (3 to 9) in an African country during their transport to Europe. Some had already fallen ill while in Africa. Other had reportedly died from fever before reaching Europe.

Malaria in Chinese immigrants highlighted a new route being used by traders of "human cargo," which bypassed the traditional route through Central Asia and Eastern Europe. A single country, Ivory Coast, was the transit country for almost all patients. The clustering of cases, despite variable time in transit, suggested that the illegal immigrants arrived in Europe in groups when the entry conditions were more favorable. Although Italy was the final destination, at least some entered through France, which also had reports of *P falciparum* cases in Chinese immigrants (F. Legros, Centre National de Référence de l'Epidémiologie du Paludisme, France, personal communication, 2003).

**Summary**

When using all its advantages of clinical vigilance, direct communication, and fast feedback, a clinical surveillance network can be remarkably effective in detecting sentinel events and in translating the new information into modifications of clinical practice. Travelers have great advantage when serving as surveillance tools for imported diseases. They travel widely and potentially expose themselves to all types of infectious diseases, they are very mobile, and they return during the incubation period of most diseases to a medical system that is capable of achieving fast and definitive diagnosis. Clustering of infections in returnees can be used immediately to warn outbound travelers of a particular risk and to increase their protection. In addition, travelers can also serve as "canary birds" for disease outbreaks in developing countries that might not be able to provide facilities for fast diagnosis. Information derived from returning travelers can be invaluable for the host country if channeled back to the medical authorities. TropNetEurop screening for increases in unexpected notifications has proved to be a sensitive early warning tool for the detection of increased transmission rates in endemic countries.

For the future, it is hoped that traditional surveillance systems and recently introduced networks will be able to cooperate more fully. All systems have strengths and weaknesses and can gain from information provided by each other. Linkage of existing networks, which avoids duplication of work and fully exploits the information potential of all combined systems, should be targeted.

## References

[1] PubMed 2004. Available at: http://www.ncbi.nlm.nih.gov/entrez/query.fcgi. Accessed June 6, 2004.
[2] NaTHNac 2004. Available at: http://www.nathnac.org/. Accessed June 6, 2004.
[3] FluNet 2004. Available at: http://oms.b3e.jussieu.fr/flunet/. Accessed June 6, 2004.
[4] Hutchinson E, Joseph C, Bartlett C. EWGLI: a European surveillance scheme for travel associated Legionnaires' disease. Euro Surveill 1996;1:37–9.
[5] DoDGeis 2004. Available at: http://www.geis.ha.osd.mil/aboutGEIS.asp. Accessed June 6, 2004.
[6] Talan D, Moran G, Mower W, et al. EMERGEncy ID NET: an emergency department-based emerging infections sentinel network. Ann Emerg Med 1998;32:703–11.
[7] Freedmann D, Kozarsky P, Weld L, et al. GeoSentinel: the global emerging infections sentinel network of the International Society of Travel Medicine. J Travel Med 1999;6:94–8.
[8] TropNetEurop 2004. Available at: http://www.tropnet.net. Accessed June 6, 2004.
[9] Jelinek T, Behrens R, Björkmann A, et al. European network on imported infectious disease surveillance (TropNetEurop). European Quality Assurance News 2000;11:170–2.
[10] Jelinek T, Schulte C, Behrens R, et al. Clinical and epidemiological characteristics among travellers and immigrants with imported falciparum malaria in Europe: sentinel surveillance data from TropNetEurop. Clin Infect Dis 2002;34:572–6.
[11] Anonymous. Surveillance of malaria in European Union countries. Euro Surveill 1998;3:45–7.
[12] Anonymous. Yearbook of tourism statistics. Madrid, Spain: World Tourism Organization; 1999.
[13] Anonymous. Yearbook of tourism statistics. Madrid, Spain: World Tourism Organization; 2000.
[14] Jelinek T, Nothdurft HD, Löscher T. Malaria in non-immune travelers: a synopsis of history, symptoms and treatment in 160 patients. J Travel Med 1994;1:199–202.
[15] Matteelli A, Colobini P, Gulletta M, et al. Epidemiological features and case management practices of imported malaria in northern Italy 1991–1995. Trop Med Int Health 1999;4:653–7.
[16] Nüesch R, Scheller M, Gyr N. Hospital admissions for malaria in Basel, Switzerland: an epidemiological review of 150 cases. J Travel Med 2000;7:95–7.
[17] Anonymous. International travel and health. Geneva: World Health Organization; 2003.
[18] Mühlberger N, Jelinek T, Behrens R, et al. Age as a risk factor for severe manifestations of falciparum malaria in non-immune patients: observations from TropNetEurop and SIMPID surveillance data. Clin Infect Dis 2003;36:990–5.

[19] Jelinek T, Mühlberger N, Harms G, et al. Imported dengue fever in Europe: sentinel surveillance data from TropNetEurop. Clin Infect Dis 2002;35:1047–52.
[20] Anonymous. Dengue, USA (Hawaii). Available at: http://www.promedmail.org/20010922.2296 ed: ProMED-mail, 2001. Accessed August 17, 2004.
[21] Lange WR, Beall B, Denny SC. Dengue fever: a resurgent risk for the international traveler. Am Fam Physician 1992;45:1161–8.
[22] Melissant CF, Kauffmann RH. Infection with dengue virus. Neth J Med 1992;41:272–4.
[23] Wittesjo B, Eitrem R, Niklasson B. Dengue fever among Swedish tourists. Scand J Infect Dis 1993;25:699–704.
[24] Chippaux A, Poveda JD. Imported dengue in France (1989–1993): conditions to be met for assuring an accurate etiological diagnosis. Bull Soc Pathol Exot 1993;86:402–5.
[25] Hasler C, Schnorf H, Enderlin N, et al. Imported dengue fever following a stay in the tropics. Schweiz Med Wochenschr 1993;123:120–4.
[26] Pick N, Potasman I. Dengue fever. Harefuah 1995;129:30–2.
[27] Anonymous. Imported dengue—United States, 1992. MMWR Morb Mortal Wkly Rep 1994;43:97–9.
[28] Anonymous. Imported dengue—United States, 1991. MMWR Morb Mortal Wkly Rep 1992;41:731–2.
[29] Anonymous. Imported dengue—United States, 1993–1994. MMWR Morb Mortal Wkly Rep 1995;44:353–6.
[30] Jelinek T, Corachan M, Grobusch M, et al. TropNetEurop: emergence of falciparum malaria among European tourists to the Dominican Republic. Emerg Infect Dis 2000;6:537–8.
[31] Anonymous. Malaria in the Americas, 1996. Epidemiol Bull 1997;18:1–8.
[32] Castellanos P. Malaria, imported—Europe ex Dominican Rep. (03). ProMED, 1999. Available at: www.promedmail.org. Archive No. 19991217.2173. Accessed November 20, 2004.
[33] Jelinek T, Bisoffi Z, Bonazzi L, et al. Cluster of African trypanosomiasis among travellers to the Serengeti. Emerg Infect Dis 2002;8:634–5.
[34] Ponce de Leon S, Lisker-Melman M, Kato-Maeda M, et al. *Trypanosoma brucei rhodesiense* infection imported to Mexico from a tourist in Kenya. Clin Infect Dis 1996;23:847–8.
[35] Ripamonti D, Massari M, Arici C, et al. African sleeping sickness in tourists returning from Tanzania: the first 2 Italian cases from a small outbreak among European travelers. Clin Infect Dis 2002;34:e18–22.
[36] Bisoffi Z, Matteelli A, Aquilini D, et al. Illicit trade in humans and risks of disease spread: recurrent clusters of malaria in Chinese illegal immigrants to Europe through Africa. Emerg Infect Dis 2003;9:1177–8.
[37] Shen J, Zhang S, Xu B, et al. Surveillance for low-level malaria. Trans R Soc Trop Med Hyg 1988;92:3–6.

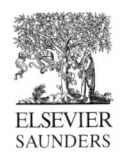

# Challenging Scenarios in a Travel Clinic: Advising the Complex Traveler

Kathryn N. Suh, MD, FRCPC[a,b,*], Maria D. Mileno, MD[c,d]

[a]*Division of Infectious Diseases, Children's Hospital of Eastern Ontario, 401 Smyth Road, Ottawa, ON K1H 8L1, Canada*
[b]*Department of Paediatrics, University of Ottawa, Ottawa, ON, Canada*
[c]*The Miriam Hospital, 164 Summit Avenue, Providence, RI 02906, USA*
[d]*Department of Medicine, Brown Medical School, Providence, RI, USA*

As the spectrum of international travelers continues to expand, travel health professionals are faced with the challenges of counseling a diverse group of travelers, including those at extremes of age, pregnant women, and travelers with children and with underlying medical conditions. With appropriate planning and advice, most people can experience safe and rewarding travel.

Travelers, especially complex or high-risk travelers, should seek pretravel advice as far in advance as possible. Along with a discussion of immunizations, malaria prophylaxis, and an approach to the management of traveler's diarrhea (TD), additional advice regarding supplemental health insurance, accidents and injury, motion sickness, jet lag, extremes of temperature and sun exposure, and food and water safety should be provided. An emergency medical bracelet (eg, Medic Alert) can provide priceless information for the traveler who may lose consciousness (eg, travelers with diabetes, epilepsy, cardiac disease). A list of medical services abroad can be obtained in advance from several sources including the International Association for Medical Assistance to Travelers (www.iamat.org) and Travax EnCompass (www.shoreland.com). Medical care with English-speaking physicians can be arranged in advance if required. International SOS (www.internationalsos.com) and Medex (www.medexassist.com) also provide emergency medical assistance for travelers in many countries.

---

* Corresponding author. Division of Infectious Diseases, Children's Hospital of Eastern Ontario, 401 Smyth Road, Ottawa, ON K1H 8L1, Canada.
  *E-mail address:* ksuh@cheo.on.ca (K.N. Suh).

Special considerations regarding immunization of complex travelers must be addressed. Routine immunizations should be updated. Measles-mumps-rubella (MMR), varicella, and yellow fever (YF) vaccines are live viral vaccines and are contraindicated in most individuals with underlying immune deficiencies. Live vaccines should either be given simultaneously or be separated by at least 28 days; inactivated vaccines may be given before, after, or at the same time as live vaccines. Contraindications to available vaccines can be found at www.cdc.gov/nip/recs/contraindications.htm. Travelers with medical contraindications may be exempted from YF immunization, required by many countries in South America and Africa (www.cdc.gov/travel/yb/outline.htm#2). Immunoprophylaxis should be considered for the following diseases, depending on the traveler's age, duration of travel, destination, and specific exposure risks: hepatitis A and B, Japanese encephalitis (JE), meningococcal disease, rabies, and *Salmonella typhi*. JE poses an extremely low risk to most travelers to Asia, with an estimated risk of 1 case per 5000 travelers per month in travelers to endemic areas including China, Korea, Japan, Southeast Asia, and the Indian subcontinent [1]. Meningococcal disease is a low risk to most travelers [2] except those to epidemic and endemic regions, particularly sub-Saharan Africa between December and June. Typhoid vaccine is recommended for prolonged travel to developing countries [3]. Because a significant proportion of cases occurs in short-term travelers, however, immunization is appropriate for any travelers to high-risk destinations (India, Nepal, Africa, and Central and South America) [4], and travelers at risk of severe consequences from typhoid fever. The seasonality of influenza differs depending on the destination; in the tropics influenza occurs year-round, and in the Southern Hemisphere between April and September. Cholera vaccine is not recommended for travelers by the Centers for Disease Control and Prevention [5] and is no longer available in the United States.

Emerging resistance patterns of malaria and the potential side effects or contraindications of antimalarial agents can make it difficult to advise complex travelers venturing to malarious areas. Personal protective measures and appropriate chemoprophylaxis must always be recommended.

Given the risks of bacteremia from TD in some immunocompromised travelers, food and water safety is of paramount importance in preventing TD and certain other infections. Although antibiotics for self-treatment of TD can be used safely, chemoprophylaxis is not usually recommended.

This article examines specific issues related to complex travelers by presenting illustrative scenarios and discussing relevant issues in detail.

### Scenario 1: traveling with young children

A family of five is planning a 6-week vacation in Africa in July, 3 months from their visit. The three healthy children will be 9 years, 4 years, and 8 months of age at departure. They are traveling first to Cape Town, South

Africa, and will visit Kruger National Park. They will also visit Madagascar and Kenya before returning to South Africa and then coming home. They anticipate spending some time in remote areas.

*What advice should be provided regarding travel preparation for their children? What special issues must be considered when traveling with children?*

Travel can be enriching and quite suitable for some families with small children. Children may be more tolerant to disruptions in regular schedules, environment, time changes, and jet lag, yet more precautions are needed because they are more susceptible to accidents, extremes in temperature, and some travel-related infections (eg, TD, rabies). The consequences of infections, such as TD and malaria, may also be more severe in children.

Notarized documentation of the child's status may prove invaluable if both parents cannot travel with their children. For the child traveling without either parent, a letter signed by both is recommended. For the child traveling with one parent, a letter signed by the nontraveling parent, or documentation of custody rights (or death of the other parent) is recommended [6]. Inability to produce documentation if requested in the United States may result in travel delays while the child's status is ascertained; in other countries, entry may be denied.

Air travel is safe for healthy children of any age, including newborns [5]. With time or appropriate therapy, most underlying medical conditions can be improved sufficiently to permit travel. Children with chronic medical conditions (eg, cardiopulmonary diseases, otolaryngologic disorders) should be assessed to determine if air travel is safe and if any additional requirements (eg, supplemental oxygen) should be arranged before flight. The Federal Aviation Agency recommends that all children less than 40 lb who fly, regardless of age, use an appropriate Federal Aviation Agency–approved safety restraint; this requires a separate ticket for the child [7].

*Immunizations*

Recommended immunizations should be updated (available online at www.cdc.gov/nip/recs/child-schedule.htm). Effective Fall 2004, influenza immunization is also recommended for all healthy children between 6 and 24 months of age. Some routine immunizations can be administered early and using an accelerated schedule, if required (Table 1). DTaP, inactivated poliovirus, and *Haemophilus influenzae* type b vaccines can be given as early as 6 weeks of age. Note that infants may respond poorly to some vaccines for several reasons, including the relative immaturity of the immune system in early life and interference of maternal antibodies with the vaccine response [8,9].

At least three doses of tetanus toxoid and pertussis vaccine are recommended before travel [5]. MMR vaccine is not routinely recommended for children less than 12 months because of suboptimal immune response [8],

Table 1
Accelerated schedules for recommended childhood immunizations[a]

| Vaccine | Dose and route | Minimum age at first dose | Minimum interval between subsequent doses[b] | Comments |
|---|---|---|---|---|
| DTP or DTaP | 0.5 mL IM | 6 wk | 4 wk (see comments) | First three doses can be given at 4-wk intervals to achieve minimum of three doses before travel; fourth dose at ≥12 mo of age, provided ≥6 mo have elapsed since third dose |
| Polio (inactivated) | 0.5 mL IM or SC | 6 wk | 4 wk (see comments) | Three doses of IPV recommended before travel; fourth dose recommended at 4–6 y but can be given at 18 wk of age |
| Haemophilus influenzae type b | 0.5 mL IM | 6 wk | 4 wk (see comments) | PRP-OMP: usually two doses at 2, 4 mo of age; HbOC or PRP-T: usually three doses at 2, 4, 6 mo of age; third (PRP-OMP) or fourth dose required at 12–15 mo regardless of vaccine used |
| MMR (live) | 0.5 mL SC | 6 mo | See comments | May be contraindicated in some immunosuppressed children; for children 6–12 mo, monovalent measles vaccine preferred (0.5 mL SC; 12–15 mo and 4–6 y MMR still required |

| | | | | |
|---|---|---|---|---|
| Pneumococcal (conjugate) (Prevnar) | (0.5 mL SC or IM) | 6 wk | 4 wk (see comments) | First three doses can be given at 4-wk intervals; fourth dose at 12–15 mo; for all children 2–23 mo (and for high-risk children 2–5 y) |
| Hepatitis B | 5 μg (Recombivax) 10 μg (Engerix) | Birth | 4 wk before 2nd 3 mo before 3rd | Infants born to HBsAg-positive mothers also require hepatitis B IG |
| Influenza | 0.25 mL IM (6–35 mo) 0.5 mL IM (>3 y) | 6 mo | See comments | Children <9 y receiving for the first time require two doses at least 4 wk apart |
| Varicella zoster (live) | 0.5 mL SC | 12 mo | See comments | May be contraindicated in some immunocompromised children; children ≥13 y require two doses at least 1 mo apart |

*Abbreviations:* DTaP, diphtheria-tetanus-acellular pertussis; DTP, diphtheria-tetanus-pertussis; HBsAg, hepatitis B surface antigen; IG, immune globulin; IM, intramuscular; IPV, inactivated polio virus; SC, subcutaneous.

[a] Whenever possible, children should be immunized according to the recommended immunization schedule (available online at www.cdc.gov/nip/recs/child-schedule.htm). The accelerated schedule should only be used when time does not allow the recommended schedule to be followed.

[b] Refers only to those doses required to complete primary series.

but children aged 6 to 12 months who are traveling to areas where measles remains common (Africa, southeast Asia, Europe) should be immunized [5]. Monovalent measles vaccine is preferred; MMR can also be given but does not negate the requirement for two doses of MMR immunization after age 12 months. Immune globulin (IG) interferes with the response to measles and MMR (and varicella) vaccines for at least 3 months after IG administration. Children who require hepatitis A IG (those who cannot be immunized) should receive measles or MMR vaccine at least 2 weeks before receiving hepatitis A IG.

Contraindications to and minimum age for travel immunizations are shown in Table 2. Bacille Calmette-Guérin, although widely used in children in tuberculosis-endemic areas, is not recommended for children before travel [10]. Tick-borne encephalitis vaccine is safe for use in infants and children and routinely administered to children living in endemic areas (central and eastern Europe); however, it is not available in the United States [11]. YF vaccine is absolutely contraindicated less than 6 months of age and not recommended before 9 months of age because of the increased risk of postvaccinal encephalitis in infants [12]. Although the overall risk of this complication is low (<1 in 8 million), 16 of the 25 reported cases associated with YF vaccine between 1945 and 2002 have occurred in children less than 7 months of age (0.5 to 4 cases per 1000 immunized infants) [12,13]. In general, travel to active YF areas should be avoided in children less than 9 months old; if travel is essential, vaccination can be considered in consultation with the Centers for Disease Control and Prevention (telephone 404-498-1600).

Hepatitis A is prevalent in many parts of the world. Maternal hepatitis A antibody may interfere with vaccine response in infants [14], and for this reason immunization is not recommended for children as young as 12 months of age [11]. Children born to seropositive mothers can respond well to vaccine at 1 year of age, however, and infants born to seronegative mothers respond at even younger ages, so that in many other countries hepatitis A vaccine is recommended for children greater than or equal to 12 months of age [11]. The risk of hepatitis B in pediatric travelers is greatest in those who visit endemic areas for prolonged periods. For children requiring hepatitis A and B immunizations, the combined vaccine is safe to use [15]. In the United States, however, this vaccine is licensed only for those 18 years of age or older; in other countries (eg, Canada) a pediatric formulation is licensed for use in children greater than 1 year. JE vaccine is not recommended in children less than 1 year of age because safety and efficacy data are lacking [1]. An accelerated schedule is not recommended in children, although it is tolerated in healthy adults.

Response to the quadrivalent polysaccharide *Neisseria meningitidis* vaccine is suboptimal in children less than 2 years [16], although a partial antibody response may be generated to serotype A in children greater than 3 months. Conjugate vaccines for serogroups C and A-C, available outside the United States, are safe and highly immunogenic [17], with estimated vaccine efficacy in infants of 92% [18]. Children less than 2 years cannot be offered complete protection against all vaccine serotypes of *N meningitidis*.

Children are at greatest risk of acquiring rabies. They may not avoid stray animals or report animal contact. Bites occur more often on the trunk and face and are more severe than in adults. Immunization is appropriate if exposure to rabid animals is likely to occur (Africa, Asia, India, Central and South America), or if safe postexposure management is not readily accessible. Vaccine-adverse events are uncommon. Pre-exposure immunization averts the need to find expensive (and often unavailable) rabies IG urgently in the event of an exposure. Regardless of immunization status, a thorough assessment is still required if exposure or a bite has occurred.

Two typhoid vaccines are available in the United States. The injectable polysaccharide vaccine, Typhim Vi, is poorly immunogenic in children less than age 2 years. Ty21a, the live attenuated oral vaccine, is more cumbersome to administer and can only be given to children greater than or equal to 6 years of age. The protective efficacy of either vaccine is 70% at most and falls with decreasing age [19,20].

*Malaria*

Malaria can be more severe in young children, who are more vulnerable to insect exposures. Permethrin (or deltamethrin) applied to clothing and bed nets is extremely safe for use in infants and children. Children less than 2 months of age are relatively immobile and can be protected largely by using permethrin-impregnated clothing and mosquito nets. N, N-diethyl-meta-toluamide (DEET) is the most effective mosquito repellant and can be applied safely (as directed) to children over 2 months of age [5]. Thirty-five percent DEET is the suggested maximum concentration recommended for use in adults and children, although concentrations of up to 50% are safe if applied properly. Concern regarding increased neurotoxicity (seizures) in children is based on a handful of case reports associated with excessive application, and has not been borne out in a large population-based study in the United States [21]. DEET should be washed off when children come indoors.

Pediatric (weight-based) dosing for antimalarial chemoprophylaxis is outlined in Table 3. Chloroquine, mefloquine, primaquine, and atovaquone-proguanil (AP) are available in the United States as tablets only, but can be crushed and the appropriate dose encapsulated. Chloroquine, mefloquine, and AP taste bitter; the use of a once-weekly agent (if possible) and addition of syrup, jam, or pudding to the powder may facilitate administration.

Chloroquine is safe and well tolerated in children of any age. In Europe, pediatric tablets (125 mg, 75 mg chloroquine base) and suspension are available. Crushing the adult tablets may be easier using generic chloroquine [22]. Where chloroquine-resistant *Plasmodium falciparum* is prevalent, mefloquine should be used regardless of age and weight [5], although it is not Food and Drug Administration approved for use in children less than 15 kg. Adverse

Table 2
Travel vaccines: minimum age, dose and schedule, and contraindications

| Vaccine | Dose | Earliest age at first dose | Minimum interval before subsequent doses[b] | Contraindications[a] or Comments |
|---|---|---|---|---|
| Cholera | — | — | — | Not recommended |
| Hepatitis A | 0.5 mL IM | 24 mo (United States) | 6 mo | Same volume for VAQTA or HAVRIX pediatric formulations; minimum age in many other countries is 12 mo; give ≥ 2 wk before departure |
| Hepatitis A IG | 0.02–0.06 mL/kg IM | Birth | — | Vaccine preferred; use only if immunization cannot be administered (can also be given simultaneously with vaccine)<br>Travel <3 mo: 0.02 mL/kg<br>3–5 mo: 0.06 mL/kg<br>>5 mo requires repeated dosing |
| Japanese encephalitis | 0.5 mL SC on days 0, 7, 30 | 1 y | 7 d (day 0, 7, 14) | Complete series at least 10 d before departure; accelerated schedule not recommended in children |
| Meningococcal (polysaccharide) | 0.5 mL SC | 2 y | — | Suboptimal efficacy under age 2 (see text) |
| Meningococcal (conjugated) (eg, Menjugate, Neis Vac-C) | 0.5 mL IM | 2 mo | 4 wk | Not yet available in the United States; children <12 mo require three doses (usually at 2, 4, 6 mo of age); children ≥12 mo require one dose only |

| | | | |
|---|---|---|---|
| Rabies | 1 mL IM on days 0, 7, and 21 or 28 | Birth | Same volume regardless of vaccine used (PCEC, HDCV or RVA); intradermal route not recommended |
| Typhoid, inactivated (Typhim Vi) | 0.5 mL IM | 2 y | — |
| Typhoid (*live*, Ty21a) | 1 capsule every other day × four doses | 6 y | Contraindicated in immunosuppressed children; must be stored refrigerated and taken on an empty stomach |
| Yellow fever (*live*) | 0.5 mL SC | 6 mo | Contraindicated in immunosuppressed children (waiver); not recommended <9 mo of age (waiver, or do not travel) |

*Abbreviations:* HDCV, human diploid cell vaccine (rabies); IM, intramuscular; PCEC, chick embryo culture vaccine (rabies); RVA, rabies vaccine adsorbed; SC, subcutaneous.

[a] Includes known sensitivity to any component of the vaccine.
[b] Refers to those doses required to complete primary series; subsequent booster doses not included.

Table 3
Pediatric dosing for antimalarial chemoprophylaxis

| Agent | Pediatric dose | Duration |
|---|---|---|
| Atovaquone-proguanil[a] | <11 kg: no data<br>11–20 kg: one quarter adult tab or one pediatric tab daily<br>21–30 kg: half adult tab or two pediatric tabs daily<br>31–40 kg: three quarters adult tab or three pediatric tabs daily<br>>40 kg: one adult tab daily | Starting 1 d before entering malaria-endemic area, daily during exposure, and for 1 wk after departure |
| Chloroquine (base)<br>(150 mg base = 250 mg salt)[b] | 5 mg/kg (max 300 mg) po weekly | Starting ≥1 wk before entering malaria-endemic area, weekly during exposure, and for 4 wk after departure |
| Doxycycline | <8 y: contraindicated<br>≥8 y: 1.5 mg/kg (max 100 mg) daily | Starting 1 d before entering malaria-endemic area, daily during exposure, and for 4 wk after departure |
| Mefloquine (base)<br>(228 mg base = 250 mg salt)[b] | <5 kg: no data; 5 mg/kg<br>5–9 kg: one eighth tab weekly<br>10–19 kg: one quarter tab weekly<br>20–30 kg: half tab weekly<br>31–45 kg: three quarters tab weekly<br>>45 kg: one tab weekly | Starting ≥1 wk before entering malaria-endemic area, weekly during exposure, and for 4 wk after departure |
| Primaquine (base)<br>(15 mg base = 26.3 mg salt) | 0.5 mg/kg (max 30 mg) daily | Starting 1 d before entering malaria-endemic area, daily during exposure, and for 1 wk after departure |

[a] Atovaquone-proguanil (Malarone) pediatric tablets contain 62.5 mg atovaquone and 25 mg proguanil per tablet; adult tablets contain 250 mg atovaquone and 100 mg proguanil per tablet.
[b] Generic chloroquine tablets and mefloquine tablets are scored.

effects are primarily gastrointestinal; neuropsychiatric side effects are less common in children [23]. Children with known seizure disorders, pre-existing cardiac conduction defects, and neuropsychiatric disorders should not take mefloquine. Febrile seizures before age 5 years and attention deficit disorder have been suggested as contraindications to mefloquine [22], although no data support this. In mefloquine-resistant areas doxycycline can be used in children 8 years of age and older; permanent discoloration of teeth may occur if used in younger children. AP is Food and Drug Administration approved for use in children weighing 11 kg or more only, but should also be considered in children less than 11 kg traveling to drug-resistant areas, in whom other agents are contraindicated, not tolerated, or ineffective [22]. It is relatively expensive and must be administered daily, but is effective and well tolerated in children [24]. Primaquine can be used safely in children intolerant to other agents once G6PD deficiency has been ruled out. Standby therapy should not be routinely recommended for children.

*Traveler's diarrhea*

TD in children is best defined as a twofold increase in volume of loose stool. The risk of acquiring TD and the severity of illness seem to be greatest in children less than 3 years of age [25]. General food and water safety is the most important preventive measure. If infants are formula-fed, safe water (boiled or bottled) should be used for preparing formula.

Chemoprophylaxis of TD is not recommended [26]. Parents need careful instruction about when and how to treat TD. TD is usually self-limited; treatment consists mainly of rehydration with a glucose- and electrolyte-containing solution. Antidiarrheal agents, such as loperamide, should be avoided given the severe adverse effects (eg, ileus, toxic megacolon, and respiratory depression) that have been reported with use in children, and its possible detrimental effects on illness caused by invasive pathogens [26]. Early administration of antibiotics may be beneficial, provided bloody diarrhea and severe illness are absent. Short courses of fluoroquinolones (FQs), although not Food and Drug Administration approved for use in children less than 16 years, are safe and should be considered the treatment of choice for TD in children [27]. Azithromycin is safe in children and demonstrates good in vitro activity against most bacterial TD pathogens [28]. It is particularly useful for treatment of TD in Thailand and other areas of southeast Asia, where FQ-resistant *Campylobacter* infections are prevalent [29]. Cefixime may be effective in children, but should only be considered if a FQ or azithromycin cannot be used, and does not treat *Campylobacter* infections. Antibiotic doses for children are listed in Table 4.

*Summary recommendations*

Routine immunizations should be updated. The 8 month old should receive a measles (or MMR) vaccine 2 to 4 weeks before hepatitis A IG is

Table 4
Pediatric dosing for empiric antimicrobial therapy of traveler's diarrhea

| Agent | Pediatric dose | Comments |
|---|---|---|
| Amoxicillin | 15–20 mg/kg (max 500 mg) po tid × 3 d | Limited effectiveness because of widespread resistance |
| Azithromycin | 10 mg/kg (max 500 mg) po on day 1, then 5–10 mg/kg (max 500 mg) on days 2 and 3 | May be used as first-line therapy (or ciprofloxacin); especially useful for travel to Thailand and Southeast Asia because of high rates of fluoroquinolone-resistant *Campylobacter* |
| Cefixime | 8 mg/kg (max 400 mg) po daily × 3 d | Use only if azithromycin and fluoroquinolone contraindicated; does not cover *Campylobacter* |
| Ciprofloxacin | 10–15 mg/kg (max 500 mg) po bid × 3 d | Not Food and Drug Administration approved for use in children <16 years; however, may be recommended as first-line therapy (or azithromycin) |
| Trimethoprim-sulfamethoxazole (TMP-SMX) | 4–6 mg TMP (maximum 160 mg TMP) po bid × 3 d | Limited effectiveness because of widespread resistance |

given. The 4 year old can receive his second MMR before departure; the 4 and 8 year olds should be immunized against hepatitis A. All should receive influenza immunizations (if available), and the two younger children in particular should be given rabies vaccine. The 8 month old should not receive YF vaccine (a waiver should be written), but the two older children should for travel to rural Kenya. Typhim Vi vaccine can be recommended for the two older children.

DEET and permethrin should be used for all three children. Adequate time must be spent outlining the safety and correct use of these agents. Mefloquine or AP should be recommended for malaria chemoprophylaxis; doxycycline may be used in the 9 year old. A 3-day course of azithromycin or ciprofloxacin can be prescribed for TD treatment.

### Scenario 2: the elderly traveler

An elderly couple in their mid-70s would like to return home to India to visit family. They have lived in the United States for the past 30 years. He is in generally good health apart from rheumatoid arthritis; he takes infliximab and nonsteroidal anti-inflammatory drugs, and uses a cane to walk. His wife is healthy with no underlying medical problems.

*Is it safe for this couple to travel, and if so what advice should be provided to them?*

Older travelers may be less tolerant of the rigors of travel, and may suffer from fatigue, jet lag, insomnia, and constipation. Acclimatization to heat, cold, or altitude may be more prolonged. Dehydration, hyperthermia, and hypothermia may occur more readily and with greater consequences.

An overall physical assessment should be performed by the individual's physician to determine fitness to travel, and to identify medical problems that may prohibit travel entirely or require further investigation or management before travel. A conditioning program can be beneficial if the trip is expected to be arduous.

Older travelers should allow ample time for transportation and transfers, and inform the air carrier in advance of the need for assistance and other special services that are required (porters, wheelchairs). Mobility aids should be accommodated at no extra cost. Aisle or bulkhead seats may be preferable.

Air travel is safe if the relative hypoxia of flight is well tolerated. This excludes those with underlying medical conditions including pneumothorax; unstable angina; recent myocardial infarction; and recent thoracic, cardiac, abdominal, or middle ear surgery. Most medical emergencies in air travelers occur on the ground; in-flight emergencies are relatively rare [30]. Unforeseen emergencies, such as sudden cardiac events, do occur, often in travelers with no prior cardiac history. Medical emergencies in the older traveler are most often related to accidents or injury; slower reaction times, auditory or visual impairment, and medication side effects may contribute to their increased occurrence in older individuals.

Risk factors for venous thromboembolic disease in travelers include advanced age (>75 years); a prior history of venous thromboembolic disease; malignancy; prolonged immobility; and hyperestrogenic and hypercoagulable states [31]. Long-haul flights may further increase this risk. Measures that can reduce the risk of venous thrombosis include regular contraction of calf muscles during flight (periodically walking the aisles or, if this is not safe or feasible, flexing the ankles) and adequate hydration. Compression stockings or aspirin or other anticoagulants may be appropriate in travelers with significant risk factors for venous thrombosis [31].

*Immunizations*

Recommendations are unaltered by older age. Specific precautions and recommendations for travelers, such as this man taking infliximab, and those with other causes of immune suppression, are shown in Table 5. Responses to immunization may take longer and be less robust in the older traveler, but data relating to vaccine efficacy and immunogenicity in this population are lacking. Tetanus is rare in adequately immunized individuals, and deaths occur mainly in the elderly [32]. Pneumococcal (23-valent)

Table 5
Immune suppression[a] and immunizations

| Type of immune suppression | Cautions | Suggestions |
|---|---|---|
| Travelers with solid organ transplants | Avoid traveling <1 y posttransplant | Pneumococcal, meningococcal, and *H influenzae* type b vaccines. Hepatitis B and influenza vaccines pretransplant. |
| Travelers with hematologic malignancies | No live virus vaccines <3 mo after last therapy | Pneumococcal and *H influenzae* type b vaccines, ideally 2 wk before suppressive therapy. DTaP, Td, influenza, IPV as indicated. MMR and varicella if not severely immunosuppressed. |
| Congenital immune disorders | No live vaccines | Intravenous immunoglobulin is used in the management of a number of these disorders but the benefit only lasts for 2–3 wk. |
| Drug-induced immunosuppression | No live vaccines if taking >20 mg/d steroids for >2 wk | Vaccinate 1 mo after last dose of steroid therapy. |
| Other immunosuppressive drugs/therapy[a] | No live vaccines; suppression may last up to 3 mo from last dose; can use double dose for hepatitis B vaccine | Vaccinate >1 mo after last dose. If vaccinated while receiving immunosuppressive therapy or in the 2 wk preceding therapy, revaccinate ≥3 mo after therapy is discontinued. |
| Autoimmune disorders: multiple sclerosis | | Immunize as normal |
| Chronic diseases and drugs associated with immune defects | No live vaccines with significant immunosuppression | Pneumococcal, influenza, *H influenzae* type b, hepatitis B vaccines. |
| Hyposplenism | | Pneumococcal, meningococcal, *H influenzae* type b, and influenza vaccines. Prophylactic antibiotics. |

*Abbreviations:* DTaP, diphtheria-tetanus-acellular pertussis; IPV, inactive poliovirus; MMR, measles-mumps-rubella; Td, tetanus-diphtheria.

[a] Immune suppression includes the following immunosuppressive agents and procedures: alkylating agents; cyclophosphamide; tumor necrosis factor blocking drugs (infliximab, etanercept); plasma exchange; methotrexate (including low dose); 6-mercaptopurine and azathioprine; cyclosporine and tacrolimus; total lymphoid irradiation; antilymphocyte globulin.

and influenza immunizations are recommended for all adults 65 years of age and older. Most adults from temperate zones are immune to varicella, but immunization should be considered if they are seronegative.

The risk of severe disease and death from YF increases with age. Vaccine side effects (local reactions, headache, and myalgias) seem to be less common in older recipients. Postvaccinal encephalitis is rare in adults, but the risk of vaccine-related viscerotropic disease, characterized by severe multiorgan failure, increases with age [33]. Although the absolute risk is still relatively small (for those >65 years, 1 in 50,000), consideration should be given to providing a medical waiver to older travelers when immunization is required for entry but no risk of YF exists.

Many older travelers who have lived in or traveled to hepatitis A–endemic areas are immune to this disease; serologic screening may be cost-effective in these circumstances. Typhoid vaccine is advisable given the increased morbidity and mortality of typhoid fever with advancing age. Excluding YF vaccine, there is no evidence that older travelers suffer more adverse effects from travel vaccines than younger travelers, but data are lacking in this population.

*Malaria*

Malaria risk in older travelers must not be trivialized. The severity of disease and mortality from malaria both increase with age. DEET and permethrin are safe to use and should be encouraged. Age alone is not a contraindication to the use of any chemoprophylactic agent. Chloroquine can rarely cause permanent retinal damage and hearing loss if used in the presence of existing visual and auditory impairments, respectively. Cardiac conduction defects are more prevalent in older travelers and are contraindications to mefloquine use. AP is well tolerated based on the small number of subjects greater than 65 years included in studies to date.

*Traveler's diarrhea*

TD may be poorly tolerated in older travelers, especially those who may be severely affected by resulting fluid and electrolyte imbalances. There is no evidence that chemoprophylaxis of TD is of value in the elderly. Antidiarrheal agents should be used with caution, because they may cause rebound constipation and paralytic ileus. Older FQs remain the antibiotics of choice for self-treatment of TD in most destinations.

*Summary recommendations*

Provided there are no absolute contraindications to travel, this couple can travel safely to India. They may need extra time and assistance during travel, given the husband's arthritis and use of a cane. Review measures to reduce the risk of venous thromboembolic disease, and reinforce the need for adequate hydration with the husband's ongoing need for nonsteroidal anti-inflammatory drugs. He should ensure that he has a more than adequate supply of medication for the duration of travel, and carry this with him. It may be prudent also to carry a copy of a recent EKG and prescriptions. Were he to develop a severe infection (eg, tuberculosis), effective treatment would require discontinuation of his immunosuppressive agent.

Update immunizations, including influenza and pneumococcal vaccines. It is worthwhile to test for hepatitis A and varicella antibodies before immunization. YF vaccine is not indicated. Inactivated typhoid vaccine should be offered. The need for other travel vaccines should be based on their anticipated exposures.

The need for malaria prophylaxis must be stressed. This couple, like many immigrants from malaria-endemic regions, may believe themselves to be immune to malaria especially if they have had it before [34]. Chloroquine-resistant *P falciparum* is common in India, and for this reason mefloquine (alternatively, AP or doxycycline) should be recommended. Because of the high prevalence of *Plasmodium vivax* malaria in India, G6PD testing can be performed in the event that primaquine is required for terminal prophylaxis of this infection.

Food and water safety may be problematic if they are staying with relatives and eating locally prepared foods. Ciprofloxacin is appropriate for empiric therapy of TD.

### Scenario 3: the diabetic traveler

A 66-year-old retired lawyer seeks advice to prepare for travel to Beijing, China, where he will give a presentation about his book. He will travel there eastbound nonstop from Boston and then will present in, Egypt, Turkey, Uzbekistan, and Hong Kong in addition to Beijing. He continues to fly east from Beijing to complete his travel itinerary passing through the west coast of the United States. Other plans include walking tours in several cities. He has used an antihypertensive agent daily for 6 years and just began taking metformin for type II diabetes, although he admits he had uncontrolled fasting blood sugars ranging from 138 to 156 mg/dL for several years despite dietary changes. He has never taken such a long air flight. He recently began a new exercise program of walking and just purchased new shoes for the trip.

*What questions should we ask about his current pattern of blood sugar monitoring? What are his risks of hypoglycemia and how can they be avoided? How would insulin administration change if needed? What other risks are there?*

It is most important for this patient to carry an adequate supply of everything required for diabetes care (and any other medical conditions) on his person during travel, including an additional 50% supply of medications and food, meals, glucose tablets, and glucagon in case of unforeseen transportation delays [31]. He should carry a letter from his physician in his passport outlining the diagnosis; treatment requirements; and the need to carry medication, needles, and syringes. Travelers can check the American Diabetes Association website (www.diabetes.org) and with the airline carrier to confirm the airline's policy with regard to carrying diabetes medication and supplies, given some of the newer security measures taken since 9/11.

*Management of diabetes*

Individualized advice by expert personnel regarding insulin management during travel is best, provided a simplified approach is offered. Tight glucose control, an important goal for all diabetics, runs the risk of hypoglycemic episodes while crossing multiple time zones. A safer approach is to advise the traveler to accept higher than normal glucose readings during travel. More frequent blood glucose monitoring is the best way to avoid the serious consequences of hypoglycemia and to determine insulin needs [35]. Keeping track of elapsed time during travel is the most challenging part. Instruct individuals to take their blood glucose measurements every 4 to 6 hours while en route and crossing multiple time zones, even if they are not accustomed to such frequent monitoring. Travelers on oral hypoglycemics do not require additional doses and should take their medication according to local time; however, care should be taken to avoid missing meals. Omitting the evening dose on eastbound flights results only in tolerably elevated blood glucose levels and helps avoid hypoglycemia, rather than taking doses too close together. For insulin users, north-south travel and crossing less than six time zones also requires no adjustment of insulin dosing schedules [36]. Crossing greater than or equal to six time zones while traveling eastward leads to a shortened day, and less insulin is required. Sane et al [37] suggest decreasing the daily dose of insulin by 2% to 4% per hour of time shift during eastward flights, and increasing dosing by the same amount for westward flights. Good examples of individualized insulin regimens are available at www.diabetesmonitor.com. Cultural and religious issues may include fasting as an important part of the traveler's plans and such risks should be drawn out and addressed during the consultation.

Insulin preparations vary, and advances in diabetes care with availability of prefilled syringes and cartridges can ease administration and storage during travel. In particular, active traveling diabetic patients can benefit from short-acting insulin Lispro because of its convenience and short-acting property. Details on these preparations can be found in additional excellent resources [31,35,36].

*Other issues*

Prevention strategies and early antibiotic treatment of routine problems can help avoid life-threatening syndromes in diabetic persons. Appropriate self-medication strategies for several issues should be set in place before travel. Diligent foot care is of paramount importance. Advise frequent changes of socks to reduce persistent pressure points and avoidance of new shoes. New shoes may cause blisters, thereby creating portals of entry for bacteria and increasing the risk of cellulitis or more serious infections of underlying soft tissue or bone. Examination of feet each night, along with management of foot injuries with appropriate antibiotics on hand if there is a possible early infection to avoid both severe local infection (eg, pyomyositis) and systemic infection, should be reinforced. Urinary tract infections in diabetic women are common and a 2-week supply of FQs should be offered for the occurrence of such infections.

It is important to ask about any recent surgery. For example, for 1 year after laser treatments the diabetic retina may not respond well to hypoxia from prolonged air flights requiring pressurized cabins. Remind the traveler to seek advice from his or her ophthalmologist regarding the risk of recent eye treatments.

Although not a specific risk to diabetic travelers per se, preventive measures against venous thromboembolic disease should also be reviewed.

*Immunizations, malaria, and traveler's diarrhea*

The usual vaccines and discussion of prevention of food- and water-related illness and malaria, and empiric treatment for TD, should be offered as for any traveler. Note that a diabetic individual might be more likely to require health care abroad and this strongly increases the importance of hepatitis B immunization. Emphasize that safe drinking water may also reduce *Helicobacter pylori* seroconversion rates [38], and this infection has been associated with increased insulin requirements and poor diabetes control particularly in diabetic children [39].

*Summary recommendations*

Diabetic travelers require no changes in pretravel preparation regarding immunizations, malaria prevention, or TD. Dissuade this traveler from wearing new shoes. Review interventions to reduce his risk of venous thromboembolic disease developing during flight. A significant impact can be made by reviewing diabetes care and medication (oral hypoglycemic agents or insulin) adjustments; avoidance of hypoglycemic episodes; and the risks and prevention of minor injuries. He should be advised not to miss meals during travel, and to omit his evening dose of metformin on the flights leading up to Beijing and following; he should resume his regular dose and schedule on arrival, according to local time. Some of his other flights are shorter and may not require this adjustment.

**Scenario 4: the pregnant traveler**

A healthy 26-year-old woman and her partner are leaving on a 2-month trip to Thailand. Most of their trip, apart from their flight to Bangkok, is unplanned; they had intended to trek and camp most of the time. The couple has just learned she is pregnant. They are scheduled to leave in 2 months, at which time she will be approximately 14 weeks pregnant.

*They are reluctant to cancel their trip. What advice should pregnant travelers receive and what specific precautions need to be addressed? Are there any circumstances that warrant postponing travel?*

Travel during pregnancy is safe provided no medical contraindications to travel exist, and the destination and type of travel do not pose significant harm to mother or child. The pregnant woman should be thoroughly assessed by her obstetrician regarding her safety to travel. The presence of significant medical or obstetric conditions may be contraindications to travel (Box 1). In general, it is preferable to avoid using medications and immunizations during the first trimester, based largely on theoretical risks to the developing fetus, and to avoid travel during the last 4 to 6 weeks of pregnancy.

The safest time to travel is during the second trimester. The risk of miscarriage is greatest early on, and obstetric complications (preeclampsia, preterm labor) are more likely during the third trimester. Travel during the third trimester may also be more uncomfortable. Airline travel itself is not harmful to the pregnancy [40] and is usually permitted until the thirty-fifth (international) or thirty-sixth (domestic) week of gestation.

Additional issues worthy of discussion include the use of high SPF sunscreen to avoid excessive facial pigmentation of pregnancy; treatment of

---

**Box 1. Some possible contraindications to travel during pregnancy**

*Obstetric contraindications*
- Extremes of maternal age
- Multiple gestation this pregnancy
- Vaginal bleeding this pregnancy
- Gestational diabetes mellitus or hypertension, ever
- Miscarriage, preterm labor, or premature rupture of membranes, ever

*Medical contraindications*
- Valvular heart disease or other cardiac disease
- Other medical conditions: pulmonary or kidney disease, diabetes, severe anemia
- History of thromboembolism

*Factors at travel destination*
- Extreme altitude
- Risk of YF, measles (live viral vaccine recommended)
- Mefloquine-resistant *P falciparum* malaria
- Epidemics of other infectious diseases
- Natural disasters, civil unrest

vaginal yeast infections; and the use of urine dipsticks and blood pressure cuffs for self-monitoring, especially during the third trimester. The possibility of unforeseen complications requiring health care abroad should be considered. Clear plans on when and how to seek emergency medical assistance should be established.

*Immunizations*

The risks and benefits of immunizations during pregnancy must be carefully weighed. Factors to consider include the woman's risk of illness, the likelihood of adverse fetal outcomes if the mother becomes ill, and the risks of the vaccine. Immunizations should be delayed until after the first trimester if possible. Serologic studies (eg, for varicella, hepatitis A or B) may be reasonable in some women to assess the need for active immunization.

In general, inactivated vaccines are safe and live vaccines are contraindicated during pregnancy. Tetanus and diphtheria toxoids and influenza vaccine can be administered routinely [41]. MMR and varicella are not recommended, but inadvertent administration during pregnancy has not been associated with an increased rate of adverse outcomes. If MMR is required and the risk of measles is significant, consideration should be given to delaying travel until MMR can be administered. Inactivated polio vaccine may be used if needed.

The safety of YF vaccine given during pregnancy is unknown. The risks of immunizing a pregnant woman are probably outweighed by the risk of disease if travel cannot be avoided [12], although serious consideration should be given to avoiding travel to active YF areas. If the risk of YF infection is small but proof of immunization is required, a medical waiver can be provided. Immunizations against hepatitis A and B, JE, meningococcal disease, rabies, and typhoid fever (inactivated) may be administered during pregnancy if the risk of acquiring these infections warrants. There are no safety data for JE or hepatitis A vaccines given during pregnancy. An effective alternative to hepatitis A immunization is hepatitis A IG.

*Malaria*

Malaria during pregnancy can have serious adverse outcomes to both mother and fetus. Pregnant women traveling to malarious areas should be informed of these risks and consider postponing travel, particularly when the destination includes mefloquine-resistant areas; traveling after pregnancy with the newborn may be an option. If travel during pregnancy cannot be avoided, personal protective measures are essential and antimalarial prophylaxis is mandatory.

Permethrin (or deltamethrin) and DEET are both safe for use during pregnancy. DEET does cross the placenta in small amounts, but has not been associated with an increased risk of adverse events in the fetus when used as directed. Chloroquine is safe during pregnancy. Mefloquine prophylaxis is not associated with increased rates of stillbirth or congenital malformations when used during the second and third trimesters. Postmarketing surveillance suggests that administration during the first trimester is also safe [42]. Doxycycline and primaquine are contraindicated. AP is not currently recommended because of the lack of safety data.

*Traveler's diarrhea*

Reduced gastric acidity during pregnancy may predispose to gastrointestinal illness. Listeriosis and toxoplasmosis may have significant effects on the pregnancy and developing fetus, and hepatitis E is of concern given its high mortality (up to 30%) in pregnant women. Boiling water is the most effective and safest means of purification. Iodinization of water should be avoided because of the risk of congenital goiter. Meats should be well cooked and all dairy products (including cheeses) should be pasteurized.

Bismuth and salicylate-containing products (eg, Pepto-Bismol) carry the risks of congenital malformations and fetal bleeding, respectively. Loperamide may be used if necessary. Effective antimicrobial choices are limited. Fluoroquinolones are contraindicated, although inadvertent exposure during pregnancy has not been associated with adverse outcomes. Azithromycin is safe in pregnancy (Food and Drug Administration category B). Cefixime is also safe during pregnancy but has not been proved effective in treatment of TD in adults.

*Breast-feeding and travel*

Breast-feeding during travel should be encouraged. In addition to its immunologic advantages, breast-feeding eliminates the need for preparing formula with potentially contaminated water.

Neither live nor inactivated vaccines are contraindicated during breast-feeding; they should be administered as otherwise indicated to both mother and child. Rubella is the only live virus known to be excreted into breast milk [43], but no vaccines administered to breast-feeding mothers are known to affect the health of the infant. There are no data regarding the use of live intranasal influenza vaccine with breast-feeding.

DEET is safe for use; ensure that the infant does not ingest it. All antimalarial agents are excreted into breast milk, but concentrations achieved are insufficient for protection of the infant, who must also be given appropriate antimalarial prophylaxis. Doxycycline is believed to be safe for use in breast-feeding mothers [5]. Although the concentration of primaquine in breast milk is unknown, the Centers for Disease Control and Prevention recommend that infants be tested for G6PD deficiency before primaquine is used. Similarly, caution is recommended when AP is considered during breast-feeding of infants less than 11 kg, because of lack of safety data.

For therapy of TD, amoxicillin, cephalosporins, trimethoprim-sulfamethoxazole, and azithromycin are safe for use while breast-feeding.

Fluoroquinolones may be used if necessary, without cessation of breast-feeding, because the risks to the infant are considered to be low [44].

*Summary recommendations*

The pregnant couple needs counseling regarding the risks of travel during pregnancy, particularly considering their destination. They may wish to postpone their trip; at very least they need to plan their itinerary carefully, attempting to avoid travel to mefloquine-resistant malaria zones. The physical aspects of travel during pregnancy should be reviewed; even women who feel well may not anticipate the effects that a pregnancy may have on travel.

Routine immunizations should be updated, excluding MMR. YF vaccine is not indicated. Hepatitis A IG or vaccine should be given. Hepatitis B is endemic in Thailand and it is appropriate to immunize her, in case she requires medical care while abroad. JE is hyperendemic in northern Thailand and sporadic cases occur in the south of the country; vaccination is reasonable if her risk warrants it. Typhoid vaccine (inactivated) should be recommended given the high prevalence of antimicrobial resistant *S typhi* in Thailand and the potential consequences of illness during pregnancy. Rabies vaccine should be offered if she may be at risk.

Malaria in Thailand is limited to the country's borders with Cambodia and Myanmar (Burma) (mefloquine-resistant *P falciparum*) and Laos (mefloquine-susceptible *P falciparum*). There is no safe and effective chemoprophylaxis for mefloquine-resistant falciparum malaria during pregnancy, and travel to the Cambodian and Burmese border regions should be discouraged. Mefloquine could be safely used for travel to eastern Thailand (Laotian border region), because she will be in her second trimester. For other areas of Thailand, malaria prophylaxis is not indicated.

For self-treatment of TD in pregnancy, and more so in Thailand, azithromycin, 500 mg orally daily for 3 days, is appropriate. Less effective but safe alternatives in mid-pregnancy include amoxicillin, trimethoprim-sulfamethoxazole, or cefixime. Acetaminophen rather than aspirin should be used to control fever.

**Scenario 5: travelers with HIV and AIDS**

A 44-year-old HIV-infected businessman with a CD4 count of 426 cells/mm$^3$ plans a 2-month trip to Africa with his partner, a 50-year-old man with AIDS (CD4 260 cells/mm$^3$). Both were diagnosed 1 year ago and are receiving antiretroviral agents with good control and they tolerate their therapies well. Apart from *Pneumocystis carinii* pneumonia as an AIDS-defining illness in the 50-year-old, no other opportunistic processes have occurred. Their plans include relief work with AIDS orphans for 1 month in Durban, South Africa, followed by trips to Kruger National Park and to Kenya for safari.

*What increased risks present in light of their HIV disease? What drug interactions must be avoided? Which vaccines are contraindicated?*

One consideration strictly related to HIV-infected persons who travel is the country-specific entry restriction; these vary greatly [45]. None exists at their destinations for their purposes of travel.

*Immunizations*

Susceptibility to and frequency and severity of many infectious diseases are increased in persons with HIV [35]. Vaccine-preventable diseases should be avoided and for most vaccines it is safe to immunize HIV-infected persons. Live vaccines are not recommended if the CD4 count is below 200/mm$^3$ [46]. Inactivated vaccines are safe in both children and adults, and yet immune responses may depend on the quality and number of CD4 cells, especially if less than 300/mm$^3$ [47,48]. Vaccines are not likely to offer benefit to persons who have less than 100/mm$^3$. Some experts recommend vaccinating 3 to 6 months after initiation of highly active antiviral therapy to allow maximal improvement in both number and function of CD4 cells [44].

There is controversy over YF vaccine use. Most agree that persons with CD4 counts greater than 400/mm$^3$ tolerate the vaccine safely, and with good efficacy. Other authors consider vaccination for HIV-infected persons with CD4 counts greater than 200/mm$^3$ who may be at substantial risk [46,49].

*Malaria and other infections*

Malaria can be more severe in HIV-infected individuals, with increased density and duration of parasitemia, and prolonged fever. There is also evidence that HIV is activated and replication increases in the presence of *P falciparum* [50]. Acquisition of other HIV-1 subtypes is a possibility during unprotected sex or needle sharing in other geographic regions [51]. Little information is available on the drug resistance profiles of subtypes other than B, the most common type in the United States (Table 6). Prudent behavior and avoidance of medical care abroad that incurs blood transfusions are sufficient to reduce this risk and should be discussed.

*Traveler's diarrhea*

There are increased risks of worsened disease from numerous pathogens, such as *Cryptosporidia*, *Isospora*, *Microsporidia*, and *Cyclospora*, and of bacteremia caused by *Campylobacter* and *Salmonella*. Filtration using a pore size of less than 1 μm may not remove all bacteria, and viruses and *Microsporidia* may be too small to be removed by this degree of filtration. Purification by boiling is adequate for elimination of all important enteric pathogens. Although some bacterial spores, such as those of *Clostridia* spp, may be resistant to boiling, they are not generally water-borne and boiling remains the most reliable method of water treatment.

Table 6
Geographic distribution of human immunodeficiency virus subtypes

| Country | Predominant subtypes (approximate %) |
| --- | --- |
| Brazil | B (80%), F (14%), C (3%) |
| China | B (41%), E (32%), reports of C and D |
| Haiti | B (most) |
| India | C (80%–95%), B (2%–10%), A (2%) |
| Malawi | C (most) |
| Peru | B (98%) |
| South Africa | C (most) |
| Thailand | CRF01_AE (80%–95%), B (5%–20%) |
| United States | B (most) |
| Vietnam | E (most) |
| Zimbabwe | C (70%), B (12%), A (12%), D (7%) |

AACTG A5175 supported in part by the Adult AIDS Clinical Trials Group of the National Institute of Allergy and Infectious Diseases Cooperative Agreement (AI38858), CFDA #93.856 and the General Clinical Research Center Units funded by the National Center for Research Resources.

*Adapted from* AACTG Protocol A5175: a phase IV, randomized, open-label evaluation of the efficacy of once-daily PI & once-daily non-NRTI - containing therapy combinations for initial treatment of HIV-1 infected individuals from diverse areas of the world. Appendix 1, p. 104.

*Drug interactions*

Numerous antiretroviral agents are available for treatment of HIV disease and consideration should be taken to avoid the impact of drug interactions. For example, mefloquine and protease inhibitors are both metabolized by cytochrome P-450 [52]. Inducers or inhibitors of P-450 might be expected to alter drug levels of these agents. Mefloquine has been shown to decrease ritonavir levels, yet there is less interaction between mefloquine and either nelfinavir or indinavir [52–54]. Ritonavir has little effect on mefloquine. Efavirenz (Sustiva) is an antiretroviral agent that may worsen the neuropsychiatric effects of mefloquine, although there are no data. By itself efavirenz can cause dizziness, altered consciousness, altered thinking, abnormal dreams, sleepiness, confusion, memory loss, and hallucinations [55].

Atovaquone can increase drug levels of the nucleoside reverse transcriptase inhibitors, such as stavudine and zidovudine, although it is unknown whether this is associated with increased toxicity. There are few data regarding proguanil and the antiretrovirals [56]. Abacavir can cause a hypersensitivity reaction similar to other drug eruptions (eg, photosensitivity from doxycycline), which can lead to fatal Stevens-Johnson syndrome if not discontinued promptly. Doxycycline can also lead to candidiasis, which can be an underlying problem for HIV-infected individuals. These challenges warrant discussion and planning for safe travel with HIV infection.

The best advice is to start antimalarials in advance of travel and monitor for adverse reactions. Short alterations in drug levels are unlikely to have a profound adverse effect on the progression of HIV disease. Review of other known drug interactions [46] is recommended before providing prescriptions for empiric treatment.

*Summary recommendations*

Both travelers could be vaccinated against YF. They should definitely receive both hepatitis A and B vaccines if not yet done, and inactivated typhoid vaccine. Pneumococcal vaccine every 5 to 6 years and yearly influenza vaccines are routine recommendations as are standard diphtheria and tetanus updates, and should be offered if required. Persons born before 1957 or with a history of measles infection or those who have a positive titer should be safe from acquiring new measles. These travelers will be working with children, and may well be at substantial risk of acquiring measles or meningococcal disease and may need these vaccines. Malaria prophylaxis and especially personal protective measures to avoid mosquitoes and other insects (eg, sandflies that transmit leishmaniasis) are of great importance. Consider AP as an antimalarial for persons on antiretroviral agents given its tolerability, and have the patient try concomitant use for a few days before departure.

Discussion of water and food safety and the approach to boiling and filtering water may make a great impact. Persons on short trips with very poor immune systems reflected by CD4 counts of less than or equal to 200/ $mm^3$ may benefit from daily ciprofloxacin, 500 mg daily, although antimicrobial prophylaxis for TD is not routinely recommended for HIV-infected travelers [57].

Tuberculin skin testing (purified protein derivative) before and after travel should be performed in both individuals to detect a potentially deleterious co-infection with tuberculosis. If the CD4 count is less than 100/ $mm^3$, consider prophylaxis with isoniazid during travel, regardless of the purified protein derivative result.

**Scenario 6: transplanted, asplenic, and cancer chemotherapy survivors**

A 21-year-old college graduate presents for travel advice for an upcoming 3-week trip to Ghana before entering medical school. Her plans include volunteer work at a hospital and she will be living with the family of friends while there. She reports that she is in good health currently but had undergone an autologous hematopoietic stem cell transplant as part of the treatment of osteogenic sarcoma 20 months ago. She is not currently on immunosuppressants. She had "lots of shots and blood transfusions" but her vaccination records were left at her college and are not available for review.

*Which immunizations should be completed before travel and how effective will they be? Is her risk for malaria the same as that of other travelers? Are opportunistic infections a risk for her? How does her risk compare with the asplenic and cancer chemotherapy patient?*

Transplant recipients are unique travelers and represent a small but significant population of high-risk travelers. Solid organ transplant recipients have defects in cell-mediated immunity because of continued need for immunosuppressants, which place them at risk for the usual and opportunistic pathogens. One retrospective survey of solid organ transplant recipients who have traveled revealed that 63% went to hepatitis A–endemic regions yet only 5% received the hepatitis A vaccine, and half traveled to dengue- and malaria-endemic areas yet less than 25% adhered to mosquito prevention measures [58]. Only 66.3% sought pretravel health information, mostly from their transplant physician.

Persons who have undergone allogeneic hematopoietic stem cell transplantation are more severely immunosuppressed than are solid organ recipients and are considered functionally asplenic [35]. Hematopoietic stem cell transplantation recipients are presumed immunocompetent at or beyond 24 months following transplantation if they are not on immunosuppressive therapy and do not have graft-versus-host disease.

Although risks of infections post-transplant more often relate to reactivation of dormant pathogens, such as herpes viruses, outbreaks caused by diseases such as histoplasmosis have been reported in travelers, and transplant recipients may have more risk for exposure to opportunistic pathogens.

*Immunizations*

Antibody titers to vaccine-preventable diseases including tetanus, polio, measles, mumps, rubella, and encapsulated organisms decline during the 1- to 4-year period following allogeneic and autologous hematopoietic stem cell transplantation unless the recipient is revaccinated. A vaccination strategy for hematopoietic stem cell transplantation patients is outlined in Table 7, and advice for solid organ transplant recipients is shown in Table 8. Influenza vaccination of family members and close or household contacts is strongly advised during each influenza season starting before the hematopoietic stem cell transplantation and continuing through at least 24 months afterward to prevent influenza exposure in transplant recipients [59]. Vaccinations given to recipients within 6 months of hematopoietic stem cell transplantation are unlikely to be effective [59]. In general live vaccines should be avoided in transplant recipients receiving immunosuppressants, but hepatitis A and B, inactivated typhoid and polio vaccines, and meningococcal vaccines are safe to use and very important in preventing travel-associated infections. More data are needed regarding responses to revaccination.

Table 7
Recommended vaccinations for hematopoietic stem cell transplant recipients, including allogeneic and autologous recipients

| Vaccine or toxoid | Time after HSCT | | |
|---|---|---|---|
| | 12 mo | 14 mo | 24 mo |
| DTaP: children aged <7 y | DTaP or DT | DTaP or DT | DTaP or DT |
| DTaP: children aged ≥7 y | Td | Td | Td |
| Hib conjugate | Hib conjugate | Hib conjugate | Hib conjugate |
| Hepatitis B | Hepatitis B | Hepatitis B | Hepatitis B |
| PPV | PPV | — | PPV |
| Hepatitis A | Not routinely; can safely be offered to travelers | | |
| Influenza | Lifelong, seasonal administration, beginning before HSCT and resuming at ≥6 mo after HSCT | | |
| Meningococcal | Not routinely; can safely be offered to travelers | | |
| IPV | IPV | IPV | IPV |
| Rabies | Not routinely; can safely be offered to travelers | | |
| Typhoid | Inactivated vaccine can safely be offered to travelers | | |
| Live-attenuated vaccines | | | |
| MMR | — | — | MMR |
| Varicella vaccine | Contraindicated for HSCT recipients | | |
| Yellow fever vaccine | Controversial, few data, avoid | | |

For these guidelines, HSCT recipients are presumed immunocompetent at ≥24 mo after HSCT if they are not on immunosuppressive therapy and do not have graft-versus-host disease.

*Abbreviations:* DT, diphtheria toxoid; DTaP, diphtheria toxoid-tetanus toxoid-acellular pertussis; Hib, *Haemophilus influenzae* type b; HSCT, hematopoietic stem cell transplant; IPV, inactivated polio; MMR, measles-mumps-rubella; PPV, 23-valent pneumococcal polysaccharide; Td, tetanus-diphtheria toxoid.

Table 8
Recommendations for administration of vaccines before and after solid organ transplant

| Vaccine | Recommended for use after transplantation | Reimmunization required after transplantation[a] | Assessment of immunity required after vaccination |
|---|---|---|---|
| *Live attenuated* | | | |
| Varicella | No | No | Yes |
| Measles | No | No | Yes |
| Mumps | No | No | No |
| Rubella | No | No | Yes[b] |
| Bacille Calmette-Guerin | No | No | Yes |
| *Inactivated* | | | |
| Polio | IPV only | Yes | No |
| Acellular pertussis | Yes | Yes | No |
| Diphtheria | Yes | Yes | No |
| Tetanus | Yes | Yes | No |
| Hepatitis B | Yes | Yes[c] | Yes |
| *Neisseria meningitidis* | Yes[d] | Yes | No |
| Rabies | Yes[e] | Yes | No |
| Hepatitis A | Yes | Yes[c] | Yes |
| Influenza | Yes | Yes | No |
| *Streptococcus pneumoniae* | Yes | Yes | No |

*Abbreviations:* IPV, inactivated polio vaccine.

[a] Immunization schedule should be reinstituted once immunosuppression is decreased (typically 6 mo to 1 y after transplantation). Once resumed, immunizations should follow the recommended schedule.

[b] Documentation of immunity recommended for women of childbearing age.

[c] Decision to reimmunize should be based on assessment of serologic response to the vaccine.

[d] Recommended for college-age students and others at risk.

[e] Recommended for those at risk because of avocation or vocation.

## *Malaria and traveler's diarrhea*

Recommendations for malaria prevention are unchanged in this group, and must be thoroughly addressed. Dietary choices are important for hematopoietic stem cell transplantation patients in particular, especially those recently transplanted. Meats should be well cooked. Raw eggs, or any foods containing them, and raw seafood should be avoided because of the risks of acquiring *Salmonella* and *Vibrio* infections, respectively [60].

## *Asplenic travelers*

Considerations for the asplenic individual include greater concern about overwhelming postsplenectomy sepsis [60]. Although the risk of overwhelming postsplenectomy sepsis is lifelong, most episodes present within the first 2 years after splenectomy. Vaccinations against *Streptococcus pneumoniae*, *H influenzae* type b, and meningococcus are indicated. In addition to the usual approach to malaria prevention and enteric precautions, such individuals benefit from carrying an additional course of an antibiotic, such as cephalexin or cefadroxil, for skin and soft tissue infections, and an FQ, such as ciprofloxacin, for prompt use in case of TD. Alternatively, a newer-generation FQ that also covers gram-positive organisms, such as levofloxacin, can be used for both skin and soft tissue infections and TD. Newer FQs may also be appropriate for empiric treatment of fever given the increased prevalence of penicillin-resistant *S pneumoniae* [61]. Empiric treatment of all diarrheal episodes in asplenics is warranted because of the potential risk of bacteremia caused by *Salmonella* and *Campylobacter* spp. Azithromycin has dual benefit, as a treatment for upper respiratory infections and in treatment of FQ-resistant *Campylobacter* species [60].

*Summary recommendations*

Regarding the previously mentioned transplanted traveler, the following recommendations are certain: malaria prophylaxis and mosquito avoidance are highly recommended; complete repeat tetanus-diphtheria and hepatitis B series; one MMR should be given at 24 months posttransplant; hepatitis A, inactivated typhoid and polio, meningococcal, and influenza vaccines are all safe. Her risks of acquiring YF and of vaccine side effects are concerning; it may be preferable that she find a hospital in South Africa or another region to work in, so as to avoid any risk of adverse events [12]. Theoretically, by 24 months she is considered immunocompetent to withstand the vaccine and may benefit; successful response to YF vaccine has been documented 2 years after bone marrow transplantation for myeloma [62]. The bottom line is, no one knows whether she is more likely to have an adverse experience with YF vaccine and a waiver can be written. Educate her about how serious YF is, and have her consider whether she can change her plans. She has not undergone a splenectomy, and her immune status may well be intact.

This approach also holds for the leukemic patient in remission and others who have completed chemotherapy, except that live virus vaccines need to be avoided until after at least 3 months following completion of chemotherapy [31]. It is likely that responses to travel-related vaccines and other immunizations will be poor. Empiric antibiotics should be used for diarrhea or if travelers become febrile while abroad.

**Scenario 7: travelers with seizure disorders**

A 25-year-old woman is part of a four-member team participating in a 2-week adventure race in Brazil, Bolivia, and Paraguay, hiking, orienteering, and paddling her way through the wilderness. She is generally in good health. Your medical history reveals a seizure disorder present since age 14, which is well controlled with phenytoin. She has not had a seizure in over 18 months.

*In addition to the usual precautions you would advise for travel to South America, what specific advice should be provided in light of the history of epilepsy?*

Routine recommendations for travelers with seizure disorders do not differ from those for other travelers. Flight attendants should be informed, and emergency medications with instructions for use carried with the traveler. Seizure thresholds may be reduced at high altitudes but this should not cause problems for travelers adherent to their anticonvulsant regimens. Diving is absolutely contraindicated, however, as the risk of seizures and of death from underwater seizures is increased. The traveler should be aware of the risks of drowning and accidental deaths as a consequence of seizures during high-risk activities [63].

*Drug interactions*

Potential drug interactions with anticonvulsants must be reviewed carefully. For this traveler, malaria is a credible risk. Chloroquine-resistant *P falciparum* is present in most malarious areas of South America including this adventurer's destinations. Mefloquine is contraindicated in travelers with known seizure disorders, as is chloroquine [64]. Appropriate antimalarial chemoprophylaxis in the epileptic traveler, regardless of antimalarial resistance patterns, is then limited to either doxycycline (which coincidentally may offer protection against leptospirosis, also a risk to this traveler), AP, or primaquine. Proguanil can be used for prevention of chloroquine-susceptible *Plasmodia* infections only, but is not available in the United States.

Carbamazepine, phenytoin, and phenobarbital can increase the metabolism of doxycycline, reducing the latter's effectiveness as an antimalarial agent. Doubling the dose of doxycycline (to 100 mg orally twice a day) may overcome this problem if doxycycline is the preferred chemoprophylactic agent [64]. Alternatively, AP can be used; significant drug interactions with anticonvulsants have not been reported.

Ciprofloxacin and other FQs may reduce phenytoin levels; use of azithromycin for TD may solve this problem. Salicylate-containing medications may interact with valproate and phenytoin (increased anticonvulsant levels). Other potential drug interactions should be verified before prescription of other medications.

*Summary recommendations*

The usual precautions for travelers should be applied. For malaria prophylaxis in this instance, either doxycycline (100 mg twice a day) or AP should be recommended. Given the other possible side effects of doxycycline (photosensitivity, vaginal candidiasis), AP may be preferable. Phenytoin and ciprofloxacin may interact, and an alternate agent for TD should be used. Other drugs that may be prescribed for this trip are unlikely to interact with phenytoin.

## Summary

With adequate preparation and in consultation with a travel medicine expert, most travelers today can travel safely regardless of their age and health status. The few instances when it is prudent to alter travel plans or postpone travel altogether are not to be taken lightly. For the most part, however, most complex travelers can enjoy a healthy and rewarding travel experience.

## References

[1] Centers for Disease Control and Prevention. Inactivated Japanese encephalitis virus vaccine: recommendations of the Advisory Committee on Immunization Practices (ACIP). MMWR Morb Mort Wkly Rep 1994;42(RR-01):1–22.
[2] Memish ZA. Meningococcal disease and travel. Clin Infect Dis 2002;34:84–90.
[3] Centers for Disease Control and Prevention. Typhoid immunization: recommendations of the Advisory Committee on Immunization Practices (ACIP). MMWR Morb Mort Wkly Rep 1994;43(RR-14):1–7.
[4] Steinberg EB, Bishop R, Haber P, et al. Typhoid fever in travelers: who should be targeted for prevention? Clin Infect Dis 2004;39:186–91.
[5] Centers for Disease Control and Prevention. Health information for international travel 2003–4. Atlanta, (GA): US Department of Health and Human Services, Public Health Service; 2003.
[6] US Customs and Border Security. www.cbp.gov/xp/cgov/travel. Accessed 5 June 2004.
[7] Federal Aviation Agency. www.faa.gov/passengers/childsafetyseats.cfm. Accessed 4 June 2004.
[8] Ratnam S, Chandra R, Gadag V. Maternal measles and rubella antibody levels and serologic response in infants immunized with MMR II at 12 months of age. J Infect Dis 1993;168: 1596–8.
[9] Siegrist CA. Mechanisms by which maternal antibodies influence infant immune responses: review of hypotheses and definition of main determinants. Vaccine 2003;21:3406–12.
[10] Stauffer WM, Kamat D. Traveling with infants and children. Part II: Immunizations. J Travel Med 2002;9:82–90.
[11] Mackell SM. Vaccinations for the pediatric traveler. Clin Infect Dis 2003;37:1508–16.
[12] Centers for Disease Control and Prevention. Yellow fever vaccine: recommendations of the Advisory Committee on Immunization Practices (ACIP), 2002. MMWR Morb Mort Wkly Rep 2002;51(RR-17):1–11.
[13] Monath TP. Yellow fever. In: Plotkin SA, Orenstein W, editors. Vaccines. 3rd edition. Philadelphia: WB Saunders; 1999. p. 858–63.
[14] Fiore AE, Shapiro CN, Sabin K, et al. Hepatitis A vaccination of infants: effect of maternal antibody status on antibody persistence and response to a booster dose. Pediatr Infect Dis J 2003;22:354–9.
[15] van der Wielen M, van Damme P, Collard F. A two dose schedule for combined hepatitis A and hepatitis B vaccination in children ages one to eleven years. Pediatr Infect Dis J 2000;19: 848–53.
[16] Reingold AL, Broome CV, Hightower AW, et al. Age-specific differences in duration of clinical protection after vaccination with meningococcal polysaccharide A vaccine. Lancet 1985;326:114–8.
[17] MacLennan JM, Shackley F, Heath PT, et al. Safety, immunogenicity, and induction of immunologic memory by a serogroup C meningococcal conjugate vaccine in infants: a randomized controlled trial. JAMA 2000;283:2795–801.

[18] Balmer P, Borrow R, Miller E. Impact of meningococcal C conjugate vaccine in the UK. J Med Microbiol 2002;51:717–22.
[19] Engels EA, Lau J. Vaccines for preventing typhoid fever. Cochrane Database Syst Rev 2000; CD 001261.
[20] Centers for Disease Control and Prevention. Typhoid immunizations: recommendations of the Advisory Committee on Immunization Practices (ACIP). MMWR Morb Mort Wkly Rep 1994;43(RR-14):1–14.
[21] Bell JW, Veltri JC, Page BC. Human exposures to N, N-diethyl-m-toluamide insect repellents reported to the American Association of Poison Control Centers 1993–1997. Int J Toxicol 2002;21:341–52.
[22] Stauffer WM, Kamat D, Magill AJ. Traveling with infants and children. Part IV: Insect avoidance and malaria prevention. J Travel Med 2003;10:225–40.
[23] Luxemberger C, Price RN, Nosten F, et al. Mefloquine in infants and young children. Ann Trop Paediatr 1996;16:281–6.
[24] Lell B, Luckner D, Ndjave M, et al. Randomised placebo-controlled study of atovaquone plus proguanil for malaria prophylaxis in children. Lancet 1998;351:709–13.
[25] Pitzinger B, Steffen R, Tschopp A. Incidence and clinical features of traveler's diarrhea in infants and children. Pediatr Infect Dis J 1991;10:719–23.
[26] Stauffer WM, Konop RJ, Kamat D. Traveling with infants and young children. Part III: travelers' diarrhea. J Travel Med 2002;9:141–50.
[27] Tupasi TE. Quinolones in the developing world: state of the art. Drugs 1999;58:55–9.
[28] Gomi H, Jiang ZD, Adachi JA, et al. In vitro susceptibility testing of bacterial enteropathogens causing traveler's diarrhea in four geographic regions. Antimicrob Agents Chemother 2001;45:212–6.
[29] Kuschner R, Trofa AF, Thomas RJ, et al. Use of azithromycin for the treatment of *Campylobacter* enteritis in travelers to Thailand, an area where ciprofloxacin resistance is prevalent. Clin Infect Dis 1995;21:536–41.
[30] Cummins RO, Schubach JA. Frequency and types of medical emergencies among commercial air travelers. JAMA 1989;261:1295–9.
[31] McCarthy AE. Travelers with pre-existing disease. In: Keystone JS, Kozarsky PE, Freedman DO, et al, editors. Travel medicine. Edinburgh: Mosby; 2004. p. 241–7.
[32] Centers for Disease Control and Prevention. Tetanus surveillance: 1998–2000. MMWR Morb Mort Wkly Rep 2003;52(SS-03):1–8.
[33] Martin M, Weld LH, Tsai TF, et al. Advanced age as a risk factor for illness temporally associated with yellow fever vaccination. Emerg Infect Dis 2001;7:945–51.
[34] Bacaner J, Stauffer B, Boulware, et al. Travel medicine considerations for North American immigrants visiting friends and relatives. JAMA 2004;291:2856–64.
[35] Mileno MD, Bia FJ. The compromised traveler. Infect Dis Clin North Am 1998;12:369–412.
[36] Diabetes Monitor. www.diabetesmonitor.com. Accessed 7 July 2004.
[37] Sane T, Koivisto VA, Nikkanen P, et al. Adjustment of insulin doses of diabetic patients during long distance flights. BMJ 1990;301:421–2.
[38] Glynn MK, Friedman CR, Gold BD, et al. Seroincidence of *Helicobacter pylori* infection in a cohort of rural Bolivian children: acquisition and analysis of possible risk factors. Clin Infect Dis 2002;35:1059–65.
[39] Begue RE, Mirza A, Compton T, et al. *Helicobacter pylori* infection and insulin requirement among children with type 1 diabetes mellitus. Pediatrics 1999;103:e83.
[40] Freeman M, Ghidini A, Spong CY, et al. Does air travel affect pregnancy outcome? Arch Gynecol Obstet 2004;269:274–7.
[41] American Academy of Pediatrics. Immunization in special circumstances. In: Pickering LK, editor. Red Book: 2003 Report of the Committee on Infectious Diseases. 26th edition. Elk Grove Village (IL): American Academy of Pediatrics; 2003. p. 66–9.
[42] Vanhauwere B, Maradit H, Kerr L. Post marketing surveillance of prophylactic mefloquine (LARIAM) use in pregnancy. Am J Trop Med Hyg 1998;58:17–21.

[43] American Academy of Pediatrics. Rubella. In: Pickering LK, editor. Red Book: 2003 Report of the Committee on Infectious Diseases. 26th edition. Elk Grove Village (IL): American Academy of Pediatrics; 2003. p. 536–41.
[44] Bar-Oz B, Bulkowstein M, Benyamini L, et al. Use of antibiotic and analgesic drugs during lactation. Drug Saf 2003;26:925–35.
[45] Aidsnet. www.aidsnet.ch/index.php?newlang=english under "Immigration Clauses". Accessed 7 July 2004.
[46] Castelli F, Pizzocolo C. The traveler with HIV. In: Keystone JS, Kozarsky PE, Freedman DO, et al, editors. Travel medicine. Edinburgh: Mosby; 2004. p. 257–66.
[47] Thisyakorn U, Pancharoen C, Ruxrungtham K, et al. Safety and immunogenicity of preexposure rabies vaccination in children infected with human immunodeficiency virus type 1. Clin Infect Dis 2000;30:218.
[48] Thaithumyanon P, Punnahitananda S, Thisyakorn U, et al. Immune responses to measles immunization and the impacts on HIV-infected children. Southeast Asian J Trop Med Public Health 2000;31:658–62.
[49] Tattevin P, Depatureaux AG, Chapplain JM, et al. Yellow fever vaccine is safe and effective in HIV-infected patients. AIDS 2004;18:835–7.
[50] Whitworth J, Morgan D, Quigley M, et al. Effect of HIV-1 and increasing immunosuppression on malaria parasitaemia and clinical episodes in adults in rural Uganda: a cohort study. Lancet 2000;356:1051–6.
[51] Ramos A, Hu DJ, Nguyen L, et al. Intersubtype human immunodeficiency virus type 1 superinfection following seroconversion to primary infection in two injection drug users. J Virol 2002;76:7444–52.
[52] Khaliq Y, Gallicano K, Tisdale C, et al. Pharmacokinetic interaction between mefloquine and ritonavir in healthy volunteers. Br J Clin Pharmacol 2001;51:591–600.
[53] Schippers EF, Hugen PW, den Hartigh J, et al. No drug-drug interaction between nelfinavir or indinavir and mefloquine in HIV-1-infected patients. AIDS 2000;14:2794–5.
[54] Colebunders R, Nachega J, van Gompel A. Antiretroviral treatment and travel to developing countries. J Travel Med 1999;6:27–31.
[55] Schlagenhauf P, Beallor C, Kain KC. Malaria chemoprophylaxis. In: Keystone JS, Kozarsky PE, Freedman DO, et al, editors. Travel medicine. Edinburgh: Mosby; 2004. p. 137–56.
[56] Tessier D. Immunocompromised travelers. In: Schlagenhauf P, editor. Travelers' malaria. Hamilton, ON: BC Decker; 2004. p. 324–35.
[57] Centers for Disease Control and Prevention. Guidelines for preventing opportunistic infections among HIV-infected persons—2002. Recommendations of the US Public Health Service and the Infectious Diseases Society of America. MMWR Morb Mort Wkly Rep 2002;51(RR-8):1–52.
[58] Boggild AK, Sano M, Humar A, et al. Travel patterns and risk behavior in solid organ transplant recipients. J Travel Med 2004;11:37–43.
[59] Rolston KV, Wingard JR. Managing infections in patients with hematologic malignancies. New York: Academy for Heathcare Education; 2003. p. 1–22.
[60] Mileno M. Preparation of immunocompromised travelers. In: Keystone JS, Kozarsky PE, Freedman DO, et al, editors. Travel medicine. Edinburgh: Mosby; 2004. p. 249–55.
[61] Watson DAR. Pretravel health advice for asplenic individuals. J Travel Med 2003;10:117–21.
[62] Gowda R, Cartwright K, Bremmer JA, et al. Yellow fever vaccine: a successful vaccination of an immunocompromised patient. Eur J Haematol 2004;72:299–301.
[63] Committee on Sports Medicine and Fitness. Medical conditions affecting sports participation. Pediatrics 2001;107:1205–9.
[64] Richens A, Andrews C. Clinical practice: antimalarial prophylaxis in patients with epilepsy. Epilepsy Res 2001;51:1–4.

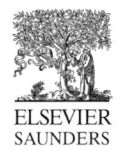

# Risk Assessment and Disease Prevention in Travelers Visiting Friends and Relatives

Sonia Y. Angell, MD, MPH, DTM&H[a],*, Ron H. Behrens, MB, ChB, MD, FRCP[b]

[a]Cardiovascular Disease Prevention and Control, New York City Department of Health and Mental Hygiene, 2 Lafayette Street, 20th Floor, CN-46, New York, NY 10007, USA
[b]Travel Clinic, Hospital for Tropical Diseases, London School of Hygiene and Tropical Medicine, Capper Street, London WC1E 6AU, UK

Travelers from the developed world to a developing country for the purpose of visiting friends and relatives (VFRs) have long been considered at potentially high-risk. Never before, however, has this objective for travel abroad reached such high volume as in recent years. Excluding travel to Canada and Mexico, in 2002 United States residents included VFR as a purpose for their travel in 44% of their 26 million airplane trips made abroad [1]. During the same year, 13% of the 59 million visits from the United Kingdom to destinations abroad were made for this reason, reflecting an annual growth rate of 4.3% per year from 1998 to 2002 [2]. Disparities in the rates of disease or number of VFR travelers with reported, preventable travel-related illnesses as compared with those who travel for other purposes, such as tourism, have been documented. A closer look at this growing population of travelers, the contributors to their disease risk, and opportunities to prevent illness is warranted.

Those diseases for which VFR travelers are at greater risk when compared with travelers for other purposes include but are not limited to malaria, hepatitis A and B, typhoid fever, routine childhood vaccine preventable diseases, and tuberculosis. For example, the GeoSentinel global surveillance data on returned travel patients shows that VFR travelers present with malaria as their diagnosed illness at eight times the rate of

---

This work was completed while Dr. Angell was a fellow in the Robert Wood Johnson Scholars Program, University of Michigan, Ann Arbor, Michigan.
* Corresponding author.
E-mail address: sangell@health.nyc.gov (S.Y. Angell).

tourists [3]. VFR travelers from the United Kingdom to West Africa are 10 times more likely to develop malaria than are tourists [4].

VFR travelers are largely composed of foreign-born immigrants and their children, and their travel destinations are their countries of origin. This population of potential travelers makes up an increasing proportion of the general population of many developed countries. Eight percent of the United Kingdom's 58 million people are now from minority ethnic groups [5]. In the United States, 56 million people (one fifth of the country's population) are either foreign-born or are children of foreign-born parents [6]. Both in the United States and in the United Kingdom, most new immigrants now come from developing countries. In the United States, most are from Latin America and Asia [6]. In 2003, 30% of the United Kingdom's new citizens were from Africa, and 24% were from the Indian subcontinent [7].

## Understanding visiting friend and relative traveler morbidity

A detailed understanding of contributors to VFR traveler morbidity is complicated by terminology. On review of the literature, relevant key words that variably capture this population of travelers include not only VFR but others, such as "immigrant," "migrant," "ethnic minority," "semi-immune," and "foreign-born." The definition of VFR is not standardized. In its most basic form, VFR simply describes a traveler's self-reported reason for travel. This article focuses on the VFR traveler who travels from a so-called "developed nation" to a less developed country to visit friends and family.

High VFR traveler risk for illness is most commonly explained by characteristics considered typical of VFR travel as compared with travel to the same country for such purposes as tourism or business. VFR travelers more likely go to destinations not developed for tourism, often with poor public health infrastructure and higher transmission of local pathogens. Environment-related characteristics of VFR travel include longer durations of visits [2], more remote destinations, the use of local water sources, and the consumption of foods that are cooked in homes. VFR travelers are likely to have close contact with the local population and may use local health, entertainment, and social facilities. VFR travelers' children, who were often born in resource-rich regions, may be at particular risk of morbidity during travel, because they lack the pre-existing immunity to travel-related disease that their parents may have gained through early childhood exposure. Because of such travel characteristics, the risks of exposure to disease for the VFR traveler may approach that of the local population, unless the risk of infection is influenced by innate immunity to disease, or if travelers use preventive environmental and personal measures to reduce exposure. Because many of the diseases for which VFR travelers are at risk are preventable through currently available measures, understanding VFR traveler morbidity requires a much closer look at those factors influencing their access to preventive care, including immunizations.

Travel medicine clinics have developed largely around a self-referral system. VFR travelers are less likely to seek predeparture services, despite their often sophisticated knowledge of disease in a destination country [8]. Although limited travel-related services may typically be accessed in the primary care setting, travel-specific immunizations and medications remain largely uncovered by public and private health insurance plans. For example, in the United Kingdom, National Health Insurance does not cover the costs of antimalarials and most travel-specific vaccinations. As a group, foreign-born individuals within the United States, and ethnic minorities in the United Kingdom, are more likely to be poor [5,9]. With limited resources, their out-of-pocket uncovered cost of travel-related services may act as a major inhibitor and barrier to access.

Provider-related factors may also contribute to decreased care delivery, including difficulty in communicating because of language differences and the lack of culturally appropriate care [10]. Primary care providers might also bypass screening for high-risk travel, and may lack adequate travel medicine knowledge, resulting in improperly prescribed medications [11,12].

When travel medicine services are delivered, VFR travelers may be less likely to follow provider recommendations than non-VFR travelers, suggesting that current methods of provider-to-patient risk communication may be less effective in this population. Traditionally, travel medicine counseling includes a focus on disease risk, followed by recommended interventions. The health behavior–health education "health belief model" supports this approach [13]. By first increasing the individual traveler's sense of perceived susceptibility and severity of disease, their perceived sense of personal threat is increased, theoretically increasing adherence to provider-recommended behavioral changes.

This focus on risk during counseling may be less effective in VFR travelers who come to clinics with pre-established travel-related health beliefs that are often based on personal experience in the destination country [14]. In this case, the provider's emphasis on disease threat in the destination country may be in direct conflict with the VFR traveler's expectations. Hence, they may discount provider recommendations.

## Tools for provider intervention

### A new approach to counseling

Although the health belief model remains relevant, in VFR travelers more time spent on recommended preventive behaviors may prove more efficacious. Within the theory, these so-called "cues to action" include providing strategies for disease prevention, exploring with the traveler those potential barriers to adherence, and proposing alternatives. For example, after providing instruction on malaria risk, modes of transmission, and its symptoms, the provider may spend most of the time discussing the practical aspects of applying repellent and hanging nets. Similarly, providing cues for remembering to take weekly medications by renaming a day of the week as a reminder may increase adherence (eg, "malaria Monday" or similar wordplay in the traveler's native language). In sum, sensitivity to the VFR traveler's unique relationship with the destination country, and how it may affect their reception of provider recommendations, is critical.

*Visiting friend and relative traveler risk assessment*

Many VFR travelers repeat their journey at some later time. Primary care provider screening for future travel during the patient's initial visit allows adequate lead time to plan for patient needs and to coordinate care with other providers as necessary.

The framework for VFR traveler risk assessment is no different than that for all travelers. Up-to-date reports of diseases in the destination country should be checked at recognized sources, such as the Centers for Disease Control and Prevention (CDC) website, www.cdc.gov, or the World Health Organization's International Travel and Health website, http://www.who.int/ith/. Providers should clarify the anticipated itinerary, accommodations, and the likelihood of high-risk activities, including the use of local health care facilities. Other reasons for travel should be explored. These may include undergoing medical procedures that are unavailable; not covered by insurance; or are cost prohibitive in their country of residence, such as dental procedures, cosmetic surgery, or even organ transplants.

*General recommendations*

Because VFR travel may be of long duration, providers must ensure that sufficient amounts of regular medications with written prescriptions and other necessary equipment are provided. Those with comorbidities should carry summary information about their medical conditions and management plans. Translation of the document into the language of the destination country is ideal, but usually not necessary. Patients anticipating medical care, dental procedures, or parenteral injections while abroad should receive risk counseling on blood-borne diseases, wound infections, and appropriate vaccinations. Providers should discuss sexually transmitted disease prevention and the use of condoms. Noninfectious disease risks should also be covered including motor vehicle safety.

Adult VFR travelers who may not seek care for themselves often seek predeparture care for their children [12,14]. Beyond care provision for this very important group of high-risk children, providers should take advantage and make use of this interface to counsel or refer VFR traveler adults for their own travel medicine care.

To illustrate some unique VFR traveler risks, a discussion of some infectious diseases for which VFR travelers are at recognized risk follows. It is not exhaustive, because risk varies by country. Providers are referred to existing specialist travel medicine sources for a general review to ensure that comprehensive travel-related care is provided.

## High-risk diseases in travelers visiting friends and relatives

### Routine childhood vaccine-preventable diseases

Both outbreaks and continuous transmission of diseases that should be prevented by routinely recommended vaccines persist globally and travel contributes to their persistence [15]. For example, wild poliovirus remains endemic in six countries. Nigeria, India, and Pakistan accounted for a high percentage of all cases in 2003 [16]. Recent outbreaks in 10 African countries, previously considered disease-free, are the result of exported disease from Nigeria [17].

Despite the broad availability of vaccines in developed regions, disparities in coverage exist within countries between various subsets of their populations. In the United States, the foreign-born and subsequent American-born generations rank among those with the lowest rates of routine immunization [18–20].

Vaccination histories should be assessed carefully at the first primary care visit. Recommended childhood vaccinations are not consistent across all countries, and the number of immunizations required to complete each series may also differ. Those vaccinations typically recommended include diphtheria, tetanus, polio, and measles-mumps-rubella for everyone, and pneumococcal, *Haemophilus influenzae* type B, and pertussis for children. The importance of hepatitis A and B and varicella vaccination in the VFR traveler is discussed later. For travelers lacking certain immunizations, providers should be aware of minimum time intervals between doses and so-called "accelerated vaccination schedules" in case of short notice of departures [21].

### Hepatitis B

Hepatitis B is transmitted through contaminated blood or blood products, sexual-activity with an infected partner, and potentially skin lesions. Although infection is cleared in most cases, 6% of adults and 25% of children develop chronic infection with possible complications, such as chronic liver disease, cirrhosis, and hepatocellular carcinoma [22].

More than 2% of the population within all socioeconomic groups has evidence of chronic or active hepatitis B infection in virtually all developing regions (Fig. 1) [23]. Although relatively new, the hepatitis B vaccine is now routinely recommended for children in almost all of these countries. For example, in the Dominican Republic, where greater than 8% of the population is estimated to have chronic or active infection, hepatitis B vaccination has been included in their childhood national vaccination program since 1997 [24]. By 2002, an estimated 63% of children had been vaccinated.

The vaccine is recommended for all children born in the United States, and required for all immigrants less than 19 years of age applying for permanent resident status [25]. Yet, disparities in the levels of hepatitis B vaccination among American foreign-born children as compared with American-born children exist, 74% compared with 90%, respectively [18]. It is likely that a significant number of VFR travelers, both adults and children, remain unvaccinated.

The CDC recommends hepatitis B vaccination for all travelers going to destinations where greater than 2% of the population is seropositive for the hepatitis B surface antigen, and for travelers who anticipate "...sexual contact or who will have daily physical contact with the local population; or who are likely to seek medical, dental, or other treatment in local facilities; or any combination of these activities during their stay" [23]. Although specific indications for immunization vary by country, with few exceptions nonimmune VFR travelers are candidates for vaccination.

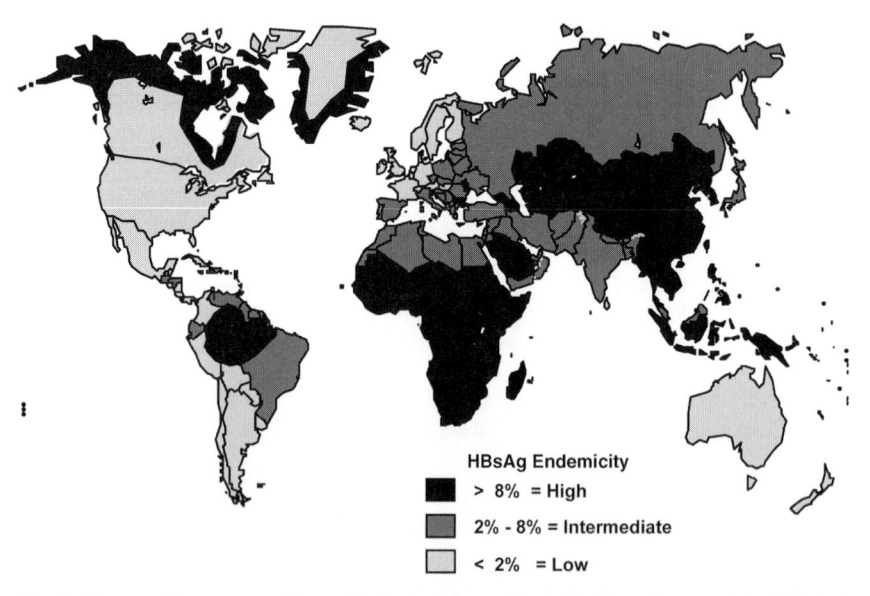

Fig. 1. Geographic pattern of hepatitis B prevalence. Hepatitis B surface antigen (HBsAg) positivity as a percent of the country's total population. (*Adapted from* World Health Organization. Available at: http://www.who.int/emcdocuments/hepatitis/docs/whocdscsrlyo20022/disease/world_distribution.html; with permission.)

## Hepatitis A

Transmission of this RNA picornavirus occurs by fecal contamination of water or food. The hepatitis A virus is responsible for roughly 50% of acute hepatitis cases in the United States; travel is a risk factor in 10% of reported cases [26]. Similarly, in the United Kingdom travel accounts for approximately 10% of cases and most of these cases are associated with travel to the Indian subcontinent [27]. Young VFR travelers to this region are at the greatest risk for disease, and have been shown to be eight times more likely to develop hepatitis A than travelers for other purposes [28].

Infected VFR travelers could contribute to the local transmission of hepatitis A on their return to their homes in developed countries. A Dutch study demonstrated distinct hepatitis A virus strains infecting children returning from visits to countries (largely Morocco) of parental origin [29]. These same strains were subsequently identified in siblings, nontraveling Dutch-origin schoolmates, and their parents.

Although only one third of the United States population has evidence of prior hepatitis A virus infection, 90% of children born in developing countries are likely to be seropositive by age 10 [26]. Prevalence in developing countries varies by region, however, and improved health and sanitation in some geographic and upper socioeconomic pockets has resulted in delaying the age of infection to adolescence or adulthood [30,31]. Although studies in developed countries indicate that seropositivity is strongly associated with foreign birth and older age at immigration, the assumption that foreign-born VFR travelers are likely immune may be increasingly less accurate. Although an American-based study of foreign-born travelers, largely from Africa, showed that 95% were hepatitis A virus seropositive [32], a Holland-based study of Turkish and Moroccan children less than 16 years old showed that only 47% of those foreign-born children had evidence of prior hepatitis A virus infection [33].

Based on such epidemiology, adult VFR travelers born in developed countries, and all child VFR travelers without a history of disease or vaccination, should be considered for immunization. The approach to immunizing adult VFR travelers born in endemic areas is less straightforward. It requires balancing the cost of hepatitis A virus screening for seropositivity against the cost of proceeding directly to hepatitis A virus vaccination, while considering the epidemiology of disease in the traveler's specific place of origin.

## Typhoid fever

An estimated 33 million cases of typhoid fever occur each year in the endemic regions of Africa, Central and South America, and Southeast Asia. In the United Kingdom, travel to the Indian subcontinent accounts for 70% to 90% of all cases of travel-associated disease [27]. In the United States,

Indian subcontinent travel has been associated with an incidence rate 18 times higher than travel to any other destinations [34] and high rates of typhoid fever are reported in children [35].

Among United States residents, VFR travelers are at the greatest risk. From June 1996 to May 1997, 80% of cases occurred in recent travelers, and half of these cases were among VFR travelers; only 4% occurred in tourists [35]. Vaccine had been administered before travel in only 4% of all cases. A second CDC study showed that, between 1994 and 1999, 80% of all travel-related cases of typhoid fever reporting a single reason for travel occurred in VFR travelers, compared with just 3% of cases occurring in tourists [36].

One reason to consider typhoid vaccination is that the medical treatment of travel-related typhoid fever has become increasingly challenging. Multidrug resistant strains are now widespread throughout the world, and they are the normal in such areas as India and other parts of Southeast Asia, including Vietnam, South Africa, and Pakistan [34,37–39]. Resistance to ciprofloxacin is also emerging, and has been associated with treatment failures [40].

Prevention of typhoid fever in travelers starts with education about food and water hygiene. Disease is rarely reported among those who are vaccinated, and immunization is recommended for those going to recognized high-risk areas. It should be noted that immunization itself actually provides only 50% to 80% protection, and it is of limited duration, 2 to 5 years depending on the type of typhoid vaccine received [23]. Put simply, vaccination is not a substitute for food and water precautions.

*Varicella*

Compared with children between the ages of 1 and 4 years, adults have 25 times the risk of death from chickenpox, and can suffer complications, such as pneumonia, encephalitis, and hemorrhage. Before the introduction of varicella immunization in the United States, approximately 20% of adult deaths caused by varicella occurred among the foreign-born [41]. Although some developed countries include varicella as a routinely recommended vaccination, the World Health Organization does not prioritize its inclusion within national programs in developing countries.

In most nontropical and developed countries, most adults are immune. In the United States, greater than 90% of the population is seropositive, most a result of childhood infection. In rural tropical areas, infection is less common and the age of infection delayed [42–44]. Adults and children who have emigrated from tropical regions to developed countries often remain susceptible to this disease.

Vaccination of nonimmune adults prevents the serious complications associated with adult disease. Assurance of immunity for all VFR travelers also prevents potential exportation of disease from a developed country to susceptible communities in tropical areas, especially important if the travel destination also has a high prevalence of HIV infection.

The cost-effectiveness analysis of first screening VFR travelers for varicella-zoster viral antibodies, as opposed to providing immediate varicella vaccination, requires knowledge of baseline seroprevalence within the population of origin [44,45]. In the case of immigrants with a history of multiple past residencies, this may be difficult to assess. A conservative approach is to consider all travelers as candidates for vaccination if they do not have a reliable history of disease or varicella immunization. Those less than 12 years of age, without contraindications, should receive immunization. In adult candidates for vaccination, it is likely cost effective to proceed with serologic screening first [23].

## Malaria

Returned VFR travelers make up the largest proportion of malaria cases reported in many developed countries. In 2002, they accounted for 45% of civilian cases of malaria in the United States [46], 63% in France [3], and 50% of all malaria cases in the United Kingdom. United Kingdom resident VFR travelers visiting West Africa have an attack rate of 1% compared with 0.1% in tourists and 0.3% in business travelers (Table 1) [4].

Two thirds of the United Kingdom's malaria cases reported occurs in London. Most are found within well-defined geographic regions (Fig. 2) [27] with rates of up to 42.3 per 100,000 residents [47]. In an East London study,

Table 1

Rates and relative risks of all species of malaria imported to the United Kingdom among visiting friends and relatives and tourist-business travelers (1999–2001)

| Country and regional malaria rates[a] | Traveler groups cases per 10,000 visits | | Relative risk of malaria |
|---|---|---|---|
| | VFR's | Tourist and business | VFR vs tourist and business travelers |
| Kenya | 13 | 6 | 2 |
| Tanzania | 16 | 11 | 1 |
| Uganda | 107 | 26 | 4 |
| **East Africa** | **45** | **14** | **3.2** |
| Ghana (rate) | 63 | 24 | 3 |
| Nigeria (rate) | 91 | 14 | 6 |
| **West Africa** | **77** | **19** | **4.1** |
| India (rate) | 1.30 | 0.39 | 3 |
| Pakistan (rate) | 3.05 | 0.17 | 18 |
| **Indian subcontinent** | **2.18** | **0.28** | **7.8** |

Imported malaria cases provided by Malaria Reference Laboratory (Health Protection Agency).

Overseas traveler figures provided by International Passenger Survey. Travel Trends 2002: A report on the International Passenger Survey. http://www.statistics.gov.uk/downloads/theme_transport/TTrends02.pdf.2003.

[a] Imported cases per 10,000 visits.

*Data from* Phillips-Howard PA, Radalowicz A, Mitchell J, et al. Risk of malaria in British residents returning from malarious areas. BMJ 1990;300:499–503.

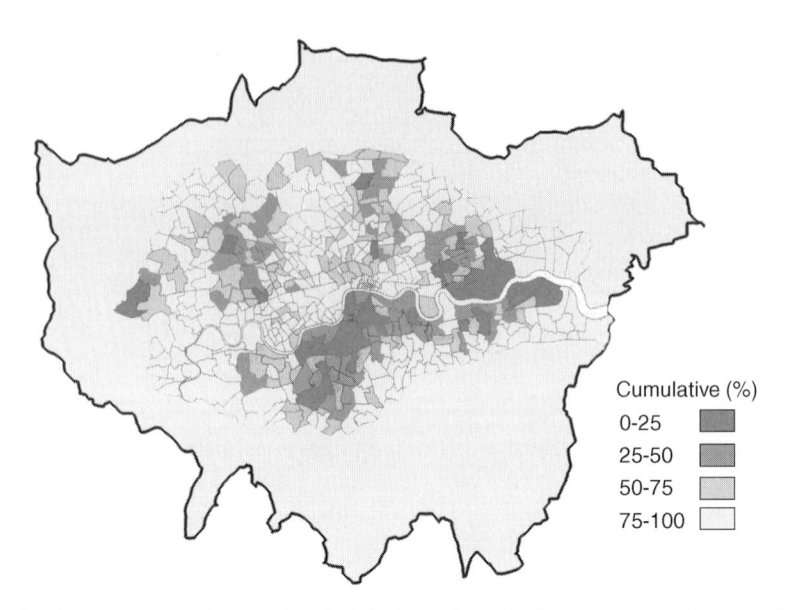

Fig. 2. Cumulative map of reported malaria in Central London by electoral ward between 1992 and 2001 highlighting the distribution of ethnic groups within Central London (unpublished data).

VFR travelers returning from West Africa accounted for 82% of childhood cases [48]. When screened, 25% of malaria case siblings also had infection with *Plasmodium falciparum*. This finding suggests that some infected travelers may be virtually asymptomatic, and that rates may actually be higher than reported.

The high volume of VFR travelers exposed to malaria by traveling in endemic regions (Fig. 3) partly explains their morbidity; however, lower rates of chemoprophylaxis use when compared with travelers for other purposes, such as tourism, has also contributed. In a 1987 study of malaria imported into the United Kingdom, 28% of VFR travelers had used malaria chemoprophylaxis; in contrast, 75% of tourists had done so [49]. Low rates of use have also been reported in other studies, including those from the United Kingdom (46%–48%) [4], Canada (31%) [11], Italy (8%) [50], and a pan-European review (24%) [51].

One possible reason for low chemoprophylaxis use among VFR travelers is the burden of cost. In a predominantly ethnic minority United Kingdom community the 1995 removal of state subsidies for malaria prophylaxis payment was associated with a dramatic decrease in prescriptions issued for malaria prevention and a subsequent increase in malaria cases when compared with preceding years [52].

Low rates of chemoprophylaxis usage may also be influenced by lower perceptions of personal risk among VFR travelers. This impression may be based on their prior personal experience of mild clinical disease. Studies

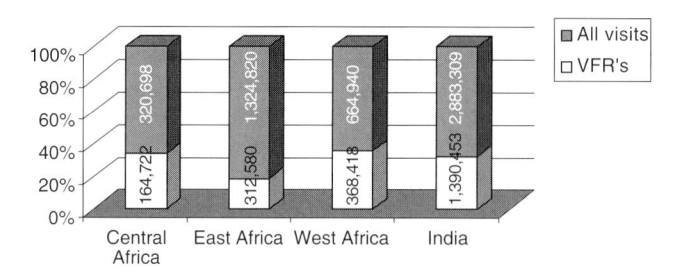

Fig. 3. Number of visits by British residents to Africa, VFRs as a proportion of all travellers 1988 to 1998.

suggest that immunity to severe and fatal malaria disease is maintained for long periods of time, even in the absence of immunity boosting through malaria reinfection [53]. Protection is not complete, however, as demonstrated by the number of VFR travelers who return from travel ill, some with severe and fatal malaria.

Even when taking antimalarial prophylaxis, high rates of inappropriate drug use have been observed among all groups of travelers, but especially among VFR travelers. In a Canadian departure lounge study, only 7% of travelers had been prescribed an appropriate antimalarial drug regimen [11]. French VFR travelers departing from Paris were twice as likely to be taking unsuitable chemoprophylaxis compared with tourists on package holidays [54]. In addition to provider prescribing errors [11], medication costs may also contribute to this problem. There is evidence that removal of the drug subsidy for antimalarials in the United Kingdom resulted in travelers selecting cheaper, but inappropriate antimalarial drug regimens [55].

Providers have an important role to play in malaria prevention. Up-to-date information on patterns of drug resistance and recommended prophylaxis in destination countries should be consistently accessed before prescribing antimalarials. Providers should have frank discussions regarding medication costs. If travelers plan to purchase less expensive drugs abroad, providers should address the potential risks, including acquiring malaria caused by delaying the initiation of predeparture therapy, or the possibility of purchasing lower-quality drugs abroad. VFR traveler perceptions of immunity should be explored; both culturally and linguistically appropriate information and education should be provided. In communities with high burdens of disease, community and school-based interventions might be considered.

*Tuberculosis*

Tuberculosis is endemic in most of the developing world. Eighty percent of the world's cases are concentrated in 22 countries and India contains nearly one third of them [15]. Urban centers and crowded living situations are ideal settings for the spread of *Mycobacterium tuberculosis*.

In the United States, rates of active tuberculosis disease continue to decrease in most populations, although less rapidly among the United States foreign-born. This rate difference has resulted in a doubling of the ratio of foreign-born to American-born tuberculosis rates, increasing from 4.2 in 1992 to 8.4 in 2002 [56]. In the United Kingdom, minority ethnic populations have an increasing burden of tuberculosis relative to the white population. In 1998, the estimated annual incidence rate of tuberculosis was increasing in the black African population (210 cases per 100,000), while decreasing in the Indian subcontinent population (121 cases per 100,000), and also decreasing in the United Kingdom white population (4.8 cases per 100,000) [57].

The relationship between postimmigration travel and tuberculosis has not been examined in large population studies; however, there is evidence that tuberculosis contributes to morbidity in VFR travelers. A study of Dutch travelers to countries highly endemic for tuberculosis for a median of 23 weeks put the risk of infection for non–health care workers at 2.8 cases per 100,000 person years, a rate close to that of local populations in endemic areas [58]. A California study of 953 children showed that those who had traveled to high-prevalence tuberculosis countries in the preceding year were 3.9 times more likely to have a positive skin test for infection as compared with those children who had not traveled [59]. In over half of those trips abroad, children had stayed with their grandparents. A United Kingdom study of over 1000 active tuberculosis cases in individuals with ethnic origin from the Indian subcontinent, and no known contact with active disease, found that 22% had visited the Indian subcontinent before their reports of illness. Of the United Kingdom–born travelers to the Indian subcontinent, 60% had traveled within 3 years of illness, and of the non–United Kingdom born travelers, 68% had traveled to the Indian subcontinent within the 3 years [60].

In the United States, definitive expert panel recommendations for tuberculosis screening of those who take repeated short-term visits to high-prevalence regions do not exist. The tuberculin skin test is the most common screening tool for latent tuberculosis infection in the United States; however, its use is compromised by poor test specificity and sensitivity. Those with a history of prior bacille Calmette-Guérin may test positive, especially after repeat tuberculin skin test, because of the booster effect [61,62].

There are several options for managing risk of tuberculosis in frequent travelers. These include careful assessment for symptoms, with treatment to follow in the event of active disease [63]; tuberculin skin test once before travel and then again on return [64–66]; vaccination with bacille Calmette-Guérin (not available in the United States or recommended by the CDC); and chest radiograph screening. None are ideal for frequently returning VFR travelers.

No matter which of the screening methods is chosen, both the provider and traveler need to be aware of increased tuberculosis risk and have a high suspicion for active disease when new symptoms develop. The response to potential symptoms of tuberculosis should include prompt screening with tuberculin skin testing, sputum smears, and chest radiography.

## Summary

Although VFR travelers are at risk for acquiring infections and experiencing illness while traveling, many of these diseases are preventable. A comprehensive approach to decreasing their travel-related morbidity requires continued surveillance, data collection, systematic analysis, and action.

A review of the literature provides few examples of interventions designed specifically to address VFR travel needs. Given the geographic and cultural diversity of these populations, models grounded in health behavior theory provide the best potential for clinically relevant replication. Outreach aimed at improving knowledge and care-seeking behaviors among VFR travelers may be facilitated through community-based campaigns in areas with large foreign-born populations.

In developed countries, policies must be reviewed to ensure that travel-related services are accessible, affordable, and appropriate for these diverse populations. In the clinical setting, providers must develop culturally appropriate methods of communicating with traveling populations to influence behavior. In particular, primary care providers should take an active approach through screening for high-risk travel, and increasing their competency in travel medicine. Special attention should be given to illness that is prevented by routine childhood immunization (eg, varicella, measles, and hepatitis B); by disease prevented by travel vaccines (eg, typhoid fever and hepatitis A); and disease that can be prevented by careful avoidance measures or compliance with preventive medication (eg, malaria and tuberculosis).

With increased immigration from developing to developed regions and widely affordable travel, the number of VFR travelers is expected to increase. As such, increased efforts to prevent VFR traveler morbidity serve the individual while also contributing to global public health.

## Acknowledgments

The authors acknowledge the contribution to the content of this paper from Angell S, Cetron M. Health disparities among travelers visiting friends and relatives abroad. Ann Intern Med, in press, 2005. The authors also thank Sonya DeMonner, MPH, and Namrata Shah for their assistance with graphics and referencing; Joel Howell, MD, for his review of the manuscript; and the Robert Wood Johnson Clinical Scholars Program for their support.

# References

[1] Office of Travel and Tourism Industries. Office of Travel and Tourism Industries publication: 2002 profile of US resident traveler visiting overseas destinations. Reported from: Survey of International Air Travelers. Available at: http://tinet.ita.doc.gov/view/f-2002-101-001/index.html?ti_cart_cookie=20040203.085507.08935. Accessed December 14, 2004.

[2] National statistics travel trends 2002: a report on the International Passenger Survey. Available at: http://www.statistics.gov.uk/downloads/theme_transport/TTrends02.pdf. Accessed January 14, 2004.

[3] Leder K, Black J, O'Brien D, et al. Malaria in travelers: a review of the GeoSentinel surveillance network. Clin Infect Dis 2004;39:1104–12.

[4] Phillips-Howard PA, Radalowicz A, Mitchell J, et al. Risk of malaria in British residents returning from malarious areas. BMJ 1990;300:499–503.

[5] National Statistics. People and migration. Available at: http://www.statistics.gov.uk/CCI/nugget.asp?ID=764&Pos=6&ColRank=1&Rank=176. Accessed August 28, 2004.

[6] Schmidely AD. Current population reports. Series P23–206. In: US Census Bureau, editor. Profile of the foreign-born population in the United States: 2000. Washington: US Government Printing Office; 2001. p. 25.

[7] National Statistics. Persons granted British citizenship, United Kingdom, 2003. Available at: http://www.homeoffice.gov.uk/rds/pdfs04/hosb0704.pdf. Accessed December 14, 2004.

[8] Scolari C, Tedoldi S, Casalini C, et al. Knowledge, attitudes, and practices on malaria preventive measures of migrants attending a public health clinic in northern Italy. J Travel Med 2002;9:160–2.

[9] National Statistics. Ethnicity, low income. Available at: http://www.statistics.gov.uk/CCI/nugget.asp?ID=269&Pos=1&Co1Rank=1&Rank=374. Accessed December 14, 2004.

[10] Smedley BD, Stith Y, Nelson AR. Unequal treatment: confronting racial and ethnic disparities in health care. Board on Health Sciences Policy, Institute of Medicine. Washington: The National Academies Press; 2003.

[11] dos Santos CC, Anvar A, Keystone JS, et al. Survey of use of malaria prevention measures by Canadians visiting India. Can Med Assoc J 1999;160:195–200.

[12] Backer H, Mackell S. Potential cost-savings and quality improvement in travel advice for children and families from a centralized travel medicine clinic in a large group-model health maintenance organization. J Travel Med 2001;8:247–53.

[13] Janz N, Champion V, Stecher V. The health belief model. In: Glanz K, editor. Health behavior and health education: theory, research, and practice. 3rd edition. San Francisco (CA): Josey-Bass; 2002. p. 45–66.

[14] Leonard L, VanLandingham M. Adherence to travel health guidelines: the experience of Nigerian immigrants in Houston, Texas. J Immigr Health 2001;3:31–45.

[15] World Health Organization. Archives by disease: communicable disease surveillance & response-WHO. Available at: http://www.who.int/disease-outbreak-news/disease/bydisease.htm. Accessed December 14, 2004.

[16] Global Progress. Polio eradication World Health Organization. Available at: http://www.polioeradication.org/progress.asp. Accessed December 14, 2004.

[17] AFRICA. Polio hits Darfur as experts warn of largest epidemic in recent years: UN office for the Coordination of Humanitarian Affairs. Available at: http://www.plusnews.org/report.asp?ReportID=41825&SelectRegion=Africa. Accessed December 20, 2004.

[18] Strine TW, Barker LE, Mokdad AH, et al. Vaccination coverage of foreign-born children 19 to 35 months of age: findings from the National Immunization Survey, 1999–2000. Pediatrics 2002;110(2 Pt 1):e15.

[19] Centers for Disease Control and Prevention. Racial/ethnic disparities in influenza and pneumococcal vaccination levels among persons aged > or = 65 years—United States, 1989–2001. MMWR Morb Mortal Wkly Rep 2003;52:958–62.
[20] Centers for Disease Control and Prevention. Vaccination coverage by race/ethnicity and poverty level among children aged 19–35 months—United States, 1996. MMWR Morb Mortal Wkly Rep 1997;46:963–7.
[21] Catch-up immunization schedule for children and adolescents who start late or who are >1 month behind. Available at: http://www.cdc.gov/mmwr/preview/mmwrhtml/mm5301-Immunizationa1.htm#tab. Accessed December 14, 2004.
[22] Tagle M, Schiff ER. Hepatitis. In: Guerrant RL, Walker DH, editors. Essentials of tropical infectious diseases. New York: Churchill Livingstone; 2001. p. 544.
[23] Centers for Disease Control and Prevention. Health information for international travel 2003–2004. Atlanta: US Department of Health and Human Services, Public Health Service; 2003.
[24] World Health Organization. WHO vaccine preventable diseases: monitoring system. Available at: http://www.who.int/vaccines-documents/GlobalSummary/GlobalSummary.pdf. Accessed December 14, 2004.
[25] Centers for Disease Control and Prevention. Technical instruction to panel physicians for vaccination requirements. Available at: http://www.cdc.gov/ncidod/dq/pdf/TI.pdf. Accessed December 14, 2004.
[26] Centers for Disease Control. Disease burden from viral hepatitis A, B, and C in the United States. CDC / NCID 58. 2003. Available at: http://www.cdc.gov/ncidod/diseases/hepatitis/resource/PDFs/hep_surveillance_59.pdf. Accessed December 20, 2004.
[27] Health Protection Agency. Illness in England, Wales and Northern Ireland associated with foreign travel. Baseline report to 2002. London: Health Protection Agency; 2004.
[28] Behrens RH, Collins M, Botto B, et al. Risk for British travellers of acquiring hepatitis A. BMJ 1995;311:193.
[29] Van Steenbergen JE, Tjon G, Van Den HA, et al. Two years' prospective collection of molecular and epidemiological data shows limited spread of hepatitis A virus outside risk groups in Amsterdam, 2000–2002. J Infect Dis 2004;189:471–82.
[30] Tapia-Conyer R, Santos JI, Cavalcanti AM, et al. Hepatitis A in Latin America: a changing epidemiologic pattern. Am J Trop Med Hyg 1999;61:825–9.
[31] Mall ML, Rai RR, Philip M, et al. Seroepidemiology of hepatitis A infection in India: changing pattern. Indian J Gastroenterol 2001;20:132–5.
[32] Barnett ED, Holmes AH, Harrison TS. Immunity to hepatitis a in people born and raised in endemic areas. J Travel Med 2003;10:11–4.
[33] Richardus JH, Vos D, Veldhuijzen IK, et al. Seroprevalence of hepatitis A virus antibodies in Turkish and Moroccan children in Rotterdam. J Med Virol 2004;72:197–202.
[34] Mermin JH, Townes JM, Gerber M, et al. Typhoid fever in the United States, 1985–1994: changing risks of international travel and increasing antimicrobial resistance. Arch Intern Med 1998;158:633–8.
[35] Ackers ML, Puhr ND, Tauxe RV, et al. Laboratory-based surveillance of Salmonella serotype typhi infections in the United States: antimicrobial resistance on the rise. JAMA 2000;283:2668–73.
[36] Steinberg E, Bishop R, Haber P, et al. Typhoid fever in travellers: who should be targeted for prevention? Clin Infect Dis 2004;39:186–91.
[37] Coovadia YM, Gathiran V, Bhamjee A. An outbreak of multiresistant *Salmonella typhi* in South Africa. QJM 1992;82:91–100.
[38] Bhutta ZA, Naqvi SH, Razzaq RA, et al. Multidrug-resistant typhoid in children: presentation and clinical features. Rev Infect Dis 1991;13:832–6.
[39] Le TA, Lejay-Collin M, Grimont PA, et al. Endemic, epidemic clone of *Salmonella enterica* serovar typhi harboring a single multidrug-resistant plasmid in Vietnam between 1995 and 2002. J Clin Microbiol 2004;42:3094–9.

[40] Threlfall EJ. Antimicrobial drug resistance in *Salmonella*: problems and perspectives in food- and water-borne infections. FEMS Microbiol Rev 2002;26:141–8.
[41] Meyer PA, Seward JF, Jumaan AO, et al. Varicella mortality: trends before vaccine licensure in the United States, 1970–1994. J Infect Dis 2000;182:383–90.
[42] Mandal BK, Mukherjee PP, Murphy C, et al. Adult susceptibility to varicella in the tropics is a rural phenomenon due to the lack of previous exposure. J Infect Dis 1998;178(Suppl 1): 52–4.
[43] Lee BW. Review of varicella zoster seroepidemiology in India and Southeast Asia. Trop Med Int Health 1998;3:886–90.
[44] Barnett ED, Christiansen D, Figueira M. Seroprevalence of measles, rubella, and varicella in refugees. Clin Infect Dis 2002;35:403–8.
[45] Figueira M, Barnett ED, Christiansen D, et al. Cost-benefit of serotesting compared with presumptive immunization for varicella in refugee children from 3 distinct geographic regions. Pediatr Res 2000;47:261A.
[46] Shah S, Filler S, Causer LM, et al. Malaria surveillance–United States, 2002. MMWR Surveill Summ 2004;53:21–34.
[47] Cleary VA, Figueroa JI, Heathcock R, et al. Improving malaria surveillance in inner city London: is there a need for targeted intervention? Commun Dis Public Health 2003;6: 300–4.
[48] Ladhani S, El Bashir H, Patel VS, et al. Childhood malaria in East London. Pediatr Infect Dis J 2003;22:814–9.
[49] Behrens RH, Curtis CF. Malaria in travellers: epidemiology and prevention. In: Behrens RH, McAdam KPWJ, editors. Travel medicine. London: Churchill Livingstone; 1993. p. 363–81.
[50] Jelinek T, Schulte C, Behrens RH, et al. Imported Falciparum malaria in Europe: sentinel surveillance data from the European network on surveillance of imported infectious diseases. Clin Infect Dis 2002;34:572–6.
[51] Schlagenhauf P, Steffen R, Loutan L. Migrants as a major risk group for imported malaria in European countries. J Travel Med 2003;10:106–7.
[52] Badrinath P, Ejidokun OO, Barnes N, et al. Change in NHS regulations may have caused increase in malaria. BMJ 1998;316:1746a.
[53] Struik SS, Riley EM. Does malaria suffer from lack of memory? Immunol Rev 2004;201: 268–90.
[54] Semaille C, Santin A, Prazuck T, et al. Malaria chemoprophylaxis of 3,446 French travellers departing from Paris to eight tropical countries. J Travel Med 1999;6:3–6.
[55] Evans MR. Adverse events associated with mefloquine: patients may start to take cheaper over the counter regimens [letter]. BMJ 1996;313:1554.
[56] Centers for Disease Control and Prevention. Trends in tuberculosis morbidity—United States, 1992–2002. MMWR Morb Mortal Wkly Rep 2003;52:217–24.
[57] Rose AM, Watson JM, Graham C, et al. Tuberculosis at the end of the 20th century in England and Wales: results of a national survey in 1998. Thorax 2001;56:173–9.
[58] Cobelens FG, van Deutekom H, Draayer-Jansen IW, et al. Risk of infection with *Mycobacterium tuberculosis* in travellers to areas of high tuberculosis endemicity. Lancet 2000;356:461–5.
[59] Lobato MN, Hopewell PC. *Mycobacterium tuberculosis* infection after travel to or contact with visitors from countries with a high prevalence of tuberculosis. Am J Respir Crit Care Med 1998;158:1871–5.
[60] Ormerod LP, Green RM, Gray S. Are there still effects on Indian Subcontinent ethnic tuberculosis of return visits?: a longitudinal study 1978–97. J Infect 2001;43:132–4.
[61] Huebner RE, Schein MF, Bass JB. The tuberculin skin test. Clin Infect Dis 1993;17:968–75.
[62] Centers for Disease Control and Prevention. Targeted tuberculin testing and treatment of latent tuberculosis infection. MMWR Morb Mortal Wkly Rep 2000;49(RR06):1–54.
[63] Rieder HL. Risk of travel-associated tuberculosis. Clin Infect Dis 2001;33:1393–6.

[64] Anonymous. Diagnostic standards and classification of tuberculosis in adults and children.This official statement of the American Thoracic Society and the Centers for Disease Control and Prevention was adopted by the ATS Board of Directors, July 1999. Am J Respir Crit Care Med 2000;161(4 Pt 1):1376–95.
[65] Lifson AR. *Mycobacterium tuberculosis* infection in travellers: tuberculosis comes home. Lancet 2000;356:442.
[66] Hershfield ES. Medical advice for international travelers. Mayo Clin Proc 2001;76:1278–9.

# Health Risks to Air Travelers
Muhammad R. Sohail, MD[a], Philip R. Fischer, MD[b],*

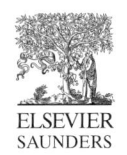

[a]*Division of Infectious Disease, Department of Medicine, Mayo Clinic College of Medicine, 200 First Street SW, Rochester, MN 55905, USA*
[b]*Department of Pediatric and Adolescent Medicine, Mayo Clinic College of Medicine, 200 First Street SW, Rochester, MN 55905, USA*

According to the Aerospace Medical Association, one billion people travel by air each year on domestic and international flights and this number is expected to double in the coming two decades [1,2]. It is estimated that in the United States alone, over 1,700,000 passengers board aircraft every day [3]. Beyond the hassles of an occasional late arrival or lost luggage, most travelers experience neither inconvenience nor adverse health consequence related to air travel. There are, however, some health risks to air travelers. Using real-life cases, concerns, and situations, this article discusses those risks and how savvy travelers can minimize air travel–associated health problems.

## Do I need to wear a face mask during my trip?

During a pretravel consultation before a trip to China in spring of 2004, a business traveler wants to know if he should wear a face mask during his return flight from Beijing to New York. "There may be [severe acute respiratory syndrome] SARS-infected patients on the flight, you know!" he explains. Are passengers at risk of acquiring respiratory infections onboard aircraft and should a face mask be recommended to help prevent such infections?

Travelers can acquire infection on commercial aircrafts in a variety of ways. Infection can be transmitted by contaminated food (*Salmonella, Staphylococcus, Vibrio* spp.); from insects that may enter the aircraft during layover at airports in endemic area (malaria); or more commonly through person-to-person transmission of respiratory infections [4]. Respiratory pathogens can spread by large droplets (which quickly fall down to the

---

\* Corresponding author.
*E-mail address:* Fischer.Phil@mayo.edu (P.R. Fischer).

ground if they fail to reach the mucous membranes) or by tiny droplet nuclei (<10 μm in diameter), which disperse widely and remain airborne for hours (measles, influenza, tuberculosis, and SARS spread by these droplet nuclei) [5,6]. Close proximity onboard commercial aircrafts can help spread these infections to fellow passengers [2]. Approximately 26% of international travelers report respiratory illness associated with their travel [7], but it is not known how much of this is caused by exposure on planes as opposed to during activities on the ground.

Cabin air in commercial aircraft is remarkably clean. Air is recycled on average 20 to 30 times an hour and recirculated air is passed through high-efficiency particulate air filters, which remove microorganisms of 0.3 to 1 μm in size including mycobacteria, fungi, and some viruses [4,8]. As a result, the concentration of microorganisms in cabin air is much lower than most city locations including shopping malls and airport terminals [9]. Despite these measures, however, in-flight transmission of respiratory infections, such as measles, influenza, tuberculosis, and more recently SARS, has been reported [4,10–12].

*Severe acute respiratory syndrome*

SARS is a novel respiratory illness, characterized by acute onset of fever, malaise, cough, and shortness of breath, which emerged in the spring of 2003. Rapid global spread of SARS-corona virus in 2003 was facilitated by international travel as illustrated by initial dissemination of the SARS outbreak from Hong Kong [13]. Although concern of transmission to fellow passengers on aircraft was raised from early on, the first documented transmission of SARS-corona virus on airplane was reported in December of 2003 [10]. In their study, three flights that carried passengers with laboratory-confirmed SARS-corona virus infection were investigated. There was strong evidence to suggest transmission of SARS-corona virus to 22 fellow passengers and crew members in one flight from Hong Kong to Beijing, which carried a symptomatic passenger. Travelers who became infected were sitting in the same row as the index case or within three rows directly in front of him (suggesting spread by aerosol and small droplets). None of the passengers in other sections of the plane acquired infection pointing against the possibility of transmission by the aircraft ventilation system. There was no evidence of transmission on flights that carried SARS-corona virus–infected passengers who were asymptomatic at the time of travel. These data suggest that the primary preventive strategy to minimize risk of in-flight transmission of SARS is to prevent symptomatic SARS patients from traveling [13].

The Centers for Disease Control and Prevention (CDC) recommends hand washing to reduce risk of transmission. Routine use of face masks or other personal protective equipment in public areas is not recommended [13]. Travelers to areas where SARS is being reported should avoid high-risk settings, such as health care facilities and live animal markets [14].

*Tuberculosis*

Increasing global travel and immigration to United States from parts of the world where tuberculosis is highly endemic increases potential for exposure and transmission of tuberculosis on commercial aircraft [12]. Although screening for tuberculosis is required for immigrants and refugees, it is not required for tourists, business travelers, and students coming to the United States [15]. Patients with active pulmonary tuberculosis may travel on commercial aircrafts without being aware of their diagnosis. The cough of a patient with tuberculosis releases droplet nuclei, which become airborne and are carried by air currents to neighboring passengers until they are cleared by the aircraft ventilation system. According to some estimates, 1 of every 26,000 airline passengers may be exposed to tuberculosis [12]. Risk is still low, however, to passengers and crew on commercial aircrafts in United States [11,12,16].

From 1992 to 1994, seven different flights that carried tuberculosis-infected passengers were investigated [11,12,16–19]. Index patients on all seven flights were highly infectious (symptomatic, sputum smear positive for acid-fast bacilli, and evidence of cavitary disease on chest radiograph). There was strong evidence of tuberculosis transmission on three flights [11,12,16]. Infection was transmitted from one flight attendant to two other crew members on one flight [16], whereas transmission from the index case to fellow passengers and flight crew was documented in another two flights [11,12]. Risk of transmission was associated with proximity to the index cases (sitting in same section of plane) and a long duration of flight (>12 hours). There was no evidence of transmission on the other four flights despite highly infectious passengers on board, suggesting that although in-flight transmission is possible, the risk is still very low.

The CDC recommends that patients should have at least three negative sputum smears for acid-fast bacilli before travel to minimize risk of transmission on aircraft [11]. If travel is essential while the patient is still infectious, a private mode of transportation should be arranged.

So what of the business traveler? He should be counseled that the risk of acquiring SARS on board is extremely low. The CDC recommends good hand washing for prevention of infection. Routine use of face masks, however, is not recommended [13].

**Do I need to arrange oxygen for my trip?**

One of your patients with chronic obstructive pulmonary disease is planning to take a trip to Hawaii. He is medically stable and does not use oxygen at home. He has read in his travel book that passengers on aircrafts may be exposed to hypoxic conditions. "Do you think I should arrange for oxygen on board, just in case"? he inquires.

Commercial jets maintain a relative cabin pressure equivalent to the atmospheric pressure at 5000 to 8000 ft during routine flights [1,6]. At this altitude, the partial pressure of inspired oxygen ($Pio_2$) drops from 150 mm Hg (sea level) to 109 mm Hg [20]. This fall in $Pio_2$ results in a drop of arterial oxygen saturation ($Sao_2$). In one study of healthy flight-crew members during 22 scheduled flights, mean nadir $Sao_2$ fell from 97% (preflight) to 88.6% at cruising altitude [21]. Most healthy travelers can compensate for this level of hypoxemia. Patients with pre-existing cardiac and respiratory conditions, however, who are hypoxemic at sea level, can develop respiratory distress with such a drop in $Sao_2$ at high altitude. Up to 10% of radio calls to ground medical staff for in-flight medical emergencies is related to respiratory problems [22]. To ensure a safe and comfortable flight for these patients, they should be evaluated for need of in-flight oxygen therapy. Recommended tests for this evaluation are summarized in Box 1.

---

**Box 1. Recommended tests to evaluate need for in-flight oxygen therapy**

1. Ability to walk 50 yards at a normal pace or climb one flight of stairs without becoming severely short of breath.
   Most practical test to evaluate fitness for commercial air travel.
2. Pulse oximetry at rest and during exertion (adequate in most cases). Patients with $Sao_2$ > 95% in room air on sea-level do not require oxygen on board, whereas those with $Sao_2$ < 92% require it. Individual in intermediate range requires some hypoxic exposure test to determine need for oxygen.
3. Arterial blood gas: single most helpful blood test because $Pao_2$ at sea-level is considered the best predictor of altitude $Pao_2$ and tolerance. $Pao_2$ < 70 in room air at sea level is an indication for in-flight oxygen therapy.
4. Hypoxia altitude simulation test: sophisticated method. $Pao_2$ is determined while patient breathes mixed gases simulating the aircraft cabin environment at 8000 ft altitude (85% nitrogen and 15% oxygen). If $Pao_2$ is <50 mm Hg, medical oxygen should be considered.
5. Exposure to hypoxia in an altitude chamber. Ideal preflight test. Also detects potential adverse effects of gas expansion. Only available in a few centers.
6. Consider departing altitude, length of flight, destination altitude, and prior history of air travel when making decision for in-flight oxygen requirement.

---

*Data from* Refs. [1,2,20,23–25].

Travelers with chronic obstructive pulmonary disease are the best studied group for flight-related problems. They are susceptible to significant in-flight hypoxemia depending on baseline Pao$_2$. Measurement of preflight forced expiratory volume in first second improves prediction of Pao$_2$ at altitude in patients with severe chronic obstructive pulmonary disease [26]. Most patients with interstitial lung disease (sarcoidosis and idiopathic pulmonary fibrosis) generally well tolerate air travel. Travel guidelines for patients with specific respiratory conditions are summarized in Table 1 [1,24,27].

What advice should you give to your patient? Certainly, he should be evaluated for a possible in-flight oxygen requirement. He should also be advised to contact the airline at least 48 to 72 hours in advance to arrange

Table 1
Travel guidelines for patients with specific respiratory conditions

| Disease | Recommendations |
| --- | --- |
| COPD: chronic bronchitis and emphysema | Arrange inflight oxygen if indicated; carry bronchodilators in hand luggage; consider PFT (FEV$_1$) in patients with severe COPD |
| Asthma | Hand carry short-acting inhalers; advise to take a course of oral steroid with them for any emergencies during trip; delay travel if labile condition |
| Interstitial lung disease (idiopathic pulmonary fibrosis and sarcoidosis) | Evaluate need for in-flight oxygen therapy |
| Bronchiectasis and cystic fibrosis | Control of lung infection with appropriate antibiotics; measures to loosen and clear secretions; adequate hydration; consider aerosolized rhDNAse to reduce sputum viscosity; medical oxygen if indicated |
| Pneumothorax | Diagnose and correct underlying etiology; delay travel until resolved |
| Pulmonary hypertension | Anticoagulation, evaluation for in-flight oxygen; restrict exercise during flight |
| Pleural effusion | Large effusion should be drained 10–14 days before flight for diagnostic and therapeutic purposes; consider repeating chest radiograph before trip |
| Neuromuscular disease (spinal cord injury, obesity hypoventilation syndrome, muscular dystrophy) | Arrange manual suctioning equipment, medical oxygen, and ventilator capabilities; some patients may require tracheostomy before trip |
| Tracheostomy | Humidification of inspired air; adequate hydration; suctioning |
| Patients on long-term home oxygen therapy | May need to increase flow rate from 1 to 2 L.min$^{-1}$ to 4 L.min$^{-1}$ |
| Recent exacerbation of any chronic respiratory disease | Delay travel until stabilized |

*Abbreviations:* COPD, chronic obstructive pulmonary disease; FEV$_1$, forced expiratory volume in 1 second; PFT, pulmonary function tests.
*Data from* Refs. [1,24,27].

oxygen onboard aircraft [25] because airlines do not allow passengers to carry their own oxygen on aircrafts out of concerns of safety and security. The patient should be provided with a prescription for in-flight oxygen and a "fitness to fly" certificate from a physician. The delivery method (face-mask versus nasal-cannula, intermittent versus continuous flow) should also be specified [28]. Airlines are not responsible for providing oxygen during airport layovers and at destination airports and travelers need to make their own arrangements.

## How long do I have to wait before I can fly?

Patients with cardiac problems represent a major group at risk for flight-related complications. Most patients with stable angina pectoris can travel safely. Individuals with acute myocardial infarction may need to delay their travel plan (Table 2) [2,25]. Previously, a delay of several weeks was recommended for patients who suffered an acute myocardial infarction. In a review of 196 adults carried on commercial aircrafts post–myocardial infarction, however, 95% were transported without incident when traveling

Table 2
Recommended travel delay for specific conditions

| Condition | Recommended travel delay |
|---|---|
| Cardiac (CABG, valve replacement) surgery | 10–14 d |
| Uncomplicated myocardial infarction | 2–3 wk |
| Complicated myocardial infarction[a] | 6 wk |
| Uncomplicated PCI | 3–5 d |
| Complicated PCI | 1–2 wk |
| Thoracic surgery | 10–14 d |
| Pneumothorax | 2–3 wk after resolution |
| Any unstable cardiopulmonary condition | Delay until stabilized |
| Stroke (CVA) | 2 wk |
| Postspinal anesthesia | 10–14 d |
| Open abdominal surgery | 1–2 wk |
| Laparoscopic abdominal surgery | 24 h (1–2 wk if intestinal lumen has been opened) |
| Colonoscopy with polypectomy | 24 h |
| Skull fracture or postneurosurgery | 1–2 wk |
| Scuba diving (one dive per day) | 12–24 h |
| Communicable diseases (including TB, SARS, measles, influenza) | Delay travel until period of communicability is over (clinical improvement, negative cultures, and so forth) |

Travel is by commercial airline flight. These are only guidelines and must be individualized based on clinical judgment and length of trip.

*Abbreviations:* CABG, coronary artery bypass grafting; CVA, cerebrovascular accident; PCI, percutaneous coronary intervention; SARS, severe acute respiratory syndrome; TB, tuberculosis.

[a] Complicated by arrhythmia, postinfarct angina, or left ventricular dysfunction.

*Data from* Refs. [1,2,29,31–33].

at least 2 weeks after the event [29]. A symptom-limited treadmill test at 10 to 14 days after myocardial infarction is a better way to assess fitness for flying than arbitrary travel restrictions [30]. Patients with an old myocardial infarction should not have any problem during air travel. Patients should be evaluated for need of in-flight oxygen. Unstable angina, decompensated heart failure, uncontrolled hypertension, uncontrolled ventricular or supraventricular tachycardia, Eisenmenger's syndrome, and severe symptomatic valvular heart disease are considered contraindications to travel by commercial air flights [1].

Postoperative patients are another group who may need to delay their travel plans after surgery. General anesthesia itself is not a contraindication for flying because cardiac depressant effects and changes in vascular systems secondary to anesthesia are rapidly reversible. Surgical procedures that result in entrapment of air in various body cavities (abdominal, chest, head, eye) can result in problems associated with expansion of gases at reduced cabin pressure at altitude (gases expand 25% at an altitude of 8000 ft). Recommended travel delay for specific surgical conditions is listed in Table 2 [1,2,29,31–33].

Travelers with permanent pacemakers and implanted cardioverter defibrillators are at low risk for flying once medically stable. Interaction with airline electronics or airport security devices is highly unlikely for the most common bipolar devices [34]. Hand-held security devices may interfere with implanted cardioverter defibrillators and travelers should carry a physician's letter specifying this hazard [33,35]. Questions about particular models should be directed to representatives of the pacemaker company. Patients should be advised to carry copies of their electrocardiogram with and without activation of their pacemaker during travel [25].

## To shock or not to shock!

Cardiovascular problems are the most common cause of air travel–related medical emergencies and deaths [6,33,36]. Almost 1000 lives are lost annually from cardiac arrest in commercial aircrafts and airline terminals in International Airlines Transport Association carriers [37]. Most of the victims do not have prior history of heart disease. Ventricular fibrillation is the most common rhythm recorded in victims of sudden cardiac arrest [38,39]. Early defibrillation is the most important predictor of success and long-term survival [40]. Chances of survival decrease by 10% for each minute defibrillation is delayed. Previously, the common practice of airlines was to continue cardiopulmonary resuscitation and divert the plane to the nearest airport. This may take 20 minutes or longer, however, even in best of circumstances. This is an unacceptable delay in view of current standards of care for sudden cardiac arrest [41]. A more logical approach is to place automated external defibrillators on board and train flight crew in their use

[42]. Onboard automated external defibrillators improve chances of survival in cardiac arrest and avoid unnecessary and futile diversions for idioventricular rhythm and asystole [6,43,44].

In the United States, American Airlines was the first to install automated external defibrillators on commercial aircrafts. In their experience from June 1997 to July 1999 [45], automated external defibrillators were used on 200 occasions. Sensitivity (ability correctly to diagnose ventricular fibrillation) and success rate (ability successfully to defibrillate) of automated external defibrillators was 100%. No inappropriate shocks were given. Rate of survival after defibrillation to discharge from hospital was 40%. Based on these data, it was estimated that use of automated external defibrillators will save 93 lives each year. Similar encouraging experience has been reported by other international carriers [41].

In June 2001, the Federal Aviation Administration mandated that all commercial air carriers with at least one flight attendant on board must carry automated external defibrillators on each aircraft by April, 2004 [6,46]. Physicians and other medical personnel who volunteer to assist during in-flight emergencies are protected from liability by the "Good Samaritan" provision of the "Airline Passenger Safety Act" of 1997 [47].

**Should I take an aspirin before traveling on airplane?**

A 35-year-old anxious woman presents for pretraveling counseling. She does not smoke but uses oral contraceptives. Her mother died with pulmonary embolism last year at age 65. She wants to know if she should take aspirin before her flight to minimize her risk of pulmonary embolism.

Air travel is now considered a well-recognized risk factor for venous thromboembolism [48–50]. The reported incidence of travel-related venous thrombosis ranges between 5% and 10% [22,31,48,51]. In a case control study of 160 patients, history of recent travel was four times more common in patients with venous thromboembolism compared with controls [49]. Most cases of travel-related deep venous thrombosis are asymptomatic and result in no clinical consequences. Pulmonary embolism is the most dreaded complication of travel-related deep venous thrombosis presenting with chest pain, dyspnea, or even sudden death. In a study of 61 cases of sudden death in passengers arriving at Heathrow airport between 1979 and 1982, pulmonary embolism was identified as the cause of death on autopsy in 18% of cases [52]. Travel-related arterial and cerebral venous thrombi have also been reported in the literature [53,54].

The term "economy class syndrome" has been used widely in the past to describe air travel–related venous thromboembolism [55]. This term, however, is misleading because the risk of venous thrombosis is not limited to travel on "economy class" of aircrafts but indeed may occur on "first class" or during travel on buses or trains [56]. Instead, use of the term "traveler's thrombosis" is probably more appropriate.

Prolonged immobility and venous stasis associated with long-haul flights are the major promoting factor for venous thromboembolism [57,58]. Risk increases with duration of flight (more common in flight of >12 hours duration, whereas rarely occurring in flights of <4 hours duration) [49,59]. Compression of the popliteal vein at the edge of a seat [60] and hemoconcentration associated with diminished fluid intake and increased insensible water loss may serve as additional risk factors [61]. Sitting at window or central seats is another potentially avoidable risk factor for air-travel–related venous thrombosis [25].

The risk of venous thrombosis is very low in travelers without pre-existing additional risk factors [60,62]. These additional risk factors include age above 50 years, clotting disorders, cardiovascular disease, malignancy, recent major surgery or trauma, history of deep venous thrombosis or pulmonary embolism, pregnancy, and use of oral contraceptives [1,22,63]. Smoking, obesity, and varicose vein may serve as additional risk factors.

Traveler's thrombosis is a potentially preventable hazard of air travel. Preventive efforts are largely focused on stimulation of circulation to prevent venous stasis. Most travelers are at low risk and only need to follow nonpharmacologic measures listed in Box 2 [1,2,33,51,64–76]. Patients with additional risk factors should seek medical advice before traveling. Physicians may recommend delaying travel plans after orthopedic surgery or trauma to lower extremities. The role of pharmacologic measures (aspirin, low-molecular-weight heparin) is controversial and their use should be limited to individuals at highest risk (malignancy, personal history of venous thromboembolism, recent major orthopedic surgery) [22,65]. Single dose of low-molecular-weight heparin 2 to 4 hours before long-haul flights (>10 hours) was associated with a significant reduction in risk of traveler's thrombosis in a randomized case-control study of 300 subjects [51,67]. Although aspirin prophylaxis has been shown to be helpful in reducing incidence of venous thrombosis and pulmonary embolism in high-risk medical and surgical patients, its role in reducing travel-related deep venous thrombosis has not yet been evaluated in prospective studies [68,69]. Travelers should be cautioned against indiscriminate use of aspirin because of potential side effects of allergic reactions and gastrointestinal bleeding [2,65].

So what should we advise to the patient? She is at low risk because her only identifiable risk factor is use of oral contraceptives. She should be counseled about nonpharmacologic measures listed in Box 2. Aspirin should not be prescribed in this case.

**Peanuts or pretzels?**

Approximately 15% of people have significant allergic disease, and about 1% of individuals have a potentially life-threatening allergy to peanuts. During travel, peanut-sensitive individuals should be reminded to be careful

> **Box 2. Measures to minimize risk of traveler's thrombosis**
>
> *Nonpharmacologic*
> 1. Bulkhead seating if available.
> 2. Wear properly fitted graduated-compression stockings especially designed for air travel. Stockings are available over-the-counter and are reusable. Wear these correctly to avoid compression in popliteal area. Stockings are contraindicated in patients with peripheral arterial disease because these may provoke ischemia in this patient population.
> 3. Avoid constrictive clothing.
> 4. Take periodic walks during the flight.
> 5. Simple, frequent, isometric calf exercises, such as flexion and extension of foot and ankle rotation exercises.
> 6. Change positions periodically while seated.
> 7. Avoid leg crossing.
> 8. Maintain adequate hydration.
> 9. Avoid excess alcohol and caffeine-containing drinks because they may cause dehydration.
> 10. Do not place hand-luggage where it may restrict movement of legs and feet.
> 11. Get off plane and walk around in air terminal at refueling stops.
>
> *Pharmacologic (may be considered for high-risk individuals)*
> 1. Aspirin: caution in patients with peptic ulcer disease or history of gastrointestinal bleeding.
> 2. Low-molecular-weight heparin.
>
> ---
> Data from Refs. [1,2,33,51,64–76].

to avoid either obvious exposure (eating free peanuts during flights) or inadvertent exposure (eating foods that might have been prepared in peanut oil). Is there, however, a risk of inadvertent exposure and a severe reaction because of "peanut dust" being circulated and recirculated in ventilated aircraft?

Peanut allergen has been identified in filters removed from aircraft [70]. This implies that significant allergen had been circulating in the aircraft air during flight. And, the filters in aircraft ventilation systems are usually changed only after 5000 hours of in-flight use. In addition, peanut reactions can occur after exposure to very small amounts of allergen [71], even by an inhalational or transcutaneous route.

Anaphylaxis is possible following a first-known peanut exposure (presumably following intrauterine or inadvertent sensitization), but most people with life-threatening reactions were already aware of their allergy and exposed themselves anyway. In addition, fatal peanut reactions are associated with both known exposure and a delay of more than 25 minutes between the onset of the reaction and the administration of epinephrine [72–74].

Travelers concerned about anaphylaxis to peanuts should be careful to avoid ingestion or handling of peanuts on airplanes (and elsewhere). They should avoid foods that might have been prepared using peanut products. They should also carry epinephrine. The epinephrine should be administered immediately on recognition of symptoms of possible anaphylaxis, and further medical care should also be sought. As new therapeutic modalities, such as those involving monoclonal IgE antibody become available, peanut-allergic individuals might also be candidates for desensitization treatment [75].

## Child safety seats

A flustered family tries to make sure they have not forgotten anything as they prepare for their flight. Packing a preschool-sized load of paraphernalia, they ask if they really need to use a car seat on the plane. "Isn't a lap adequate for our baby"? they ask.

It is estimated in America that a plane crash–associated death of a child could be prevented once every 2 years by the use of appropriate safety restraints. Some organizations, such as the American Academy of Pediatrics, advise that all infants have a ticketed seat on airplanes and that they be securely fastened in a child restraint seat [76].

Analysis of the costs and effectiveness of requiring infant seats on aircraft, however, suggests that the added inconvenience and cost of using safety seats in planes would stimulate enough children to travel by road rather than by air that there would actually be an increase in travel-related deaths [77].

What should be suggested for the flustered family? A safety restraint in an individual seat might save the life of the child in the rare event of a survivable plane crash, but the restraint should be approved by the Federal Aviation Administration because not all car seats provide appropriate protection for the sorts of forces that occur during air turbulence or plane crashes. For additional in-flight safety, infants should avoid aisle seats where hot drinks might spill when being passed over them. Restrained in a safety seat or not, families should also be advised to provide games or reading material and snacks for children during flights; this can help make the flight safer and more enjoyable for the whole family and for others sharing the aircraft cabin.

## Does air travel cause crib death?

A parent who works as a medical professional comes in with her family for a pretravel consultation. You have covered all the usual safety, diarrhea, malaria, and immunization information. The parent then asks, "Didn't the British prove that intercontinental travel causes crib death"?

Crib death (also called cot death or sudden infant death syndrome) is the unexplained death of a young child (usually between 2 and 6 months of age). Although some apparent sudden infant death syndrome deaths have been retrospectively identified as caused by trauma, suffocation, fatty acid oxidation defect, or cardiac dysrhythmia, true sudden infant death syndrome refers to a death for which no cause is identified, even after extensive evaluation.

Anecdotally, some infants have happened to die of apparent sudden infant death syndrome shortly after completing a transcontinental air flight [78]. This prompted British investigators to study the effect of a low-oxygen environment (15% ambient oxygen at sea level, approximating the oxygen content of a commercial aircraft during flight with the cabin pressurized to the equivalent of about 6500 ft elevation) [78]. Thirty-four young infants (mean age 3 months), 13 of who were siblings of sudden infant death syndrome victims, were exposed overnight to environments of 15% oxygen. Oxygen saturations were variable (85%–100%) but of lower mean (93%) in 15% oxygen as compared with 98% in room air. In low oxygen environments, irregular breathing (with respiratory pauses of less than 20 seconds) was more common.

This study stimulated ethical concern and clinical controversy. Nonetheless, how can one respond to the parent-professional concerned about air travel with an infant? First, there is no proof that international travel causes sudden infant death syndrome, and any association noted is only anecdotal and likely coincidental at this point. Second, hypoxic environments similar to those of commercial aircraft do stimulate infants to have lower oxygen saturations and irregular breathing. The studied infants did not drop to dangerously low oxygen levels or have true apnea, and neither the decreased oxygenation nor the respiratory irregularity were associated with any sign of clinical compromise. There has been concern about prolonged air travel for infants, and there are physiologic changes associated with air travel–like environments, but there is no clear evidence of prolonged air travel being dangerous for infants.

It seems safe to give cautious reassurance to parents traveling with infants. At the same time, they can be reminded to implement other interventions that have clearly been linked to decreased risk of sudden infant death syndrome. Parents, traveling or not, should avoid passive smoke exposure for infants, and infants should routinely sleep in a supine, rather than a prone, position [79].

### I get sick on planes!

A family expresses concern before a long-anticipated vacation. "What," they ask, "can we do to prevent motion sickness"?

Although approximately one third of the population is susceptible to motion sickness [80], most people are not bothered by the conditions of routine commercial air flights. Those with most susceptibility to motion sickness are children, pregnant women, and individuals with a personal or family history of migraine headaches.

Studies of nonpharmacologic measures to prevent motion sickness have yielded either negative or conflicting results. There is no clear evidence to support the use of biofeedback, acupressure, and ingestion of ginger [80]. Anecdotally, seating over the center (wing area) of the plane might be associated with less movement during times of turbulence, but location on a ship was not associated with any change in seasickness [81]. Lying down and avoiding reading are, as anecdotally reported, also useful for many travelers.

A variety of medications can help reduce the risk of symptomatic motion sickness. Dimenhydrinate is readily available and can be used at a dose of 1 mg/kg (50 mg for adults) approximately 1 hour before the expected risk of motion sickness; drowsiness can be a side effect. Scopolamine is effective [82] and is available in tablet form to be taken as 0.4 mg 1 hour before anticipated risk setting and repeated 8-hourly as needed for recurrent exposures. Scopolamine is also available in a patch form to be applied 6 to 8 hours before beginning a prolonged period of motion sickness risk (1.5 mg, gradual release over 72 hours). Transdermal scopolamine, however, is not approved in young children and carries a potential risk of adverse central nervous system effects including hallucinations and seizures. Another option is promethazine, taken as a 25-mg dose for adults with onset of activity approximately 2 hours after administration and continuing for 6 or more hours.

### Can I fly during pregnancy?

Other than the risks of venous stasis and thrombosis and the potential exposure to a minimal amount of cosmic radiation, is there any other reason why a pregnant woman should not travel by air? Although there is a little evidence that even commuter travel and its associated physical (and perhaps emotional) stresses is linked to earlier deliveries [83], there does not seem to be medical contraindications to air travel during an otherwise healthy pregnancy. If the woman has a history of preterm labor or of placental abnormalities, however, she should probably avoid air travel during pregnancy.

Why, then, do some airlines prohibit travel during the late stages of pregnancy? Although the trip will not likely change the chance of an unexpected delivery, an in-flight delivery adds significant inconvenience to the woman, the newborn, the other passengers, and the flight crew. For the sake of others, it seems wise to avoid a long flight near term when an airborne delivery could lead to a diversion of the flight.

The other risk of travel during pregnancy relates more to situations at the destination than to the actual flight. It seems that the costs and social stresses of a premature delivery away from home have negative impacts on the child, mother, and family [84].

Should a pregnant woman travel by air? For the sake of other passengers, she should probably refrain from travel during the final month of pregnancy when there is some chance of spontaneous labor and delivery. For her own sake, a pregnant woman is usually advised to avoid a trip during pregnancy that takes her away from the supportive network and medical care of her home setting. If she does choose to travel while pregnant, she should be advised to avoid tight-fitting clothes that might impede venous blood flow, to drink plenty of fluids during flight, to walk every hour or two during long flights, and to have contingency plans should urgent obstetric care be needed. In addition, she should be advised to carry a copy of her medical records and prenatal test results to share with any other providers who might become unexpectedly involved in her care.

## Summary

With focused pretravel counseling and intervention, travelers can be prepared to avoid many risks of in-flight problems. Travel medicine practitioners can include appropriate guidance for in-flight health and safety in discussions during pretravel visits.

## References

[1] Aerospace Medical Association Medical Guidelines Task Force. Medical Guidelines for airline travel, 2nd edition. Aviat Space Environ Med 2003;74(5 Suppl):A1–19. Available at: www.asma.org/Publication/medicalguideline.html. Accessed November 6, 2004.
[2] British Medical Association. The impact of flying on passenger health: a guide for healthcare professionals. Board of Science and Education. Available at: www.bma.org.uk. Accessed May, 2004.
[3] DeHart RL. Health issues of air travel. Annu Rev Public Health 2003;24:133–51.
[4] Wenzel RP. Airline travel and infection. N Engl J Med 1996;334:981–2.
[5] Imported case of measles on flight from Hong Kong. The City of New York: Department of Health and Mental Hygiene. Health Alert #18. August 1, 2004.
[6] Gendreau MA, DeJohn C. Responding to medical events during commercial airline flights. N Engl J Med 2002;346:1067–73.
[7] Hill DR. Health problems in a large cohort of Americans traveling to developing countries. J Travel Med 2000;7:259–66.

[8] Hocking MB. Passenger aircraft cabin air quality: trends, effects, societal costs, proposals. Chemosphere 2000;41:603–15.
[9] Wick RL Jr, Irvine LA. The microbiological composition of airliner cabin air. Aviat Space Environ Med 1995;66:220–4.
[10] Olsen SJ, Chang HL, Cheung TY, et al. Transmission of the severe acute respiratory syndrome on aircraft. N Engl J Med 2003;349:2416–22.
[11] CDC. Exposure of passengers and flight crew to *Mycobacterium tuberculosis* on commercial aircraft, 1992–1995. MMWR Morb Mortal Wkly Rep 1995;44:137–40.
[12] Kenyon TA, Valway SE, Ihle WW, et al. Transmission of multidrug-resistant *Mycobacterium tuberculosis* during a long airplane flight. N Engl J Med 1996;334:933–8.
[13] CDC. Public health guidance for community-level preparedness and response to severe acute respiratory syndrome (SARS) Version 2. Supplement E: Managing international travel related transmission risk. Atlanta: DHHS; 2004.
[14] Sampathkumar P, Temesgen Z, Smith TF, et al. SARS: epidemiology, clinical presentation, management, and infection control measures. Mayo Clin Proc 2003;78:882–90.
[15] CDC. Public Health Service. Technical instructions for medical examination of aliens. Atlanta. 1991. Available at: www.cdc.gov. Accessed November 6, 2004.
[16] Driver CR, Valway SE, Morgan WM, et al. Transmission of *Mycobacterium tuberculosis* associated with air travel. JAMA 1994;272:1031–5.
[17] McFarland JW, Hickman C, Osterholm M, et al. Exposure to *Mycobacterium tuberculosis* during air travel. Lancet 1993;342:112–3.
[18] Miller MA, Valway S, Onorato IM. Tuberculosis risk after exposure on airplanes. Tubercle Lung Dis 1996;77:414–9.
[19] Moore M, Fleming KS, Sands L. A passenger with pulmonary/laryngeal tuberculosis: no evidence of transmission on two short flights. Aviat Space Environ Med 1996;67:1097–100.
[20] Gong H Jr. Air travel and oxygen therapy in cardiopulmonary patients. Chest 1992;101: 1104–13.
[21] Cottrell JJ, Lebovitz BL, Fennell RG, et al. In-flight arterial saturation: continuous monitoring by pulse oximetry. Aviat Space Environ Med 1995;66:126–30.
[22] Nicholson AN, Cummin ARC, Giangrande PL. The airline passenger: current medical issues. Travel Med Infect Dis 2003;1:94–102.
[23] Vohra KP, Klocke RA. Detection and correction of hypoxemia associated with air travel. Am Rev Respir Dis 1993;148:1215–9.
[24] Managing passengers with respiratory disease planning air travel: British Thoracic Society recommendations. Thorax 2002;57:289–304.
[25] Possick SE, Barry M. Air travel and cardiovascular disease. J Travel Med 2004;11:243–50.
[26] Dillard TA, Berg BW, Rajagopal KR, et al. Hypoxemia during air travel in patients with chronic obstructive pulmonary disease. Ann Intern Med 1989;111:362–7.
[27] Gong H Jr, Mark JA, Cowan MN. Preflight medical screenings of patients: analysis of health and flight characteristics. Chest 1993;104:788–94.
[28] Mileno MD, Bia FJ. The compromised traveler. Infect Dis Clin North Am 1998;12:369–412.
[29] Cox GR, Peterson J, Bouchel L, et al. Safety of commercial air travel following myocardial infarction. Aviat Space Environ Med 1996;67:976–82.
[30] Ryan TJ, Antman EM, Brooks NH, et al. 1999 update: ACC/AHA Guidelines for the Management of Patients With Acute Myocardial Infarction: executive summary and recommendations. A report of the American College of Cardiology/American Heart Association Task Force on Practice Guidelines (Committee on Management of Acute Myocardial Infarction). Circulation 1999;100:1016–30.
[31] Kozarsky PE. Prevention of common travel ailments. Infect Dis Clin North Am 1998;12: 305–24.
[32] Ryan TJ, Anderson JL, Antman EM, et al. ACC/AHA guidelines for the management of patients with acute myocardial infarction: executive summary. A report of the American College of Cardiology/American Heart Association Task Force on Practice Guidelines

(Committee on Management of Acute Myocardial Infarction). Circulation 1996;94: 2341–50.
[33] Possick SE, Barry M. Evaluation and management of the cardiovascular patient embarking on air travel. Ann Intern Med 2004;141:148–54.
[34] Toff WD, Edhag OK, Camm AJ. Cardiac pacing and aviation. Eur Heart J 1992;13(Suppl H):162–75.
[35] WHO. Travel by air: health considerations. Available at: www.who.int/ith.html. Accessed May 17, 2004.
[36] Cummins RO, Chapman PJ, Chamberlain DA, et al. In-flight deaths during commercial air travel: how big is the problem? JAMA 1988;259:1983–8.
[37] Crewdson J. Code blue: survival in the sky [special report]. Chicago Tribune June 30, 1996.
[38] Herlitz J, Ekstrom L, Wennerblom B, et al. Effect of bystander initiated cardiopulmonary resuscitation on ventricular fibrillation and survival after witnessed cardiac arrest outside hospital. Br Heart J 1994;72:408–12.
[39] Greene HL. Sudden arrhythmic cardiac death: mechanisms, resuscitation and classification. The Seattle perspective. Am J Cardiol 1990;65:4B–12B.
[40] O'Rourke RA. Saving lives in the sky. Circulation 1997;96:2775–7.
[41] O'Rourke MF, Donaldson E, Geddes JS. An airline cardiac arrest program. Circulation 1997;96:2849–53.
[42] Dowdall N. Is there a doctor on the aircraft? Top 10 in-flight medical emergencies. BMJ 2000;321:1336–7.
[43] Kellermann AL, Hackman BB, Somes G. Predicting the outcome of unsuccessful prehospital advanced cardiac life support. JAMA 1993;270:1433–6.
[44] Bonnin MJ, Pepe PE, Kimball KT, et al. Distinct criteria for termination of resuscitation in the out-of-hospital setting. JAMA 1993;270:1457–62.
[45] Page RL, Joglar JA, Kowal RC, et al. Use of automated external defibrillators by a US airline. N Engl J Med 2000;343:1210–6.
[46] Federal Aviation Administration. Emergency medical equipment requirement; final rule. Federal Register 2001;66:19027–46.
[47] Aviation Medical Assistance Act. Pub L No. 105-107 (1998).
[48] Scurr JH, Machin SJ, Bailey-King S, et al. Frequency and prevention of symptomless deep-vein thrombosis in long-haul flights: a randomised trial. Lancet 2001;357:1485–9.
[49] Ferrari E, Chevallier T, Chapelier A, et al. Travel as a risk factor for venous thromboembolic disease: a case-control study. Chest 1999;115:440–4.
[50] Bagshaw M. Traveler's thrombosis: a review of deep vein thrombosis associated with travel. The Air Transport Medicine Committee, Aerospace Medical Association. Aviat Space Environ Med 2001;72:848–51.
[51] Cesarone MR, Belcaro G, Nicolaides AN, et al. Venous thrombosis from air travel: the LONFLIT3 study–prevention with aspirin vs low-molecular-weight heparin (LMWH) in high-risk subjects: a randomized trial. Angiology 2002;53:1–6.
[52] Sarvesvaran R. Sudden natural deaths associated with commercial air travel. Med Sci Law 1986;26:35–8.
[53] Pfausler B, Vollert H, Bosch S, et al. Cerebral venous thrombosis: a new diagnosis in travel medicine. J Travel Med 1996;3:165–7.
[54] Teenen RP, MacKay AJ. Peripheral arterial thrombosis related to commercial airline flights: another manifestation of the economy class syndrome. Br J Clin Pract 1992;46:165–6.
[55] Cruickshank JM, Gorlin R, Jennett B. Air travel and thrombotic episodes: the economy class syndrome. Lancet 1988;2:497–8.
[56] Hughes RJ, Hopkins RJ, Hill S, et al. Frequency of venous thromboembolism in low to moderate risk long distance air travelers: the New Zealand Air Traveller's Thrombosis (NZATT) study. Lancet 2003;362:2039–44.
[57] Sahiar F, Mohler SR. Economy class syndrome. Aviat Space Environ Med 1994;65(10 Pt 1): 957–60.

[58] Noddeland H, Winkel J. Effects of leg activity and ambient barometric pressure on foot swelling and lower-limb skin temperature during 8 h of sitting. Eur J Appl Physiol Occup Physiol 1988;57:409–14.
[59] Lapostolle F, Surget V, Borron SW, et al. Severe pulmonary embolism associated with air travel. N Engl J Med 2001;345:779–83.
[60] Landgraf H, Vanselow B, Schulte-Huermann D, et al. Economy class syndrome: rheology, fluid balance, and lower leg edema during a simulated 12-hour long distance flight. Aviat Space Environ Med 1994;65(10 Pt 1):930–5.
[61] Bettes TN, McKenas DK. Medical advice for commercial air travelers. Am Fam Physician 1999;60:801–8, 810.
[62] WHO. Consultation on air travel and thromboembolism. Geneva: World Health Organization; 2001.
[63] Rege KP, Bevan DH, Chitolie A, et al. Risk factors and thrombosis after airline flight. Thromb Haemost 1999;81:995–6.
[64] Scurr JH, Smith PD, Machin S. Deep vein thrombosis in airline passengers: the incidence of deep vein thrombosis and the efficacy of elastic compression stockings. Cardiovasc Surg 2001;9:159–61.
[65] Ansell JE. Air travel and venous thromboembolism-is the evidence in? N Engl J Med 2001; 345:828–9.
[66] Belcaro G, Geroulakos G, Nicolaides AN, et al. Venous thromboembolism from air travel: the LONFLIT study. Angiology 2001;52:369–74.
[67] Loke YK, Derry S. Air travel and venous thrombosis: how much help might aspirin be? Medscape Gen Med 2002;4:4.
[68] Pulmonary Embolism Prevention (PEP) Trial Collaborative Group. Prevention of pulmonary embolism and deep vein thrombosis with low dose aspirin: Pulmonary Embolism Prevention (PEP) trial. Lancet 2000;355:1295–302.
[69] Collaborative overview of randomised trials of antiplatelet therapy–III: Reduction in venous thrombosis and pulmonary embolism by antiplatelet prophylaxis among surgical and medical patients. Antiplatelet Trialists' Collaboration. BMJ 1994;308:235–46.
[70] Jones RT, Stark DF, Sussman JL, et al. Recovery of peanut allergens from ventilation filters of commercial airliners [abstract 961]. J Allergy Clin Immunol 1996;97:961.
[71] Hourihane JO, Kilburn SA, Dean P, et al. Clinical characteristics of peanut allergy. Clin Exp Allergy 1997;27:634–9.
[72] Sampson HA, Mendelson L, Rosen JP. Fatal and near-fatal anaphylactic reactions to food in children and adolescents. N Engl J Med 1992;327:380–4.
[73] Sicherer SH, Burks AW, Sampson HA. Clinical features of acute allergic reactions to peanut and tree nuts in children. Pediatrics 1998;102:e6.
[74] Yunginger JW, Sweeney KG, Sturner WQ, et al. Fatal food-induced anaphylaxis. JAMA 1988;260:1450–2.
[75] Leung DYM, Sampson HA, Yunginger JW, et al. Effect of anti-IgE therapy in patients with peanut allergy. N Engl J Med 2003;348:986–93.
[76] American Academy of Pediatrics. Restraint use on aircraft. Committee on Injury and Poison Prevention. Pediatrics 2001;108:1218–22.
[77] Newman TB, Johnston BD, Grossman DC. Effects and costs of requiring child-restraint systems for young children traveling on commercial airplanes. Arch Pediatr Adolesc Med 2003;157:969–74.
[78] Parkins KJ, Poets CF, O'Brien LM, et al. Effect of exposure to 15% oxygen on breathing patterns and oxygen saturation in infants: interventional study. BMJ 1998;316:887–91.
[79] Paris CA, Remler R, Daling JR. Risk factors for sudden infant death syndrome: changes associated with sleep position recommendations. J Pediatr 2001;139:771–7.
[80] Sherman CR. Motion sickness: review of causes and preventive strategies. J Travel Med 2002;9:251–6.

[81] Gahlinger PM. Cabin location and the likelihood of motion sickness in cruise ship passengers. J Travel Med 2000;7:120–4.
[82] Spinks A, Wasiak J, Villanueva E, et al. Scopolamine for preventing and treating motion sickness. Cochrane Database Syst Rev 2004;3:CD002851.
[83] Saurel-Cubizolles MJ. Daily commuting and preterm birth rate. Am J Obstet Gynecol 1992; 167:571–2.
[84] Easa D, Pelke S, Loo SW, et al. Unexpected preterm delivery in tourists: implications for long-distance travel during pregnancy. J Perinatol 1994;14:264–7.

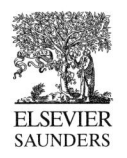

# On the Medical Edge: Preparation of Expatriates, Refugee and Disaster Relief Workers, and Peace Corps Volunteers

Michael V. Callahan, MD, MSPH, DTM&H[a],*,
Davidson H. Hamer, MD[b,c]

[a]*Biodefense and Mass-Casualty Care Center for Integration of Medicine and Innovative Technologies, Division of Infectious Diseases, Massachusetts General Hospital, 65 Landsdowne Street, Suite 200, Boston, MA 02139, USA*
[b]*Center for International Health and Development, Boston University School of Public Health, 5th floor, 85 East Concord Street, Boston, MA 02118, USA*
[c]*Gerald J. and Dorothy R. Friedman School of Nutrition Science and Policy, Tufts University, 150 Harrison Avenue, MA 02111, USA*

Travelers to remote destinations and other environs with austere medical services include adventure travelers; expedition teams; employees of petroleum, mining, and construction companies; scientists; members of the armed service and intelligence communities; and disaster or humanitarian relief workers. Each of these groups faces health threats that vary depending on itinerary; duration of travel (which may be long-term in the case of expatriates); environmental factors; and risk activity. Careful attention to pretravel evaluation and education of these special, high-risk groups can help reduce their likelihood of illness during extended international travel or overseas deployment.

To demonstrate the value of these risk-reduction activities, this article presents a series of international emergency and medical evacuation cases that establish the basis for a discussion of how careful pretravel evaluation and preparation of travelers on the edge of or beyond Western medical care can serve to reduce the risk of disease and death. The case scenarios are true stories; however, potentially identifying information has been removed to protect the confidentiality of the parties involved.

---

* Corresponding author.
  *E-mail address:* MVCallahan@partners.org (M.V. Callahan).

0891-5520/05/$ - see front matter © 2005 Elsevier Inc. All rights reserved.
doi:10.1016/j.idc.2004.10.010

*id.theclinics.com*

**Acute myocardial infarction in an expatriate in Ghana**

A 53-year-old electrical engineer with a history of hypertension, type 2 diabetes mellitus, hyperlipidemia, and coronary artery disease (status post percutaneous transluminal coronary angioplasty) was sent to work on a power plant construction site in western Ghana after a brief medical evaluation at his company in the United States before deployment. His medication regimen included metformin, glyburide, gemfibrozil, atenolol, diltiazem, enteric-coated aspirin, and isosorbide dinitrate.

Three months after deployment, he presented to the job site with complaints of dizziness, blurred vision, and intermittent substernal chest pain. On examination, he was found to have a blood pressure of 170/98 for which he was given nifedipine with improvement. He was encouraged to take his medications consistently (after the field medical officer learned that he had been poorly adherent with his complex medical regimen).

Two weeks later he presented to the infirmary with acute substernal chest pain. A 12-lead ECG suggested cardiac ischemia. The patient's symptoms responded to oxygen, sublingual nitroglycerine, beta-blockade, and morphine sulfate. The patient was monitored overnight and transported to the National Cardiothoracic Centre in Accra by means of the job site ambulance. His evaluation there revealed recrudescence of ECG changes suggestive of ischemia and laboratory tests notable for elevated creatine phosphokinase and troponin I. His symptoms resolved during treatment with intravenous nitroglycerin and heparin. Despite these symptoms, however, the patient decided to leave against medical advice. He was later found drinking in a local hotel bar and, after stabilization, was evacuated back to the United States with a medical escort on a commercial aircraft. On arrival at a teaching hospital in Los Angeles, the patient promptly underwent cardiac catheterization, which revealed diffuse left anterior descending disease for which the patient underwent stent placement with good results.

*Commentary*

This expatriate traveler was found to have ineffective pretravel screening, to be poorly adherent with his complex medical regimen while abroad, and at high risk of a significant event ultimately resulting in an acute myocardial infarction. What could have been done to prevent this event?

Long-term travelers such as this expatriate corporate employee require a more comprehensive approach to pretravel screening, immunization, personal security, and health education than the routine itinerary-specific services, immunizations, and health education offered to short-term travelers [1]. Whether it is an expatriate or an extreme traveler, the risks to health and personal security often warrant the addition of protective measures to ensure autonomy and self-reliance. Examples of such measures include prearranged in-country legal, personal security, and emergency medical services, and equipping disaster response teams, expeditions, and small at-risk groups with handheld satellite phones and advanced medical kits.

Aggressive pretravel health screening has been shown to reduce both the number of in-country medical emergencies and air medical evacuations among a group of 1770 expatriates living in rural regions of resource-poor countries [2]. Routine health screening, which is covered by health maintenance plans, is usually insufficient for the subset of travelers that spend significant time in remote environments. The physical and psychologic stresses associated with prolonged placement in austere international settings can unmask unrecognized medical or psychiatric conditions. Medical facilities in many developing countries often lack the capacity to manage complex illnesses associated with western lifestyles, such as exacerbations of chronic obstructive pulmonary disease, cardiac disease, neurologic emergencies, and complications of alcohol abuse imported by middle-aged corporate expatriates or missionaries. Medical emergencies resulting from these conditions tend to do worse as medical resources become less advanced (Fig. 1). Comprehensive pretravel medical examinations serve a critically important role in the preparation of long-term travelers to remote areas of the world by helping to identify previously unrecognized disease and allowing for treatment before travel.

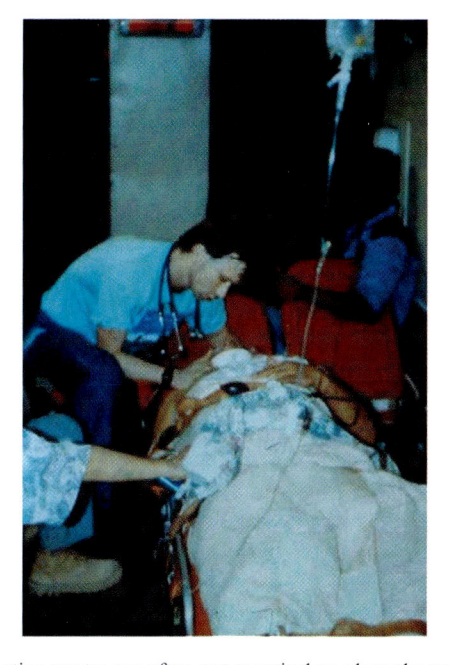

Fig. 1. Ground evacuation routes are often not practical or place the patient at increased risk for injury. Air evacuations are often necessary in medically underserved environments; these may require improvisation as in the case of this evacuation from western Ghana to the capitol city, Accra, by a Ghanaian air force plane. (Courtesy of D.H. Hamer, MD, Boston, MA.)

The components of a pretravel consultation for the expatriate include an in-depth review of the individual's medical history; a complete physical examination; and screening laboratory studies appropriate for the patients' age, health, individual risk, and the destination environment (Box 1) [3]. Careful evaluation of risk factors (eg, family history, history of alcohol or substance abuse, sexually transmitted diseases, and psychiatric illness) determine what additional tests are required. These comprehensive work-ups may identify previously unrecognized psychologic problems, inflammatory bowel conditions, malignancies, or deteriorating cardiac or pulmonary reserves. The importance of identifying drug and alcohol dependency,

---

**Box 1. Pretravel screening tests for expatriates**

*Highly recommended*
Detailed review of the individual's medical and vaccination history
Evaluation for risk factors for acute medical or psychiatric disease (eg, family history, history of alcohol or drug abuse, sexually transmitted diseases, and psychiatric illness)
Complete physical examination
Dental examination
Screening for previously unrecognized psychiatric illnesses (eg, depression)
Screening laboratory studies (eg, complete blood count, fasting glucose, lipid profile, serum creatinine, transaminases)
Chest radiograph
12-lead electrocardiogram

*Additional tests to be considered*
Urinalysis
Glucose tolerance test, hemoglobin $A_{1C}$
HIV testing
Hepatitis A, B, and C serologies
Pregnancy for women of child-bearing age
Pap smears
Purified protein derivative (tuberculin)
Maximum expiratory peak flow
Cardiac stress testing
Colonoscopy
Mammography

---

*Adapted from* Callahan MV, Hamer DH. Remote destinations. In: Keystone JS, Kozarsky PE, Freedman DO, et al, editors. Travel medicine. 1st edition. London: Elsevier Limited; 2004. p. 321–8; with permission.

depression, and other psychiatric illnesses cannot be overemphasized because these conditions are likely to be unmasked during stressful situations and unfamiliar surroundings.

Any abnormalities encountered during the comprehensive pretravel evaluation must be carefully addressed and treated before departure. In certain cases, new medical or psychiatric conditions identified during screening may preclude travel or long-term international placement because certain problems cannot be effectively managed in a health resource–poor setting. Careful consideration should be given to travelers with certain chronic diseases that are uncommon in many developing countries. Stent-stabilized coronary artery disease, cardiac dysrhythmias, brittle diabetes mellitus, and chronic obstructive pulmonary disease exacerbations are particularly difficult to manage in rural regions of developing countries. Physicians in many developing regions often lack both the experience and resources necessary for managing these routine but potentially life-threatening medical problems.

Corporate expatriates, missionaries, Peace Corps volunteers, and medical relief workers are likely to have prolonged contact with the local population, which places them at increased risk for exposure to and acquisition of tuberculosis [4]. As a consequence, these types of long-term or high-risk travelers should undergo tuberculin skin testing before and after travel.

Dental emergencies are another important cause of trip interruption and a leading reason why travelers access local medical care [5]. The primitive conditions of dental facilities may be worse than those of rural health care posts. In one series, dental problems accounted for up to 8% of medical emergencies implicated in business interruption at overseas job sites [2]. Pretravel dental examinations should be performed if there is any type of oral discomfort, a history of dental problems, and for anyone who has not been evaluated in the last year. The dentist who performs the examination should be informed that the traveler might not have access to dental care for an extended period. The dental consultant should be encouraged to perform the examination in a manner that identifies dental problems that might evolve during the planned period of overseas deployment.

In addition to the aforementioned detailed medical, dental, and psychologic evaluations, the long-term traveler should have their adult immunizations updated and should be given specialized vaccines, depending on destination, for the prevention of meningococcal meningitis, rabies, and Japanese encephalitis. Hepatitis B should be provided to all long-term travelers, especially medical relief personnel and expatriates with prolonged placement.

## Relief worker with malaria and schistosomiasis

A 28-year-old medical student took a year off from school to work for the International Rescue Committee in eastern Democratic Republic of the Congo. Before traveling to Africa, he was given yellow fever, hepatitis A, and typhoid fever vaccines and a polio booster. He had previously been fully immunized against hepatitis B. He was provided information on avoidance of vector-, food-, and water-borne disease including schistosomiasis. He was prescribed weekly mefloquine for malaria prophylaxis.

His work for the International Rescue Committee involved the implementation and management of a number of health care programs including in vivo efficacy studies of antimalarials for the war-torn lakes region of the Democratic Republic of the Congo. Several European expatriate relief workers told him that mefloquine was a bad drug that "might make him crazy." This information coupled with several months of insomnia, intense dreams, and mild dysphoria led him to discontinue taking the mefloquine. Several months later he developed falciparum malaria complicated by severe anemia. Fortunately he was able to receive effective treatment locally and did not require a blood transfusion.

The student also swam regularly in the local lakes, following the lead of the European expatriates who assured him that there was no schistosomiasis in that region. About 8 months into his stay, he developed painless terminal hematuria. After being told by his American-based advisor that he might have schistosomiasis, he had a urine ova and parasite examination done, which showed *Schistosoma haematobium* ova. To his dismay the student learned that praziquantel was not available in any of the villages in the region where he was working. Fortunately he was eventually able to obtain the medication from a medical vendor in distant regions, and was able to self-treat for urinary schistosomiasis.

*Commentary*

This student acquired both malaria and schistosomiasis during his trip. False and exaggerated information circulating among the development community contributed to his acquisition of both infections. In addition, side effects from his antimalarial also played a role in his decision to discontinue chemoprophylaxis.

Despite having received pretravel advice to avoid fresh water contact in the Democratic Republic of the Congo, this relief worker failed to heed the advice over the duration of his stay and developed urinary schistosomiasis. Although the risk of schistosomiasis is well known for certain popular destinations, such as Lake Malawi [6], the disease is widespread in sub-Saharan Africa and is more sparsely distributed in the Americas, Middle East, and Asia [7]. Unfortunately, as is often the case in expatriate communities, false information about the risks of local infectious disease risks is often spread among expatriate communities and long-term leisure travelers, increasing the risk of infections that might otherwise have been prevented. The only way to mitigate the damage that results from the spread of expatriate lore and incorrect information is to make sure all members of expatriate or relief worker communities receive consistent preventive advice before deployment. This should include education about which areas are endemic for schistosomiasis, potential acute and chronic problems that may arise if infected, and the importance of avoiding contact with fresh water [8].

This case also demonstrates the limited availability of certain medications in medically austere environments. This student spent several weeks searching for a source of praziquantel, despite the fact that schistosomiasis was a local problem. The limited or nonavailability of effective chemotherapeutic agents or postexposure prophylactic agents, such as antirabies immunoglobulin, underscores the importance of avoidance and pretravel immunization strategies for rare diseases that may be either fatal or associated with significant morbidity.

Malaria is a leading infectious cause of death and severe morbidity for expatriates. Despite the high risk of malaria in many locales, expatriates such as this relief worker often fail to incorporate antivector, personal protection behaviors, and counter-measures. Budget travelers often switch or discontinue their antimalarial prophylactic agent without consulting a specialist [1]. The risk of prophylaxis discontinuation has been shown to increase with longer overseas residence [9]. In addition, many long-term travelers become convinced that their self-selected ineffective medication is efficacious because they do not acquire malaria.

Although weekly mefloquine has been demonstrated to be highly efficacious for the prevention of malaria caused by *Plasmodium falciparum* in long-term travelers, such as Peace Corps volunteers [10], this drug has been associated with a high risk of moderate to severe events, especially neuropsychiatric events [11]. As a consequence, adherence is often suboptimal and discontinuation of this medication by long-term expatriates is common [1,9].

Alternatives to mefloquine for travel to areas with chloroquine-resistance include doxycycline, atovaquone-proguanil, and primaquine. Although doxycycline represents an inexpensive, well-tolerated, efficacious chemoprophylactic agent, long-term adherence among expatriates is often poor because of concerns about the chronic use of antibiotics and risk of photosensitivity reactions. Atovaquone-proguanil has been shown to be highly efficacious, safe, and well tolerated in medium-term travelers with use for up to 34 weeks [12,13]. The high cost of this fixed dose combination and its lack of availability in many developing countries, however, limit its use as a long-term agent for malaria prophylaxis.

Although not approved by the Food and Drug Administration for the prevention of malaria, primaquine has been shown to be efficacious for the prevention of *P falciparum* and *Plasmodium vivax* [14,15]. Primaquine has been used on a daily basis for the prevention of malaria for as long as 1 year with relatively few side effects and no evidence of worrisome hematologic or biochemical abnormalities [16]. Only individuals who have normal levels of glucose-6-phosphate dehydrogenase (G6PD) should use primaquine. In addition, there are limited efficacy data for sub-Saharan Africa.

Consequently, although primaquine seems to be a potentially useful option, more data are needed to establish both the drug's efficacy in Africa and tolerance for long-term travelers.

In circumstances where many expatriate and relief workers opt not to take long-term malaria chemoprophylaxis, several alternative approaches to the management of malaria may be considered. These include the use of malaria prophylaxis during and shortly after the rainy season, the time of most intense transmission; taking prophylactic agents only during travel to high-risk regions of an endemic country; and the intensive use of personal protection measures alone. This latter approach must be coupled with knowledge of a nearby health care provider who can perform and reliably interpret a blood smear and provide effective therapy. Although expatriates often use these different approaches, they have not been carefully studied or compared to see which are best. Because the risk of malaria varies, the best approach may depend on the country of residence. An alternative approach is to train and equip the traveler in the use of self-administered rapid diagnostic tests and stand-by therapy. This should not be done without training, however, in the use of both the test and therapy itself.

**Geologic engineer with fever, malaise, and a rapidly spreading lesion**

In May 2000, a 39-year-old employee of an American petroleum company traveled to a rural village located 9 hours north of Santiago, Chile. The village, located in a small agricultural region at an elevation of 1500 m, had no medical facilities. The expatriate traveler stayed in a screen-protected cottage. On the morning of the third day he noted a painless red-blue area approximately 3 cm in diameter on his right thigh. Within the hour, the patient reported onset of a dull ache to the thigh and mild malaise, which prompted a call to an American-based emergency travel health service. The consult physician suspected probable necrotic arachnidism (spider bite) from one of several medically significant South American spiders.

The patient was instructed to obtain a digital image of the lesion and quickly send it to the consulting physician using a nearby Internet café (Fig. 2). Initial treatment recommendations included use of cold dry compresses, mild elevation, careful demarcation of the effected area using an ink marker, and avoidance of physical activity or use of nonsteroidal anti-inflammatory or aspirin analgesia. He was instructed to collect urine in a clear container (in this case a soda bottle) to observe for color change (indicating hemolysis or myoglobinuria). He was also instructed to return to Santiago for immediate medical evaluation. The hosts were instructed to spray the cottage bedroom with insecticide after dark and to collect the dead insects and spiders for later identification. Over the next 8 hours the lesion spread significantly and in a gravitational manner, further increasing

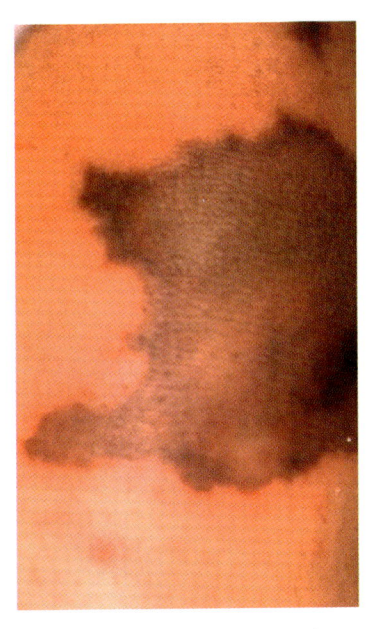

Fig. 2. *Loxosceles laeta* envenoming of the right thigh of an oil worker in Chile. Note dependent spread and red-blue color characteristic of early lesions (8–12 hours postbite). (Courtesy of M.V. Callahan, MD, Cambridge, MA.)

suspicion for necrotic loxoscelism. A private practitioner known to the American-based medical security service saw the patient on his return to Santiago. Follow-up therapy included screening for G6PD deficiency and treatment with dapsone (200 mg orally twice a day for 72 hours), clarithromycin (500 mg orally twice a day; see comments), naproxen sodium (220 mg orally three times a day), and culture of wound fluid. The lesion was covered with dry sterile dressing and the patient was advised to maintain continuous use of cold compresses for the next 3 days. At the end of the third day, the edges of the wound were well demarcated and the area had developed a large black eschar (Fig. 3). When the specimens collected from the patient's bedroom were inspected 3 days later, they were found to include seven adult Chilean violin spiders (*Loxosceles laeta*), the most venomous member of the *Loxosceles* genus.

*Commentary*

Pretravel health preparation should include education regarding local hazards and methods for reducing contact with toxic, venomous, and dangerous flora and fauna. Arguments that specific recommendations for protecting against bites and stings are impractical in the setting of the travel medicine clinic are difficult to reconcile with the experience of military personnel and special risk groups that are deployed to a variety of different

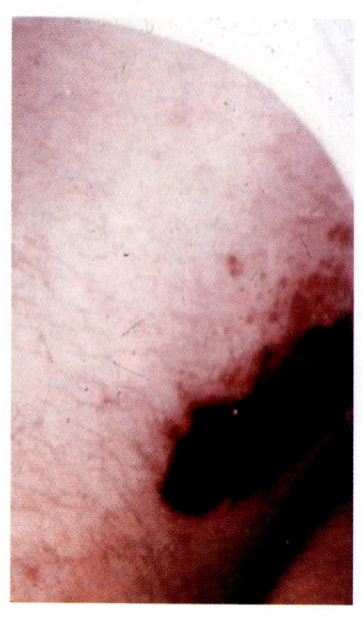

Fig. 3. The same *Loxosceles* bite at 3 days. Note the dark eschar overlying the ulcer. The patient was counseled by American physicians against using locally recommended ointments and elixirs. The ulcer healed by secondary intention and required a skin graft. (Courtesy of M.V. Callahan, MD, Cambridge, MA.)

overseas environments. These experiences have demonstrated that most undesirable encounters with toothy, venomous, and pugnacious fauna can be easily avoided using general recommendations. It should be emphasized that in far-forward and remote environments, the consequences of a bite or sting injury may be disastrous (Fig. 4).

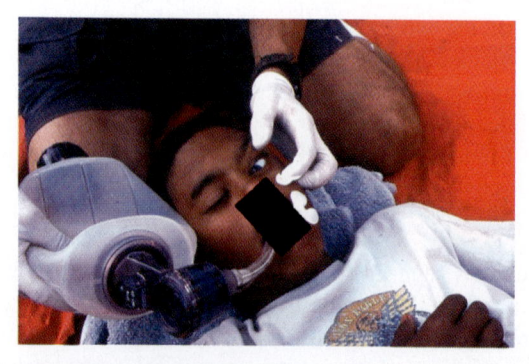

Fig. 4. Krait-bite (Bungarus) paralysis in a 9-year-old boy. Respiratory paralysis occurred within 4 hours of diplopia onset. Note bulbar palsy. Travelers should be educated about local hazards in destination environments. (Courtesy of M.V. Callahan, MD, Cambridge, MA.)

The case presented occurred in a territory known as the "gangrenous spot of Chile," a reference to the high number of necrotic skin injuries caused by *L laeta*. Precautions for avoiding contact with dangerous spiders also protect against other medically significant arthropods, such as *Scolopendra* centipedes; scorpions; and phlebotomine vectors of infectious disease (*Lutzomyia, Simulium*, and the mosquito species, *Culex, Aedes*, and *Anopheles*). Before travel to Chile, this patient received a brief pretravel medical evaluation but no specific recommendations for avoiding local environmental hazards. General advice should have included recommendations for the use of permethrin-treated sleep barriers or corralling sleeping areas within improvised barriers, such as insecticide-impregnated twine; spraying bedrooms with insecticide before sleeping; and checking bathtubs for trapped spiders and scorpions before bathing. Because a significant number of bites occur when travelers put on clothing where a spider, scorpion, or centipede has taken refuge, storing clothing in closed polyethylene bags (eg, line luggage with heavy duty garbage bags) and treating all clothing with permethrin should be considered.

This case demonstrates the importance of a differential diagnosis and the value of initial therapy of envenomation injuries The management of spider, scorpion, and arthropod envenoming requires familiarity with the range of important species, attention to a wide differential that includes etiologies both benign and catastrophic, and attentiveness to controversies in medical management. Medically significant spiders are virtually worldwide in distribution. Dangerous South American species include the Brazilian wandering spider (*Phoneutria nigriventer* and *Phoneutria fera*); six-eyed crab spiders (*Sicarius*); widow spiders (*Latrodectus*); and *Loxosceles* spiders. *Loxosceles* bites often occur at night and are initially painless, an observation that helps to implicate this species when the spider itself is not available. Systemic symptoms usually appear within 12 to 36 hours and include fever, chills, nausea, myalgias, and weakness. In severe cases, laboratory studies demonstrate hemoglobinuria, myoglobinuria, acute renal failure, and elevated creatine phosphokinase and liver enzymes. International travelers suspected of having symptomatic spider bites should seek timely medical evaluation from a qualified local health care practitioner. Local medical practices may not be effective and may interfere with tissue preservation measures or may exacerbate the damage resulting from the bite.

The medical management of *L laeta*, like all members of the genus, is both controversial and dissatisfying. Despite numerous studies, there is limited evidence that dapsone, colchicines, or even crude antivenin is of benefit after the first 12 to 24 hours. The authors have observed local complications resulting from corticosteroid treatment administered by well-intentioned medical practitioners. Both local and systemic therapy for confirmed *Loxosceles* bite is supportive. For cutaneous injuries, cold treatment is used to inhibit normothermic activity ($>20°C$) of spider venom sphingomyelinase. When available, laboratory studies include complete blood count with quantitative platelets, liver function tests, and urine chemistry with microscopic evaluation of sediment. Dapsone may be considered for select patients who are seen early providing they have neither allergies to sulfa medications or G6PD deficiency. Antivenins are likely to play a limited role in loxoscelism [17] because much of the pathology occurs early and is mediated by aberrant activation, chemotaxis, and degranulation of neutrophils. Patients with *Loxosceles* envenoming likely require pain control, antihistamines, and tetanus prophylaxis. Macrolide antibiotics may also play a role in decreasing local inflammation from necrotic loxoscelism. Following stabilization of the wound, a plastic surgeon may need to be consulted for functional or cosmetic skin grafting. In high-risk and remote medical settings and for cases where wound care is impractical or nonexistent, the normal conservative recommendation against prophylactic antibiotics is withheld.

## A climber with intermittent blindness and 24-hour history of acute psychosis

In October 1999, a member from a climbing expedition presented to the Himalayan Rescue Association (HRA) high-altitude medical clinic with mental status changes and a 24-hour history of transient bilateral blindness. The 31-year-old Swedish climber had descended with assistance from an altitude of 16,000 ft to the HRA clinic, which is located in the Khumbu village of Pheriche in Nepal at an altitude of 14,300 ft. The patient's teammates reported that, on the previous evening, the patient became delusional and combative. Descent was not possible so the team restrained the patient in his sleeping bag using duct tape and climbing webbing. No drug use or head trauma was reported and no treatment was given.

The following morning, the patient regained his normal mental status and remained lucid, suggesting he could climb down on his own. Before descent, however, the patient developed complete blindness and intermittent mild changes in sensorium. He was "short-roped" to a climbing partner and was able to down-climb for several hours to lower elevation where his vision improved. When the patient presented that evening to the HRA clinic, his work-up was suggestive of cortical blindness secondary to cryptic high-altitude cerebral edema (HACE). Subsequent physical examination was nonfocal and oxygen saturation was altitude-appropriate. Eye examination was negative. The patient was strongly advised to terminate his climbing ambitions and descend to moderate elevations.

Several days later, the patient represented to the HRA clinic in extremis characterized by a severely obtunded state, bradycardia, hypertension, and irregular respirations, consistent with Cushing's triad. The treating physician suspected HACE was responsible for increasing intracranial pressure. The patient was intubated and hyperventilated to induce hypocapnia (Fig. 5). Because he could not be transported to lower elevations, the patient was also

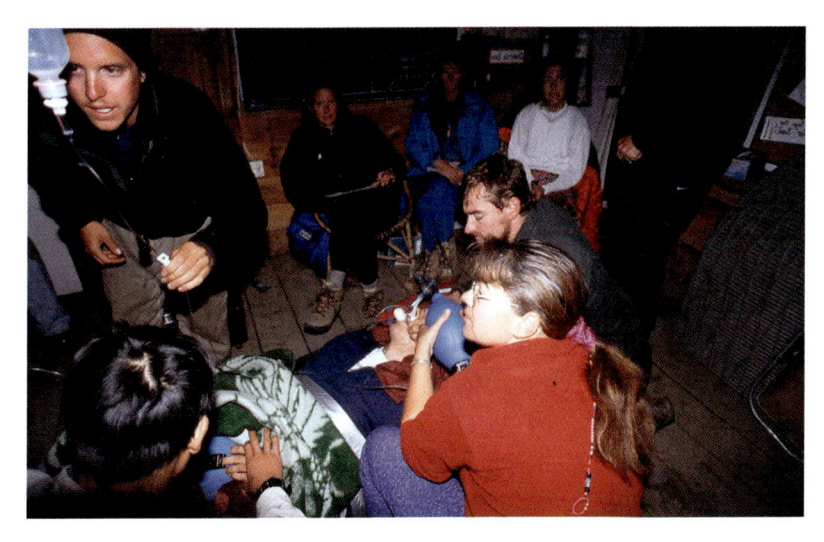

Fig. 5. High-altitude cerebral edema in a Swedish climber in Nepal. The patient was intubated and hyperventilated to reduce intercranial pressure. (Courtesy of E. Johnson, MD.)

treated with portable hyperbaric pressure using a PACBAG, a portable airtight chamber that increases internal atmospheric pressure using a foot pump (Fig. 6). After a difficult 24 hours, the patient was air evacuated by special high-altitude helicopter to Kathmandu (4000 ft elevation). Work-up

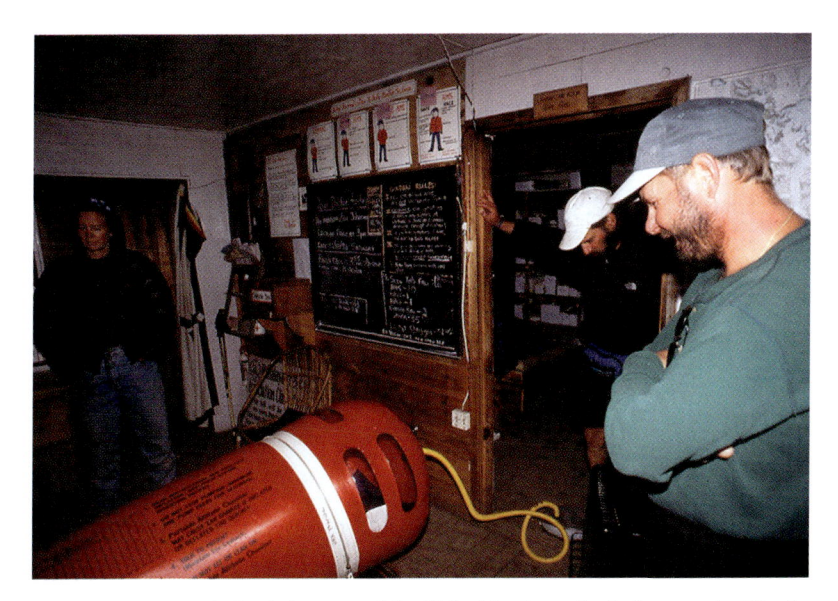

Fig. 6. New Zealand climber being treated for high altitude cerebral edema at the Himalayan Rescue Association clinic in Pheriche, Nepal. The patient is being treated with a portable hyperbaric chamber. Note foot pump. (Courtesy of E. Johnson, MD.)

included imaging CT of the head, neurology and metabolic work-up, and continued therapy for HACE. Despite a stormy course, the patient made a full recovery and communicates regularly with the HRA physician who saved his life.

*Commentary*

The differential diagnosis of mental status changes at altitude is broad (Box 2). The clinician must be familiar with unique stresses at high altitude (eg, hypobaric hypoxia, cold stress); the risk factors associated with extreme climbers (covert use of amphetamines, dexamethasone, erythropoietin, acetazolamide, and recreational drug use); and consider that tropical

---

**Box. 2. Differential diagnosis of acute mental status change in high-altitude trekkers**

Tumors of the central nervous system
Infectious diseases
Cerebral abscess (more common in local porters than western climbers)
Meningoencephalitis (vector-borne encephalitis acquired at low elevations)
Neurocysticercosis (common in South America; seizures precipitated by hypobaria)
Cerebral malaria with severe anemia (acquired at low elevations)
Systemic vascular
Subdural hematoma
Angioma
Intracranial aneurysm (unmasked by hypobaric and physiologic stress)
Vasculitis (eg, systemic lupus erythematosis)
Atheroma (causing thrombosis, embolism, and hemorrhage)
Hypertensive encephalopathy (elderly trekkers)
Medications
Alcohol, benzodiazepines, and opiates (and their withdraw)
Amphetamines (dextroamphetamine sulfate use is still common among extreme alpinists)
Cocaine (use was common among alpinists)
Other
Hypoglycemia
Asphyxia
Hypotension (multifactorial)
CO or $CO_2$ narcosis

diseases or pre-existing medical problems are likely to be unmasked by the high altitude. Altitude illness is the result of inefficient responses to low oxygen tension, which occurs following exposure to low barometric pressures at high elevations. The resultant hypobaric hypoxia results in a spectrum of altitude illnesses that include acute mountain sickness characterized by headache, anorexia, lethargy, and sleep disturbances, and the more severe syndromes of high-altitude pulmonary edema and HACE [18]. Most cases occur when alpine travelers outpace normal acclimatization during ascent (ideally 1000 ft/d above 6500 ft). Although mild acute mountain sickness may occur at 5000 ft, most problems are encountered following rapid ascent from sea level to elevations greater than 9000 ft.

Prevention of altitude illness requires careful education of alpine travelers. Many travelers intent on a high-altitude adventure are athletic and hard driving so convincing them that altitude illness effects the well conditioned and the sedentary without discrimination is a challenge. In the case previously mentioned, the patient presented with a somewhat unusual manifestation of HACE. Although mental status changes are often observed with HACE, acute psychosis is less common than impaired mental status, and high-altitude cortical blindness is almost a reportable event because of its rarity. The primary method for preventing any of the altitude illnesses, acute mountain sickness, high-altitude pulmonary edema, and HACE is slow ascent and monitoring for evidence of delayed acclimatization. The travel medicine clinician should also reinforce that the physical demands of high-altitude activities often lead to dehydration, overexertion, and cold-exposure injuries, all of which can further complicate self-evacuation or descent.

Acetazolamide (125–250 mg orally twice a day) may be considered in a subset of climbers who are on fixed itineraries and those who have previously experienced altitude illness under moderate conditions. This drug, which increases loss of renal bicarbonate resulting in a mild metabolic acidosis, which in turn allows for increased respiratory rate, is a sulfa-based diuretic. The travel medicine professional should make sure the traveler does not have sulfa allergies or underlying renal disease, and ensure that there are no interactions with other medications. Physicians experienced with the prevention and treatment of altitude illness often prescribe the long-acting calcium channel blockers, in particular nifedipine (10–30 mg orally every 4–6 h), to reduce pulmonary hypertension. The calcium channel blockers are also reasonable suggestions for those predisposed to Raynaud's syndrome, which commonly affects predisposed individuals who travel to cold mountain environments. For rapid ascent alpinists and others at risk of severe altitude illness, dexamethasone (3 mg orally every 8 h) may be prescribed as an emergency standby therapy for HACE. In addition to these medications, high-altitude climbers should consider carrying a number of other medical supplies in an emergency kit [3]. In each of the previously mentioned cases, these medical aids are no substitute for effective pretravel education by the travel medicine professional.

## Summary

Travelers to extreme environments and those who spend long periods of time in settings with limited health care resources need to have more detailed pretravel screening and education than the routine short-term traveler. Expatriates, relief workers, and Peace Corps volunteers need to receive careful pretravel medical, dental, and psychologic screening before deployment. Knowledge of special risks associated with the environment in which they will be stationed is necessary to provide effective education about ways to reduce or eliminate the risk of illness and death.

The travel medicine practitioner should also provide detailed, region-specific recommendations regarding emergency care while traveling in remote regions. Information on foreign medical facilities and practitioners should be gathered in advance and regularly updated. Many fee-for-service directories of overseas medical centers are often out of date and do not include emergency contact information. Once deployed, systems should be in place to ensure the traveler's continued personal safety and maintenance of good health. Although these systems are generally beyond the scope of work of travel medicine providers, it is important for the long-term traveler to be aware of the need to be prepared to deal with unexpected medical events. In the event of an overseas emergency, the travel medicine specialist may be called on to facilitate ground or air medical evacuation to the most appropriate medical center, to communicate treatment priorities and pertinent medical details to foreign medical providers, and to facilitate international air evacuation or repatriation if necessary. In each of these cases, the experience for the patient and the travel health professional is dramatically improved by adhering to risk-reduction measures, such as pretravel screening, pretravel health and safety education, and preparing for emergencies in advance.

## References

[1] Gamble KL, Lovell-Hawker DM. Expatriates. In: Keystone JS, Kozarsky PE, Freedman DO, et al, editors. Travel medicine. 1st edition. London: Elsevier Limited; 2004. p. 287–303.
[2] Callahan MV, Hamer DH, Bailey SA, et al. Medical emergencies in expatriates: analysis of 1770 cases [abstract FC10.04]. Presented at the Seventh Conference of the International Society of Travel Medicine. Innsbruck, Austria, May 18–22, 2001.
[3] Callahan MV, Hamer DH. Remote destinations. In: Keystone JS, Kozarsky PE, Freedman DO, et al, editors. Travel medicine. 1st edition. London: Elsevier Limited; 2004. p. 321–8.
[4] Cobelens FGJ, van Deutekom H, Draayer-Jansen IWE, et al. Risk of infection with *Mycobacterium tuberculosis* in travellers to areas of high tuberculosis endemicity. Lancet 2000;356:461–5.
[5] Kedjarune U, Leggat PA. Dental precautions for travelers. J Travel Med 1997;4:38–40.
[6] Cetron MS, Chitsulo L, Sullivan JJ, et al. Schistosomiasis in Lake Malawi. Lancet 1996;348: 1274–8.
[7] World Health Organization Expert Committee. The control of schistosomiasis. WHO technical report series No. 728. Geneva: World Health Organization; 1985. p. 17–8.

[8] Corachan M. Schistosomiasis and international travel. Clin Infect Dis 2002;35:446–50.
[9] Hamer DH, Ruffing R, Lyons S, et al. Use of antimalarial prophylaxis by expatriates at an industrial job site in West Africa [abstract C26]. Presented at the 6th Conference of the International Society of Travel Medicine. Montreal, Canada, 1999.
[10] Lobel HO, Miani M, Eng T, et al. Long-term malaria prophylaxis with weekly mefloquine. Lancet 1993;341:848–51.
[11] Schlagenhauf P, Tschopp A, Johnson R, et al. Tolerability of malaria chemoprophylaxis in non-immune travelers to sub-Saharan Africa: multicentre, randomized, double blind, four arm study. BMJ 2003;327:1–6.
[12] Petersen E. The safety of atovaquone/proguanil in long-term malaria prophylaxis of nonimmune adults. J Travel Med 2003;10(Suppl 1):S13–5.
[13] Overbosch D. Post-marketing surveillance: adverse events during long-term use of atovaquone/proguanil for travelers to malaria-endemic countries. J Travel Med 2003; 10(Suppl 1):S16–20.
[14] Shanks GD, Kain KC, Keystone JS. Malaria chemoprophylaxis in an age of drug resistance. II. Drugs that may be available in the future. Clin Infect Dis 2001;33:381–5.
[15] Baird JK, Fryauff DJ, Hoffman SL. Primaquine for prevention of malaria in travelers. Clin Infect Dis 2003;37:1659–67.
[16] Fryauff DJ, Baird KJ, Sumawinata I, et al. Randomised placebo-controlled trial of primaquine for prophylaxis of falciparum and vivax malaria. Lancet 1995;346:1190–3.
[17] Braz A, Mnozzo J, Abrev JC, et al. Development and evaluation of the neutralizing capacity of horse antivenom against the Brazilian spider *Loxosceles intermedia*. Toxicon 1999;37: 1323–8.
[18] Hackett PH, Roach RC. Current concepts: high altitude illness. N Engl J Med 2001;345: 107–14.

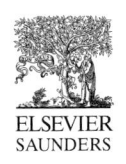

# Sexual Tourism: Implications for Travelers and the Destination Culture

Jeanne M. Marrazzo, MD, MPH[a,b],*

[a]Division of Allergy and Infectious Diseases, University of Washington, Harborview Medical Center, Mailbox 359931, 325 Ninth Avenue, Seattle, WA 98104, USA
[b]Seattle STD/HIV Prevention Training Center, Seattle, WA, USA

> But why, oh why, do the wrong people travel, When the right people stay at home? Noel Coward
> 
> —*Sail Away*

Although most people agree that travel frees the mind, fewer might spontaneously note that it also frees the body—not always in healthful ways. By providing ample opportunities for new social contacts, easing the psychologic restrictions of one's familiar sociocultural environ, and emphasizing social pleasures that often include alcohol or recreational drugs, travel can facilitate the transmission of sexually transmitted infections (STI). In the 1990s, the merciless advance of the HIV pandemic effectively emphasized the need for travelers to consider their sexual safety. Accruing evidence on recent trends in sexual risk behavior among groups traditionally at risk for HIV acquisition suggests, however, that the caution imparted by the fear of acquiring HIV is receding among some adults [1]. A new generation of travelers, especially those at risk for the most serious STI, are no exception. When key groups of travelers—particularly those who are young, sexually active, and inclined to ingest mind-altering substances—converge on travel destinations that are widely recognized for facilitating the pursuit of pleasure, sexual networks that efficiently propagate STI transmission often result. Further, disturbing trends in "old" diseases—including a resurgence of syphilis in most industrialized countries and steadily evolving antimicrobial resistance in *Neisseria gonorrhoeae* worldwide [2]—emphasize that travelers may encounter STI previously thought to be well-controlled.

---

* Division of Allergy and Infectious Diseases, University of Washington, Harborview Medical Center, Mailbox 359931, 325 Ninth Avenue, Seattle, WA 98104.
   *E-mail address:* jmm2@u.washington.edu

## Why travel and sexually transmitted infections? Evidence to support connections and interventions

The term "sexual tourism" has been defined as travel specifically arranged to facilitate the procurement of sex for the traveler, who may be referred to in this context as a "sex tourist" [3]. Traditionally, sexual tourism in this context has referred to tours arranged for men to gain access to commercial sex workers (CSW)—typically, young women or young men working in countries in Southeast Asia [4]—and is undeniably exploitative. For this article, the term "sexual tourism" is used more broadly to connote a general attitude of pleasure-seeking subscribed to by many travelers. Although travelers undertaking long and frequent journeys, including long-distance truckers, seafarers, and military troops, have long been recognized to be at risk for STI acquisition, the diversity of people who travel for recreational and business purposes now renders risk stratification by occupation or reason for travel imprecise. This mandates that travelers be evaluated before departure with individual, patient-centered risk assessment, and that they be counseled specific to pretravel infection with asymptomatic STI, especially genital herpes, *Chlamydia trachomatis, Treponema pallidum*, HIV, viral hepatitis, and human papillomavirus, and anticipated risk of STI exposure during travel.

Numerous studies have reported that travelers engage in sex as part of travel, and that this not uncommonly occurs without the use of barrier protection (condoms) [4–8]. Descriptions of the sexual tourism habits of accessible STI clinic populations indicate, not surprisingly, a relatively high degree of unprotected sex during travel: in Norway, for example, 41% of STI clinic clients reported having sex with a new partner abroad in the prior 5 years [9]. Perhaps more intriguingly, data from settings arguably more representative of the general population report similar findings. For example, of 996 women surveyed at a family planning clinic in Sweden, 28% described casual sex during travel. Those who reported casual sex while abroad were more often single, had higher educational attainment, and reported more frequent use of alcohol or marijuana [10]. Surveys of short-term vacation travelers from Sweden, Australia, and the United Kingdom indicate that up to 60% of travelers of both sexes may engage in casual sex (defined as sex with a previously unknown partner) during a trip [8,10–13]. In general, female travelers were more likely to select partners of their own nationality, while male travelers were more likely to select partners from host country nationals and CSW. Consistent factors associated with casual sex while abroad are young age, travel without a spouse or partner, and longer duration of stay [3]. In a large telephone survey in the United Kingdom of 400 young people who had traveled abroad without a partner in the previous 2 years, travelers who reported a new sex partner while abroad were also likely to report higher numbers of partners while at home, and 25% did not use condoms during sex with a new partner encountered during travel [7]. Not surprisingly, engaging in unprotected sex while traveling is often linked to other health-adverse risk behaviors, including smoking [8].

Although several studies have examined the likelihood of sex among people living or employed in foreign or developing countries for long periods, surprisingly little of this work has been reported in the last 5 years. One survey assessed 2289 Dutch marines and naval personnel during a 6-month deployment in Cambodia. Despite an education campaign to increase awareness of STI risk and provision of freely available condoms, 45% reported sexual contact with a local CSW, although consistent condom use was reported by 89% [14]. Among Dutch workers who had been in sub-Saharan Africa for an average of 3.7 years; 31% of men and 13% of women reported engaging in sex with African nationals. Factors associated with this report were not traveling with a life partner, history of previous STI, and length of stay in Africa [15]. In a recent review of the relationship between travel and STI among residents of the United Kingdom, Rogstad [16] notes that the proportion of STI acquired abroad may actually be increasing: data from 2002 indicated that up to 21% of infectious syphilis cases may have been acquired outside of the United Kingdom.

New evidence supporting the role of travel in pushing the spread of STI across borders has focused on researchers' ability to define genetic variants of key sexually transmitted pathogens, particularly HIV-1 [17]. Spread of initial local epidemics is usually characterized by a single dominant HIV-1 group M lineage, as defined by subtypes and circulating recombinant forms. Most subtypes and circulating recombinant forms are found in central Africa, with the diversity of subtypes in other continents initially quite limited. Over time, however, HIV-1 molecular diversity has progressed in non-African continents, with numerous case reports pinpointing introduction of new subtypes and circulating recombinant forms by specific travelers returning home after acquiring the infection abroad. Of related practical concern to the traveler who returns home shortly after acquiring HIV-1 is the high efficiency with which a newly infected person can infect a susceptible sex partner [18]. HIV-1 viral load in serum and genital secretions is exceedingly high during and immediately after primary infection. These persons are highly infectious, and pose a very high level of infectious risk to unprotected, uninfected sex partners. This phenomenon has been most extensively studied among men. A probabilistic model estimated the effect of changes in viral dynamics in semen on the probability of transmission per coital act among men with acute versus long-standing HIV infection [17]. The results suggested that the viral dynamics in semen in acute infection alone could increase the probability of heterosexual transmission by 8- to 10-fold between peak (day 20 after infection, based on the model) and virologic set points (day 54 and later after infection). Depending on coital frequency, men with average semen HIV-1 loads and without STI might infect 7% to 24% of susceptible female sex partners during the first 2 months of infection, a rate that is further increased if either partner had an STI. This observation emphasizes the need for persons at risk not only to minimize potential exposure to the virus, but also for them and their health care providers to recognize potential primary HIV-1 infection syndrome and—equally important—the presence of other STI that might have been acquired simultaneously with HIV-1 [19]. Migration within continents also contributes to the spread of HIV-1 variants, as painfully demonstrated by the waves of infection that followed migration of rural dwellers to cities, and of miners' return to their home villages, especially in South Africa, Botswana, and Zimbabwe [20].

Although condoms significantly reduce the risk of STI transmission and acquisition, particularly gonorrhea, HIV, and genital herpes, condom use is determined by a complex set of factors. These include availability of condoms; familiarity and comfort with using them; sex partners' (especially men's) acceptance of their use; and, very importantly, an individual's perception of a given partner's risk of being infected [21]. Many people believe that they can reduce their risk of exposure to STI simply by confirming the absence of visual signs of genital pathology ("but he looked clean!"). Because most STI transmission (notably that of genital herpes, HIV, human papillomavirus, and *C trachomatis*) occurs from asymptomatic individuals, correcting this erroneous belief is a key component of pretravel counseling. A corollary is that most people infected with these STI are not aware of their chronic infection; 21.9% of American adults over 12 years of age are seropositive for antibodies to herpes simplex virus type-2 (HSV-2), the virus that causes most genital herpes, but only 1 in 10 are aware of their infection [22]. Similarly, most sexually active adults have evidence of prior infection with at least one type of genital human papillomavirus [23].

Current trends in sexual risk behavior and STI epidemiology are well worth noting. Many industrialized countries are presently experiencing a rise in the proportion of HIV-1 transmission occurring within the heterosexual population, particularly in inner cities among intravenous drug users, CSW, and immigrants from high-risk areas. Men engaging in unprotected sex with other men continue to be at risk, and many urban areas in the United States have experienced an alarming reversal of the trend toward protected sex among men engaging in unprotected sex with other men. Rates of early syphilis (primary, secondary, and early latent) are presently higher than at any time in the last two decades in many large American cities, notably San Francisco, Los Angeles, Seattle, and New York City [1]. Even more worrisome, about a third of the men engaging in unprotected sex with other men with early syphilis in these areas are already HIV-infected, with a median age in the early 30s. Many report having used the internet to locate new, frequently anonymous sex partners, which creates profound challenges for management of exposed sex partners and disease control efforts [24]. These disturbing developments highlight the need for pretravel risk assessment and STI-HIV screening, especially for men engaging in unprotected sex with other men [25].

Finally, travelers need to know that a person's risk of transmitting or acquiring HIV is greatly enhanced in the presence of some STI, especially genital ulcer disease and inflammatory conditions like urethritis and mucopurulent cervicitis. In fact, some investigators have proposed that genital herpes may be a principal driving force in the accelerated pace of the HIV epidemic in sub-Saharan Africa, and interventions to test this hypothesis are underway [26].

The remainder of this article presents a systematic approach, summarized in Box 1, for considering a traveler's sexual health before, during, and after the journey.

## Before travel: sexually transmitted infections and HIV risk assessment, patient-centered counseling, and immunization

### Take a sexual history

Even in the era of the global AIDS pandemic, many physicians, particularly subspecialists, do not routinely take a sexual history from their patients. Until relatively recently, medical school and residency curriculum have not emphasized this assessment. Concomitantly, few health professionals have the opportunity to acquire the skills needed to effect STI-related risk-reduction counseling, despite the fact that at least one large, randomized trial demonstrated that a single brief patient-centered counseling session reduced the risk of bacterial STI acquisition over the course of several months [27]. Travelers should undergo a thorough sexual history as part of their pretravel evaluation. This includes current sexual behaviors; sexual relationships; use of barrier protection and contraception; past history of STI; and results of most recent screening for STI, including viral hepatitis, HIV, and if appropriate, syphilis and HSV serologies. A few considered questions regarding the role of excessive alcohol or illicit drugs in the patient's approach to sex (particularly unprotected sex outside a monogamous relationship) may yield important information to address [28].

### Perform appropriate screening tests

There are three principal reasons to screen patients for STI before they travel. First, it is an opportunity to provide primary care, if appropriate, as best illustrated by screening of women for *C trachomatis* [29]. Second, detection of latent STI, especially syphilis and HIV, can direct not only timely therapy, but also informative counseling sessions targeting risk-reduction messages for the patient's anticipated sexual behavior during travel. Third, persons with no immunity to hepatitis A or B should be vaccinated, as appropriate [30].

> **Box 1. Approach to the traveler's sexual health**
>
> *Before travel: STI-HIV risk assessment, patient-centered counseling, and immunization*
> - Discuss current risk status and intentions during travel (sexual behavior, chronic viral STI, drug and alcohol use patterns)
> - Consider appropriate screening for STI (HIV, syphilis, HSV−2[a], hepatitis B, *C trachomatis*)
> - Immunize for viral hepatitis (A and B) if appropriate[b]
> - Counsel on risk-reduction behavior: partner choice (especially avoidance of commercial or exploitative sex), condoms, avoidance of nonoxynol-9 preparations, excessive alcohol or drug use
> - Emphasize patient recognition of common STI syndromes (especially primary HIV, hepatitis, urethritis, genital herpes, and proctitis)
> - Educate about emergency contraception options, HIV postexposure prophylaxis as appropriate
> - Provide condoms
> - For HIV-infected travelers, emphasize highly active antiretroviral therapy adherence and relation to reduced (but not eliminated) HIV-STI transmission
>
> *Posttravel: risk assessment and screening*
> - Know key features of STI-HIV epidemiology of traveler's destination[c]
> - Revisit the sexual history
> - Targeted examination, as indicated
> - Screening tests, if indicated, for common STI[d]
>
> ---
> [a] Serologic assays for type-specific antibody to HSV glycoprotein G are available.
> [b] See www.cdc.gov/hepatitis for specific recommendations on indications for immunization against hepatitis A and B.
> [c] Key summaries available at www.who.org.
> [d] May include HIV, syphilis, and hepatitis A and B serologies; assays for *C trachomatis* and *N gonorrhoeae* from cervix, urethra, rectum, or pharynx (depending on sites exposed).

Performance of pretravel screening diagnostic tests should be dictated by the results of the sexual history. If the pretravel assessment is occurring in the setting of primary care, it provides an excellent opportunity to assess whether young women ($\leq$25 years) or older women with risk factors have been tested for *C trachomatis* within the prior year, as recommended by the

US Preventive Services Task Force and as summarized in Box 2 [29]. Men who report sex with other men should be screened for HIV and syphilis, depending on the timing of most recent testing relative to ongoing risk behavior, and for hepatitis A and B, depending on previous immunization [25]. Newer serologic tests that detect antibody to HSV-specific glycoprotein G can reliably distinguish between prior infection with HSV-1 and -2 [31]. Although the Centers for Disease Control and Prevention (CDC) do not recommend this assay for routine screening of the general population, approximately 22% of sexually active American adults are infected with genital HSV-2, and 90% of them are unaware of their infection; further, most HSV-2 genital transmission occurs from asymptomatic partners, by subclinical shedding of the virus [22]. The CDC details groups in whom HSV-2 serologic screening should be considered (Box 3) [25], but the considerable burden of this common infection supports a discussion of the option of screening for all patients if the test is available and affordable. Further, valacyclovir has recently been shown to reduce the risk of HSV-2 genital transmission from asymptomatic infected persons to susceptible partners; patients with HSV-2 may benefit from counseling about this option [32].

---

**Box 2. Recommendations for annual screening of women for genital infection with *Chlamydia trachomatis***

All asymptomatic sexually active women ≤25 years old
Women of any age at risk for infection[a], defined as:
  Inconsistent condom use
  New sex partner in preceding 3 months
  Multiple sex partners in preceding 3 months
  Presence of mucopurulent cervicitis[b]

---

[a] Other patient characteristics acknowledged by the US Preventive Services Task Force to be associated with a higher prevalence of infection include single marital status, new male sex partner or greater than or equal to two sex partners during the preceding year, African-American race, prior history of STI, and presence of cervical ectopy. The latter four risk factors are endorsed by the American College of Preventive Medicine as formal indicators for routine screening [56]. Although individual risk depends on the number of risk markers and local chlamydia prevalence, most experts recommend using the risks listed in Box 2 as minimum criteria to consider screening in women >25 years.

[b] Although the presence of mucopurulent cervicitis (defined by the presence of mucopurulent discharge, easily induced endocervical bleeding, or edematous cervical ectopy) technically qualifies as an indication for diagnostic testing rather than screening, it is generally included in *C trachomatis* screening guidelines to emphasize the need for testing for this organism in this context.

> **Box 3. Indications for use of type-specific HSV serologic screening of adults**
>
> *Definite indications*
> - Diagnosis of genital ulcers or lesions, especially when lesions cannot be sampled or are unlikely to yield virus
> - Assessment and counseling of sex partners of persons with genital herpes
> - Screen persons at risk for HIV transmission (HIV+)
>
> *Other uses*
> - Pregnant women and partners
> - Patient request
> - Not clear whether all sexually active persons should be screened (cost versus benefit)

*Counsel patients on risk-reduction behavior*

For many physicians, STI-related risk reduction is limited to the simple provision of male condoms, usually to male patients who may or may not know how to use them correctly [21,33]. In fact, physicians can help patients identify other methods to reduce risk. Although the discussion should be individualized depending on the patient's sexual history, key elements should consistently be addressed. Patients should be encouraged to exercise cautious judgment in choosing a sex partner; in some situations, not having sex may be the safest course. At the most basic level, they should be advised to avoid commercial sex, or any sex trade that seems to be exploitative. Many studies have shown that HIV-1 infection is common among CSW: 50% to 85% of urban CSW in Africa and Thailand are HIV-infected, and prevalence of other STI may be high despite reports of consistent condom use [34]. Promotion of child prostitution has been only one horrific consequence of such findings; in many countries, the erroneous belief that sex with very young persons is safer than with older CSW is widespread. Finally, travelers should be reminded of the generally adverse effect that alcohol and other mind-altering drugs have on one's judgment. Depending on the context, quantity of alcohol ingestion is generally inversely associated with condom use, and travelers are no exception [35].

*Provide key educational messages for all patients*

Regardless of stated risk and intentions for sex during future travel, all patients benefit from education related to STI and sexual health. The role of excessive alcohol and of illicit drug use in facilitating incautious sex partner selection should be addressed. Providing travelers with basic information on the recognition of common STI syndromes, especially primary HIV, hepatitis, urethritis, genital herpes, and proctitis, can help direct timely care-seeking and potentially critical intervention. Women should be educated or reminded about emergency contraception options, and provided appropriate medication if indicated. All travelers who report current or anticipated unprotected sexual behavior, including those who might be at risk for sexual assault in countries with relatively high HIV seroprevalence, should be made aware that HIV postexposure prophylaxis exists, although its availability in such countries is likely to be limited [36].

*Provide condoms*

Although condom use is strongly recommended for every act of sexual intercourse when the STI status of a partner is unknown, protection afforded against STI is incomplete, even under the best of circumstances. In several studies of couples who were discordant for the presence of HIV-1 infection, use of condoms significantly reduced the risk of HIV-1 transmission to the uninfected partner (up to a 10-fold reduction) [37,38]. A recent Cochrane review of the available evidence concluded that consistent use of condoms (defined as using a condom for all acts of penetrative vaginal intercourse) results in an 80% reduction in HIV incidence [39].

The normal breakage rate during vaginal intercourse with properly applied high-quality latex condoms produced in the United States is about 2%; complete slippage occurs about 1% of the time [40]. Similar rates probably apply for anal intercourse, although failure rates as high as 5% have been reported. Condoms manufactured abroad may have a higher breakage rate. Improper storage conditions (heat, moisture) or oil-based lubricants (mineral oil, petroleum jelly, massage oils, body lotions, shortening, cooking oil) can weaken latex condoms and contribute to a higher breakage rate. Use beyond the expiration date also increases the likelihood of breakage.

Latex condoms offer the most reliable barrier against STI. For persons with latex allergy (approximately 1%–3% of the American population), polyurethane (plastic) condoms offer an alternative; these are thinner than latex but as strong, and unlike latex are not weakened by use with oil-based lubricants. They are, however, more costly and may require more lubrication than latex condoms. Natural membrane condoms (often called "natural" condoms or, incorrectly, "lambskin" condoms) are usually made from lamb cecum, and can have pores up to 1500 nm in diameter. Although this prevents passage of sperm, this is more than 10 times the diameter of HIV and more than 25 times that of the hepatitis B virus. Because laboratory studies support that viral STI transmission can occur with natural membrane condoms, it is generally recommended that they not be used.

Because the decision to use a male condom is ultimately made by the male partner, and because male-to-female transmission of HIV is markedly more efficient than female-to-male, development and testing of female-controlled methods for STI protection are a high priority. This is especially critical in nonindustrialized countries where women's social and political status is particularly limited, and where HIV seroprevalence among young women may approach 10 times that of age-matched men. The first female condom (Reality) became available in the mid-1990s. Its high cost relative to the male condom can present a considerable deterrent; for this reason, while recognizing that the approach is not optimal, several organizations have issued protocols for its repeated use [41]. The female condom is slightly less effective for preventing pregnancy compared with male condoms; clinical studies in small numbers of women indicate protection against trichomoniasis reinfection, implying but not yet proving similar protection against other STI. New prototypes of the female condom are under development, and it is hoped they will provide a more acceptable and affordable means of female-controlled protection from STI.

*Advise against nonoxynol-9*

Vaginal use of the spermicide surfactant nonoxynol-9 has proved to be a surprisingly ineffective intervention to reduce STI acquisition. In fact, in several studies, use of high concentrations of nonoxynol-9 increased the risk of cervical and vaginal ulceration, which is thought to have modulated the increased risk of HIV acquisition noted in nonoxynol-9 users in at least one study [42]. Subsequently, large, randomized controlled studies confirmed a lack of benefit for women who use nonoxynol-9 [43,44]. Although adverse effects of nonoxynol-9 can likely be mitigated by reduced frequency and use of low-concentration preparations, most experts recommend against its use given the small but consistent increase in HIV acquisition risk and its failure to prevent acquisition of non-HIV STI, and the CDC has recommended that condoms packaged with nonoxynol-9 be discarded. Other potentially promising microbicides are well into advanced clinical trials, and may prove to offer much-needed additional options for women seeking to protect themselves from STI [45]; however, none can be recommended at present.

*Address the importance of medication adherence in the HIV-infected traveler*

Highly active antiretroviral therapy reduces, but does not reliably eliminate, the quantity of HIV in endocervical and urethral secretions, and in semen [46]. Although appropriate highly active antiretroviral therapy regimens do not uniformly protect a partner susceptible to HIV, they very likely reduce the risk of HIV transmission. Combined with consistent and correct use of condoms, highly active antiretroviral therapy is probably a potent method of reducing (but not eliminating) the sexual transmission of HIV.

## During travel: what the patient might encounter

Unprotected sex between asymptomatic fellow travelers who originate from industrialized countries is most likely to result in infections prevalent in those home countries: genital herpes; human papillomavirus; chlamydial disease; and depending on the circumstances (sexual behavior and host country or regional prevalence), gonorrhea, HIV-1, and syphilis. Unprotected sex with host-country nationals in developing countries also offers potential exposure to diseases uncommon in Western industrialized countries, including chancroid (caused by *Haemophilus ducreyi*), lymphogranuloma venereum, and granuloma inguinale, and a much higher risk of exposure to HIV-1 in sub-Saharan Africa, India, China, the Caribbean, and some areas of Eastern Europe [47]. In addition to HIV-1, sexual transmission of HIV-2 and other viruses (primarily hepatitis B and human T-lymphotropic virus 1) are a greater risk in parts of the developing world.

Genital herpes, syphilis, chancroid, lymphogranuloma venereum, and granuloma inguinale are all causes of genital ulcer disease. All but genital herpes are bacterial genital ulcer disease and are curable with appropriate antibiotic treatment; moreover, antiviral therapy can lessen the clinical symptoms and viral shedding associated with genital herpes. Travelers should be advised of the synergistic relationship between the presence of several STI and the risk of acquiring and transmitting HIV-1. Although the presence of genital ulcers is a well-documented risk for increased acquisition of HIV-1, other factors have been increasingly recognized. These include nonulcerative, inflammatory STI (notably, trichomoniasis and gonorrhea); cervical ectopy; certain sexual practices (sex during menses, use of vaginal drying agents); and frequent vaginal use of nonoxynol-9. Incident, asymptomatic genital infection with HSV-2 probably confers significantly increased risk [48]. Lack of circumcision among men may play a major role in enhancing men's likelihood of acquiring HIV [49,50], an observation that has spurred the implementation of a randomized controlled trial of this procedure in Kenya.

Acquisition of hepatitis B infection among unvaccinated travelers is not rare, with rates estimated at 60 per100,000 journeys overall, 7.6 to 11.5 per 100 person-years among French volunteers, and 10.6 per 100 person-years among American missionaries [51]. This may occur either through sex (with particular efficiency between men engaging in unprotected sex with other men), or through sharing of unclean needles during intravenous drug use. The latter mechanism also transmits hepatitis C virus, which is inefficiently transmitted sexually to such an extent that routine screening is not recommended in the context of STI-related assessment. Hepatitis A, however,

Table 1
Recommendations for testing for major STI in returned travelers

| Etiologic agent | Commonly associated syndromes | Incubation period[a] | Recommended tests | Indications for screening | Other comments |
|---|---|---|---|---|---|
| *Chlamydia trachomatis* | Mucopurulent cervicitis, urethritis, acute dysuria syndrome, PID, proctitis, conjunctivitis | 10–14 d; best documented for acute dysuria syndrome in women | NAAT[b] | Unprotected sex during travel<br>No testing in previous year among women at risk [29]<br>Compatible clinical syndrome | Sensitivity of NAAT on first-catch urine in women approaches that for endocervical sampling<br>70%–90% of infection in women and 40%–60% in men show no signs |
| *Neisseria gonorrhoeae* | Mucopurulent cervicitis, urethritis, PID, proctitis | 3–4 d for symptomatic urethritis in men | Culture, NAAT | Unprotected sex during travel<br>Compatible clinical syndrome | 50% of infections in women and 25% in men show no signs |
| Herpes simplex virus | GUD, cervicitis | 10–14 d | Culture, antigen detection, serology | Compatible clinical syndrome | Most genital herpes acquired from asymptomatic viral shedding by infected partner |
| Hepatitis A and B | Hepatitis | 30 d (hepatitis A)<br>40–110 d (hepatitis B) | Serology | Unprotected sex during travel<br>Compatible clinical syndrome<br>For hepatitis B, IDU during travel | Hepatitis A efficiently transmitted by oral-anal sex |

| | | | | |
|---|---|---|---|---|
| Treponema pallidum (syphilis) | GUD, rash, cranial neuropathy, aseptic meningitis | 1–3 wk for primary infection, 3 wk to 3 mo for secondary infection | Serology; darkfield examination of ulcer exudate | Compatible clinical syndrome Unprotected sex during travel | Syphilis is enjoying a resurgence in industrialized countries, especially among HIV-infected MSM |
| Human papillomavirus | Genital warts, cervical neoplasia | NA | Visual examination; Pap smear | Compatible clinical syndrome | Most sexually active adults are exposed to multiple genital HPV types early in sexual experience; high likelihood of exposure pretravel |
| Lymphogranuloma venereum | Genital ulcers | 3–12 d | Chlamydia serology | Compatible clinical syndrome after travel to affected locale | Consider if exposure occurred in endemic area[c] |
| Granuloma inguinale | Genital ulcers | ~17 d (variable) | | Compatible clinical syndrome after travel to affected locale | Consider if exposure occurred in endemic area[c] |
| Chancroid (Haemophilus ducreyi) | Genital ulcers | 4–7 d | Culture on specific media | Compatible clinical syndrome after travel to affected locale | Consider if exposure occurred in endemic area[c] |

*Abbreviations:* GUD, genital ulcer disease; HPV, human papillomavirus; IDU, intravenous drug use; MSM, men who have sex with men; NA, not available; NAAT, nucleic acid amplified test; PID, pelvic inflammatory disease.

[a] Where relevant. Acquisition of most STI occurs from asymptomatic contacts, and initial infection usually causes no evident signs or symptoms.
[b] NAATs include polymerase chain reaction, transcription mediated amplification, and strand displacement assay.
[c] Incidence of LGV, granuloma inguinale, and chancroid is highly localized. See www.cdc.gov/nchstp/dstd/dstdp.html for data on American trends, and www.who.int/health_topics/sexually_transmitted_infections/en/ for links to information on other countries.

is transmitted through any fecal-oral mechanism, including oral-anal sex; this behavior should be specifically assessed as part of the sexual history, and serology obtained if reported.

Treatment provided to travelers who seek care for STI-related syndromes while abroad is dependent on both the individual traveler's resources and those of the host country. For example, public sector clinics in most nonindustrialized countries ascribe to STI syndromic management guidelines disseminated by the World Health Organization [52]. More extensive fee-for-service capabilities in the private sector are available in most countries, but access is variable, depending in part on the traveler's financial resources.

## After travel: what questions, and what tests?

The traveler who seeks care after travel often has specific concerns in mind. Those who count potential STI exposure among them may be reluctant to acknowledge this as the principal reason for a visit, especially if STI risk reduction counseling was a prominent part of the pretravel interaction. Providers can facilitate patients' admission of potential STI exposure by routinely repeating a brief sexual history in all returning travelers; specifically, ask if the patient had sex during travel, if protection was used, if any encounters created concern. Genitourinary symptoms should be incorporated into the review of systems. Providers can also prepare themselves for recognizing STI-related syndromes or inapparent infections by maintaining awareness of key STI epidemiology of major host countries. Certainly, unprotected sex in sub-Saharan Africa is an obvious red flag for exposure to HIV, but HIV seroprevalence in young, sexually active adults in other countries, notably India and China, is on the increase. Similarly, unprotected sex in Russia and the former states of the Soviet Union might raise concern for exposure to syphilis [53].

No data are available to support the cost-effectiveness of STI screening for returning travelers [54]. Screening women for common STI like *C trachomatis* is cost-effective above a prevalence of 4% to 6%, however, a level likely to be present in many young women seeking care for travel-related concerns in most areas of the United States, which have not had long-standing screening programs in place [55]. For other STI, the cost of the screening tests is either absolutely inconsequential (syphilis) or relatively low relative to the benefit of early detection (HIV, gonorrhea); providers should have a very low threshold for performing them in the returned traveler. The benefit of early detection includes not only potential therapeutic interventions for the traveler, but the interruption of future sexual transmission to partners exposed after the traveler's return. A targeted physical examination may also be indicated if the traveler reports abnormal vaginal discharge, pelvic discomfort, urethral or rectal discharge, dysuria, scrotal pain, fever, sore throat, or rash. Table 1 outlines a suggested approach for testing of specific STI in the returned traveler.

Because of the typical time frame involved, targeted HIV postexposure prophylaxis is typically not considered during posttravel follow-up, but providers should be aware of guidelines and recommendations related to this issue. HIV postexposure prophylaxis should be administered ideally within 36 hours of suspected exposure, and should be continued for 4 weeks, if tolerated. Current guidelines refer specifically to occupational HIV exposure [56], although several excellent reviews articulate the additional concerns when HIV postexposure prophylaxis is considered for sexual exposure [57,58]. European guidelines for postexposure prophylaxis of sexual exposure to HIV are under consideration [59], and guidelines from the CDC are expected soon.

## Summary

Health care providers in a variety of settings need to improve their ability—along with the capabilities of supporting laboratories, surveillance systems, and services for sex partner management—to diagnose and treat STI. Whether the travel health care sector, as such, is willing to take on the additional burden of STI-related screening and risk reduction counseling has been raised by some authors [3]. Currently, the burden of providing formalized STI care falls on the public sector; however, in the United States, most STI are actually diagnosed in the offices of private physicians [60]. Given that the United States has the highest STI rates of any industrialized country, the undeniable synergy between STI and HIV acquisition, the failure of many American providers to screen for *C trachomatis* despite clear guidelines [61], the global resurgence of syphilis and extension of resistant *N gonorrhoeae* and of HIV, and the risk behaviors consistently reported by travelers, it is hard to argue against travel specialists' joining the daunting battle against these recalcitrant infections and their often devastating consequences. Most of the relevant diagnostic tests are relatively affordable, and patient-centered risk-reduction counseling, once mastered, can be brief and easily integrated into the overall conversation about protecting oneself during travel.

## References

[1] Kahn RH, Heffelfinger JD, Berman SM. Syphilis outbreaks among men who have sex with men: a public health trend of concern. Sex Transm Dis 2002;29:285–7.
[2] Wang SA, Lee MV, O'Connor N, et al. Multidrug-resistant *Neisseria gonorrhoeae* with decreased susceptibility to cefixime—Hawaii, 2001. Clin Infect Dis 2003;37:849–52.
[3] Matteelli A, Carosi G. Sexually transmitted diseases in travelers. Clin Infect Dis 2001;32: 1063–7.
[4] Mulhall BP. Sex and travel: studies of sexual behaviour, disease and health promotion in international travelers: a global review. Int J STD AIDS 1996;7:455–65.

[5] Hawkes S, Hart GJ, Johnson AM, et al. Risk behaviour and HIV prevalence in international travellers. AIDS 1994;8:247–52.
[6] Moore J, Beeker C, Harrison JS, et al. HIV risk behavior among Peace Corps volunteers. AIDS 1995;9:795–9.
[7] Bloor M, Thomas M, Hood K, et al. Differences in sexual risk behaviour between young men and women travelling abroad from the UK. Lancet 1998;352:1664–8.
[8] Bellis MA, Hughes K, Thomson R, et al. Sexual behaviour of young people in international tourist resorts. Sex Transm Infect 2004;80:43–7.
[9] Tveit KS. Casual sexual experience abroad in patients attending an STD clinic and at high risk for HIV infection. Genitourin Med 1994;70:12–4.
[10] Arvidson M, Kallings I, Nilsson S, et al. Risky behavior in women with history of casual travel sex. Sex Transm Dis 1997;24:418–21.
[11] Arvidson M, Hellberg D, Mardh PA. Sexual risk behavior and history of sexually transmitted diseases in relation to casual travel sex during different types of journeys. Acta Obstet Gynecol Scand 1996;75:490–4.
[12] Mulhall BP. Sexually transmissible diseases and travel. Br Med Bull 1993;49:394–411.
[13] Gillies P, Slack R, Stoddart N, et al. HIV-related risk behaviour in UK holiday-makers. AIDS 1992;6:339–41.
[14] Hopperus Buma AP, Veltink RL, van Ameijden EJ, et al. Sexual behaviour and sexually transmitted diseases in Dutch marines and naval personnel on a United Nations mission in Cambodia. Genitourin Med 1995;71:172–5.
[15] Houweling H, Coutinho RA. Risk of HIV infection among Dutch expatriates in sub-Saharan Africa. Int J STD AIDS 1991;2:252–7.
[16] Rogstad KE. Sex, sun, sea, and STIs: sexually transmitted infections acquired on holiday. BMJ 2004;329:214–7.
[17] Perrin L, Kaiser L, Yerly S. Travel and the spread of HIV-1 genetic variants. Lancet Infect Dis 2003;3:22–7.
[18] Pilcher CD, Tien HC, Eron JJ Jr, et al. Brief but efficient: acute HIV infection and the sexual transmission of HIV. J Infect Dis 2004;189:1785–92.
[19] Pilcher CD, Wohl DA, Hicks CB. Diagnosing primary HIV infection. Ann Intern Med 2002; 136:488–9 [author reply: 488–9].
[20] Quinn TC. Population migration and the spread of types 1 and 2 human immunodeficiency viruses. Proc Natl Acad Sci U S A 1994;91:2407–14.
[21] Sanders SA, Graham CA, Yarber WL, et al. Condom use errors and problems among young women who put condoms on their male partners. J Am Med Womens Assoc 2003; 58:95–8.
[22] Fleming DT, McQuillan GM, Johnson RE, et al. Herpes simplex virus type 2 in the United States, 1976 to 1994. N Engl J Med 1997;337:1105–11.
[23] Koutsky LA. Epidemiology of genital human papillomavirus infection. Am J Med 1997; 102:3–8.
[24] Rietmeijer CA, Bull SS, McFarlane M, et al. Risks and benefits of the internet for populations at risk for sexually transmitted infections (STIs): results of an STI clinic survey. Sex Transm Dis 2003;30:15–9.
[25] Sexually transmitted disease treatment guidelines. MMWR Morb Mortal Wkly Rep 2002; 51(RR-6):7.
[26] Wald A, Corey L. How does herpes simplex virus type 2 influence human immunodeficiency virus infection and pathogenesis? J Infect Dis 2003;187:1509–12.
[27] Kamb ML, Fishbein M, Douglas JMJ, et al. Efficacy of risk-reduction counseling to prevent human immunodeficiency virus and sexually transmitted diseases: a randomized controlled trial. Project RESPECT Study Group. JAMA 1998;280:1161–7.
[28] Outbreak of syphilis among men who have sex with men—Southern California, 2000. MMWR Morb Mortal Wkly Rep 2001;50:117–20.

[29] Screening for chlamydial infection: recommendations and rationale. Am J Prev Med 2001; 20:90–4.
[30] Alter MJ. Epidemiology and prevention of hepatitis B. Semin Liver Dis 2003;23:39–46.
[31] Ashley RL, Wald A. Genital herpes: review of the epidemic and potential use of type-specific serology. Clin Microbiol Rev 1999;12:1–8.
[32] Corey L, Wald A, Patel R, et al. Once-daily valacyclovir to reduce the risk of transmission of genital herpes. N Engl J Med 2004;350:11–20.
[33] Overcome barriers to correct condom use. Contracept Technol Update 1999;20:31–2.
[34] Rugpao S, Wanapirak C, Sirichotiyakul S, et al. Sexually transmitted disease prevalence in brothel-based commercial sex workers in Chiang Mai, Thailand: impact of the condom use campaign. J Med Assoc Thai 1997;80:426–30.
[35] Leigh BC. Alcohol and condom use: a meta-analysis of event-level studies. Sex Transm Dis 2002;29:476–82.
[36] Katz MH, Gerberding JL. Postexposure treatment of people exposed to the human immunodeficiency virus through sexual contact or injection-drug use. N Engl J Med 1997; 336:1097–100.
[37] Davis KR, Weller SC. The effectiveness of condoms in reducing heterosexual transmission of HIV. Fam Plann Perspect 1999;31:272–9.
[38] Pinkerton SD, Abramson PR. Effectiveness of condoms in preventing HIV transmission. Soc Sci Med 1997;44:1303–12.
[39] Weller S, Davis K. Condom effectiveness in reducing heterosexual HIV transmission. Cochrane Database Syst Rev 2002; CD003255.
[40] Macaluso M, Kelaghan J, Artz L, et al. Mechanical failure of the latex condom in a cohort of women at high STD risk. Sex Transm Dis 1999;26:450–8.
[41] The safety and feasibility of female condom reuse. Report of a WHO consultation. Geneva: World Health Organization; 2002.
[42] Kreiss J, Ngugi E, Holmes K, et al. Efficacy of nonoxynol-9 contraceptive sponge use in preventing heterosexual acquisition of HIV in Nairobi prostitutes. JAMA 1992;268: 477–82.
[43] Richardson BA, Lavreys L, Martin HL Jr, et al. Evaluation of a low-dose nonoxynol-9 gel for the prevention of sexually transmitted diseases: a randomized clinical trial. Sex Transm Dis 2001;28:394–400.
[44] Roddy RE, Zekeng L, Ryan KA, et al. Effect of nonoxynol-9 gel on urogenital gonorrhea and chlamydial infection: a randomized controlled trial. JAMA 2002;287:1117–22.
[45] Recommendations for the nonclinical development of topical microbicides for prevention of HIV transmission: an update. J Acquir Immune Defic Syndr 2004;36:541–52.
[46] Quinn TC, Wawer MJ, Sewankambo N, et al. Viral load and heterosexual transmission of human immunodeficiency virus type 1. Rakai Project Study Group. N Engl J Med 2000; 342:921–9.
[47] Epidemic update AIDS: 2003. Geneva: UNAIDS; 2003.
[48] Reynolds SJ, Risbud AR, Shepherd ME, et al. Recent herpes simplex virus type 2 infection and the risk of human immunodeficiency virus type 1 acquisition in India. J Infect Dis 2003; 187:1513–21.
[49] Gray RH, Kiwanuka N, Quinn TC, et al. Male circumcision and HIV acquisition and transmission: cohort studies in Rakai. Uganda. Rakai Project Team. AIDS 2000;14:2371–81.
[50] Reynolds SJ, Shepherd ME, Risbud AR, et al. Male circumcision and risk of HIV-1 and other sexually transmitted infections in India. Lancet 2004;363:1039–40.
[51] Hall AJ. Hepatitis in travellers: epidemiology and prevention. BMJ 1993;49:382–93.
[52] Guidelines for the management of sexually transmitted infections: World Health Organization, 2003. Available at: www.who.int/reproductive-health/publications/rhr_01_10/01_10.pdf. Accessed September 15, 2004.

[53] Tichonova L, Borisenko K, Ward H, et al. Epidemics of syphilis in the Russian Federation: trends, origins, and priorities for control. Lancet 1997;350:210–3.
[54] MacLean JD, Libman M. Screening returning travelers. Infect Dis Clin North Am 1998;12: 431–43.
[55] Marrazzo JM, Celum CL, Hillis SD, et al. Performance and cost-effectiveness of selective screening criteria for *Chlamydia trachomatis* infection in women: implications for a national *Chlamydia* control strategy. Sex Transm Dis 1997;24:131–41.
[56] Updated US. Public Health Service guidelines for the management of occupational exposures to HBV, HCV, and HIV and recommendations for postexposure prophylaxis. MMWR Recomm Rep 2001;50:1–52.
[57] Katz MH, Gerberding JL. The care of persons with recent sexual exposure to HIV. Ann Intern Med 1998;128:306–12.
[58] Katz MH, Gerberding JL. Management of occupational and nonoccupational postexposure HIV prophylaxis. Curr Infect Dis Rep 2002;4:543–9.
[59] Almeda J, Casabona J, Simon B, et al. Proposed recommendations for the management of HIV post-exposure prophylaxis after sexual, injecting drug or other exposures in Europe. Euro Surveill 2004;9:5–6.
[60] Brackbill RM, Sternberg MR, Fishbein M. Where do people go for treatment of sexually transmitted diseases? Fam Plann Perspect 1999;31:10–5.
[61] Centers for Disease Control and Prevention. Chlamydia screening among sexually active young female enrollees of health plans—United States, 1999–2001. MMWR Morb Mortal Wkly Rep 2004;53:983–5.

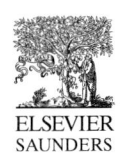

# The Impact of HIV Infection on Tropical Diseases

Gundel Harms, MD, MPH, PhD[a,*], Hermann Feldmeier, MD, PhD[b]

[a]*Institute of Tropical Medicine, Charité-University Medicine Berlin, Spandauer Damm 130, 14050 Berlin, Germany*
[b]*Institute of Infection Medicine, Department of Microbiology, Charité-University Medicine Berlin, Hindenburgdamm 27, 12203 Berlin, Germany*

In all parts of the tropics burdens of infectious tropical diseases are highest where HIV prevalence peaks. Interactions between HIV and parasitic and other pathogens must occur frequently in sub-Saharan Africa, South America and the Caribbean, and South and Southeast Asia. Knowledge about the impact of these interactions has been accumulating only recently [1].

HIV infection may alter the natural history of tropical diseases in different ways. Diagnosis and treatment may be altered and an increased pathogen burden may augment morbidity and mortality.

The impact that tropical diseases have on the course of HIV infection may also be deleterious. Many intercurrent infections increase the HIV viral load and enhance HIV disease progression and the risk of transmission of HIV to noninfected individuals. Similarly, chronic immunostimulation by pathogens, such as helminths and protozoa, may considerably accelerate the natural history of HIV infection.

Most parasitic infections can be treated effectively at low cost. On the population level, regular treatment against prevailing parasites can prevent rapid disease progression, lead to a decrease of viral load, and consequently reduce the odds of transmission of HIV. Antiparasitic treatment can be a potential tool in the fight against HIV-AIDS in the tropics.

This article reviews the known mutual interactions of HIV and major tropical diseases. The focus is on interactions of HIV with malaria, leishmaniasis, African trypanosomiasis, Chagas disease, schistosomiasis,

---

* Corresponding author.
*E-mail address:* gundel.harms@charite.de (G. Harms).

onchocerciasis, lymphatic filariasis, and intestinal helminths. Box 1 provides a review of $T_H1$-$T_H2$ balance.

## HIV and malaria

Malaria occurs throughout the tropics but 90% of the annual 300 million infections take place in sub-Saharan Africa. With more than 30 million individuals living with HIV-AIDS in sub-Saharan Africa alone, coinfection of malaria parasites and HIV has to occur frequently (Table 1).

Although earlier reports did not find any association, more recently evidence has been accumulating that HIV infection and malaria interact with one another, particularly in pregnant women and in persons with advanced HIV disease [1]. HIV-infected pregnant women have an increased incidence of malaria, not only as primigravidae but in all parities [2,3]. Dual infections during pregnancy increase the risk of adverse birth outcome, such as intrauterine growth retardation, preterm delivery, and reduction of birth weight [4]. A significant association of mother-to-child transmission of HIV with placental malaria (risk ratio 2.89) was shown [5]. This was recently confirmed by Mwapasa et al [6] who found a 2.5-fold higher peripheral HIV RNA concentration and a 2.4-fold higher placental HIV RNA concentration in HIV-infected women with placental malaria as opposed to HIV-infected women without placental malaria. Because the risk of HIV transmission increases with the level of HIV viral load in the plasma, adequate prophylaxis and treatment of malaria could have a significant impact on the transmission of HIV from the mother to the child.

Evaluations of a rural and an urban cohort of nonpregnant individuals in Uganda showed that HIV-infected patients had twice as many episodes of symptomatic parasitemia [7]. Furthermore, the incidence of malarial episodes and clinical malaria were significantly associated with falling CD4 counts and with advancing HIV disease [8]. HIV-infected adults other than pregnant women may also be more susceptible to severe malaria. In a recent study significantly more severe and complicated malaria (odds ratio 2.3) and fatal outcome (odds ratio 7.5) was observed in HIV-coinfected patients as opposed to patients with malaria only [9]. All three studies suggest that the immunodeficiency caused by progressing HIV infection impairs acquired immunity toward malaria.

Few studies have addressed the impact of malaria on the natural history of HIV. Hoffman et al [10] studied two groups of HIV-infected patients with symptomatic and asymptomatic malaria. The median plasma viral load of the patients with malaria was about sevenfold higher than in those without acute malaria. This means that acute malaria can up-regulate HIV replication and may favor progression of HIV disease.

Recently it was shown that host-parasite interactions are modified in HIV–*Plasmodium falciparum* coinfected patients treated with antiretroviral drugs [11]. Antiretroviral drugs, protease-inhibitors in particular, were shown to decrease the concentration of the endothelial receptor CD36, a receptor that binds to almost all isolates of *P falciparum* in vivo. Additionally, antiretroviral drugs seemed to impair the nonopsonic phagocytosis of parasitized erythrocytes by human macrophages. The consequences of these findings are not yet clear. A decrease in CD36 expression and a lower binding capacity of parasitized erythrocytes can be protective. The decreases in CD36-mediated sequestration can lead to a higher number of circulating parasitized erythrocytes. In this case, the binding to other receptors, such as the intercellular adhesion molecule-1, can be favored. Intercellular adhesion molecule-1 has been identified as a receptor for *P falciparum*-infected peripheral red blood cells and has been implicated in cerebral malaria. Central nervous system involvement, known as "cerebral malaria," occurs in about 1% of *P falciparum* infections and is a major cause of death [12]. In patients with cerebral malaria, intercellular adhesion molecule-1 is up-regulated on brain microvessels and on some sequestered intravascular leucocytes. Similarly, if antiretrovirals down-regulate phagocytosis of parasitized erythrocytes this might negatively affect the disease outcome.

## HIV and leishmaniasis

About 2 million new cases of leishmaniasis occur each year. Fifteen million people are estimated to be infected in tropical and subtropical regions of all continents except Australia.

The different species of *Leishmania* are transmitted by a number of phlebotomine sandflies in a specific parasite-vector association [13]. Leishmania may cause a spectrum of diseases ranging from self-healing ulcers to disseminated and fatal infections. The type of manifestation and severity of disease depend mainly on the *Leishmania* species involved but also on the host's immune responsiveness.

Leishmania-HIV coinfections have been reported from 35 countries [13,14]. Areas of major concern are those where both infections overlap with high endemicity (eg, eastern Africa, India, Brazil, and Europe) (see Table 1; Tables 2 and 3). In south-western Europe and increasingly in Brazil, transmission of both HIV and leishmania is accelerated by a second route, the sharing of needles in intravenous drug users. In HIV-leishmania coinfected individuals the clinical manifestation is mostly visceral leishmaniasis, although cutaneous forms have been described.

Leishmania and HIV mutually influence each other: the major surface protein of leishmania, a lipophosphoglycan, up-regulates HIV replication in monocytic cells and in $CD4^+$ T cells [15]. The CD4 depression in HIV infection provides a specifically favorable environment for primary infection with leishmania or for reactivation of a latent infection. With decreasing cellular immunity, and usually at CD4 counts below 200/mL, visceral

## Box 1. Review of $T_H1$-$T_H2$ balance

During an adaptive immune response CD4$^+$ T-helper ($T_H$) cell precursors develop either into $T_H1$ or $T_H2$ cells. $T_H1$ cells are essential for macrophage-dependent host responses. These helper cells produce interferon-$\gamma$, interleukin (IL)-2, and tumor necrosis factor-$\alpha$ and promote the production of opsonizing and complement-fixing antibodies, antibody-dependent cell cytotoxicity, macrophage activation, and other types of cell-mediated immunity. $T_H2$ cells orchestrate immune responses, which are independent of the activation of macrophages. These T-helper cells produce IL-4, IL-5, IL-6, IL-9, IL-10, and IL-13 and provide optimal help for adaptive humoral immune responses, including IgE and IgG1 isotype switching and growth and differentiation of eosinophils. At the same time, other cytokines produced by $T_H2$ cells, such as IL-4, IL-10, and IL-13, inhibit several macrophage functions and thereby impair the $T_H1$-type immune effector mechanisms.

Whereas IL-4 is the signature cytokine of the $T_H2$ subset, interferon-$\gamma$ is the major cytokine driving $T_H1$-type of help. The early presence of IL-4 is the most potent stimulus for $T_H2$ differentiation. This means that the inducing power of IL-4 dominates over other cytokines. If IL-4 levels reach a certain threshold, differentiation of naïve CD4$^+$ helper cells into the $T_H2$ phenotype results.

It is generally agreed that to cope with a defined pathogen a distinct balance of $T_H1$ and $T_H2$ has to develop in the infected host. Because pathogens, particularly parasites, change their antigenic make-up during development and proliferation, this balance has to be dynamic and to be tuned precisely to be effective. If $T_H1$ and $T_H2$ immune responses fail to be protective, immunopathologic sequelae develop. In leishmaniasis, for example, a predominant activity of $T_H1$ cells is required to contain the infection. If the balance is "biased" toward a $T_H2$-type of help the intracellular parasites proliferate and spread. In leprosy, a spectral disease, tuberculoid leprosy at one end of the spectrum is characterized by a preponderance of the $T_H1$ type of help and effective immune mechanisms against *Mycobacterium leprae*. Lepromatous leprosy on the other end of the spectrum is associated with an ineffective immunity caused by a shift toward $T_H2$ cells. In contrast, helminthiases are only to be controlled if a $T_H2$-type of immune responses dominates over $T_H1$ responses. This is reflected by

> high concentrations of IgE and eosinophils in the blood triggered through the release of IL-4 and IL-5, respectively.
>
> $T_H1$ and $T_H2$ cells do not derive from distinct lineages, but develop from the same precursor under the influence of genetic and environmental factors. As factors acting in the microenvironment of a naïve T-helper cell precursor the nature of the antigen and its mode of entry are of pivotal importance. *Leishmania major* parasites delivered to mice by an intranasal route fail to induce the expected $T_H1$-type of immune response and preferentially prime $T_H2$ cells. This shows that the pulmonary environment promotes the differentiation of T-helper cell precursors into $T_H2$ cells, whereas the same antigen inoculated into the skin triggers $T_H1$ immune responses.
>
> In the context of HIV infection an imbalance of T-helper responses induced by tropical parasitic diseases seems to be crucial for disease outcome. First, $T_H2$ clones are more permissive to HIV as compared with $T_H1$ clones. Second, skewing of the immune response through chronic parasitic infections toward a $T_H2$-type of help may impair the development of effective antiviral responses. Third, an increase in the cellular activation state in response to chronic or recurrent parasitic infections may enhance HIV replication by facilitating the entry of the virus into vulnerable cells, its reverse transcription, and the rate of transcription of proviral DNA.

leishmaniasis manifests like an opportunistic infection and parasites disseminate to atypical sites [1,13,14].

In coinfected individuals visceral leishmaniasis often lacks its typical characteristics: only 50% of the patients present with fever, splenomegaly, and hepatomegaly, whereas cytopenia is usually very severe [13,16–19]. Ectopic localizations of parasite multiplication are common and ulcers may be found in the gastrointestinal and respiratory tract, in the central nervous system, and in the blood [1,16–19].

Diagnosis of leishmaniasis is difficult in coinfected persons. Only 50% of the patients show the characteristic antibodies. The unusual spread of parasites into the circulation, however, may allow diagnosis from the blood [13,19]. Polymerase chain reaction of the buffy coat of the blood may detect parasite antigen in up to 100% [20].

Initially, 50% to 100% of coinfected individuals respond to treatment with pentavalent antimony ($Sb^v$) or amphotericin B in its standard preparation or in its liposomal form [13,19,21]. Side effects are significantly more frequent and pronounced, especially with $Sb^v$ [16,22]. Toxicity is lower with

Table 1
Geographic overlap of HIV and parasitic diseases in sub-Saharan Africa

| Characteristics of HIV infection | Characteristics of parasitic diseases |
| --- | --- |
| High prevalence in general population; rural and urban areas affected; high prevalence in reproductive age group; heterosexual transmission; high transmission from mother-to-child | *Malaria*: hyperendemic; all year round transmission (rural > periurban > urban); all age groups affected; small children and pregnant women most vulnerable for severe infection<br>*Visceral leishmaniasis*: prevalence varies from region to region; high endemicity in Sudan; all age groups affected<br>*Schistosomiasis*: focal distribution in rural areas; intensity of infection particularly high in children; adults of reproductive age most vulnerable for genital lesions<br>*Onchocerciasis*: patchy distribution; mass treatment has decreased infected population considerably<br>*Lymphatic filariasis*: prevalence varies from region to region; intensity of infection and development of sequels increases with age<br>*Loiasis*: limited foci near the equator<br>Sleeping sickness: focal distribution; mainly adults affected |

liposomal amphotericin B [21]. Overall, relapses occur in 25% to 80% of coinfected individuals [17,22]. The availability of highly active antiretroviral therapy (HAART) significantly reduced the incidence of visceral leishmaniasis in Italy, France, and Spain [19,23,24]. In Spain for example, HAART decreased the annual incidence of visceral leishmaniasis among local AIDS patients from 4.81 to 0.8 cases per 100 ($P < .0005$). HAART alone cannot prevent relapses of visceral leishmaniasis, however, and even if combined with secondary antileishmanial prophylaxis only partial protection against relapses is achieved [24–26]. In this context it was shown that patients receiving liposomal amphotericin B every 21 days relapsed less often (odds ratio 3.5) than those receiving no intermittent antileishmanial prophylaxis [26]. The combination of HAART and antileishmanial prophylaxis can significantly prolong survival in those affected by the fatal combination of highly pathogenic organisms.

## HIV and human African trypanosomiasis

Sleeping sickness occurs only in Africa and is caused by *Trypanosoma brucei (T b) gambiense* and *T b rhodesiense*, protozoa that are transmitted by the tsetse fly. About 60 million people are at risk of infection in 36 countries of sub-Saharan Africa and 300,000 cases have been reported annually in past years (see Table 1). Although *T b gambiense* infection

Table 2
Geographic overlap of HIV and parasitic diseases in South America

| Characteristics of HIV infection | Characteristics of parasitic diseases |
|---|---|
| High prevalence in certain urban risk groups; prevalence in general population and children rather low; considerable difference in prevalence between and within countries | *Malaria*: falciparum malaria primarily in the Amazon basin; mainly rural populations affected; small children and pregnant women most vulnerable for severe infection
*Visceral leishmaniasis*: concentrated in northeast Brazil (rural and urban); mainly children affected
*Schistosomiasis*: only *S mansoni*; limited foci in the Center and northeast of Brazil; control has reduced the infected population
*Onchocerciasis*: very small foci in native populations of the Amazon rain forest
*Lymphatic filariasis*: single foci in several states of northeast Brazil
*Chagas disease*: rural areas in Brazil, Paraguay, Bolivia |

occurs sporadically and in limited foci, *T b rhodesiense* sleeping sickness occurs in epidemics. The disease manifests itself in two phases along with dissemination of the parasites in the hemolymphatic system and, in the second phase, in the central nervous system.

Several cross-sectional studies found no evidence for an interaction of African trypanosomiasis and HIV infection [27–29]. Twelve years ago, however, Pepin et al [30] observed that HIV-1–infected patients were significantly more likely to relapse after treatment with eflornithine, indicating that HIV-infected persons may be at a higher risk for treatment failure than individuals with trypanosomal infection only. Similarly, of 18 patients treated with melarsoprol for encephalopathic trypanosomiasis, the four

Table 3
Geographic overlap of HIV and parasitic diseases in South and Southeast Asia

| Characteristics of HIV infection | Characteristics of parasitic diseases |
|---|---|
| Prevalences in general population and children still low; high prevalences in certain risks groups, (ie, intravenous drug users and sex workers); high potential for HIV outbreaks | *Malaria*: with the exception of New Guinea mainly *P vivax*; high transmission only during the rainy season; all age groups affected; small children and pregnant women most vulnerable for falciparum malaria
*Visceral leishmaniasis*: mainly eastern India, Bangladesh; predominantly adults affected
*Lymphatic filariasis*: widespread occurrence (rural and urban), all age groups affected; intensity of infection and development of sequels increases with age |

HIV-positive patients either died or had an unfavorable outcome, whereas the 14 HIV-negative patients recovered completely [31].

**HIV and Chagas disease**

Chagas disease only exists on the American continent. Sixteen to 18 million people are estimated to be infected, whereas 100 million are at risk of acquiring the infection. *Trypanosoma cruzi*, the parasite that causes Chagas disease, is transmitted by blood-sucking reduviid bugs. Transfusion of infected blood has also been a common source of infection. The southern cone countries of Uruguay, Argentina, Chile, and large parts of Brazil are now considered free of vectorial and transfusional transmission of Chagas disease (see Table 2) [32].

Chagas disease is characterized by an acute phase with high parasitemia of *T cruzi* and by a chronic phase usually without parasitemia detectable by direct microscopic examination of the blood. In HIV–*T cruzi* coinfection, however, the immunodeficiency related to HIV allows multiplication of parasites in tissues and liberation into the blood, particularly in the chronic stage [33]. Dormant *T cruzi* infection can be reactivated in immunocompromised persons and reactivation of Chagas disease in HIV-positives consistently leads to high parasitemia. In an analysis of 29 HIV-positive and 81 HIV-negative individuals with chronic Chagas disease *T cruzi* parasitemia detected by xenodiagnosis (detection of parasites after feeding of laboratory-raised triatomes on an infected individual) and blood culture was found to be significantly more frequent and higher in the HIV-coinfected subjects [34].

Although central nervous system involvement is usually never observed in chronic Chagas disease, involvement of the central nervous system is the rule in coinfected persons [35,36]. Acute fatal meningoencephalitis, tumor-like lesions, and granulomatous encephalitis have been described [37–39].

It is assumed that the persistent increase in tissue parasitism causes inflammation and accelerates the disease. Treatment of *T cruzi* infection in HIV-positive individuals should be started early, even when patients are still asymptomatic and when irreversible alterations have not yet occurred [40].

Little is known about the impact of Chagas disease on HIV disease; however, up-regulation of HIV replication by *T cruzi* was recently suggested. In an HIV-infected patient viral load increased simultaneously with exacerbation of *T cruzi* parasitemia and decreased to previous levels after antiparasitic treatment despite unchanged antiretroviral treatment [40].

**HIV and schistosomiasis**

An estimated 200 million people in the world have schistosomiasis. There are five schistosome species pathogenic for humans: (1) *S mansoni*, (2) *S haematobium*, (3) *S japonicum*, (4) *S intercalatum*, and (5) *S mekongi*, the latter two being of limited importance. *S mansoni* is widespread in Africa north and south of the Sahara, occurs in the Caribbean, and in some parts of Brazil and Venezuela. *S haematobium* is confined to Africa and the Arabian Peninsula (see Tables 1–3) [41]. Morbidity in schistosomiasis is predominantly caused by granuloma formation around eggs sequestered in different tissues and depends on the species involved, the intensity of infection, the topographic site affected, and the immune responsiveness of the host.

Recent studies showed that HIV infection may exert a deleterious effect on the natural course of schistosomiasis in different ways. In a cohort of Kenyan car washers simultaneously infected with HIV and *S mansoni*, the time until reinfection with schistosomes was shorter in coinfected- than in HIV-negative individuals. The effect became more prominent the lower was the number of CD4 T cells [42]. The same authors suggested that the lower production of $T_H2$-cytokines in coinfected individuals was responsible for lowered resistance to reinfection with *S mansoni* [43].

Treatment with praziquantel, a drug needing a functioning immune system to be effective, was not impaired in patients with *S mansoni* or *S haematobium*-HIV coinfection [44,45].

Patients infected with *S haematobium* and HIV excrete fewer eggs and also have less hematuria than those without HIV infection. By consequence, the sensitivity and positive predictive value of reported hematuria as an indication of heavy *S haematobium* infection is lower in those coinfected with HIV [45].

There is only indirect evidence that schistosomiasis has an impact on the natural history of HIV infection. Genital schistosomiasis may be a risk factor for the transmission of HIV and may predispose to increased transmission [46–49]. Genital schistosomiasis occurs in about 60% of women infected with *S haematobium* and the prevalence of genital schistosomiasis parallels that of urinary schistosomiasis [49].

Very similar to sexually transmitted infections, lesions occur in the vulva, vagina, and in the cervix [50]. Typical findings of genital schistosomiasis are thinning, erosion, and ulceration of the epithelium, particularly in the cervix [47,49]. These lesions reflect a break in the integrity of the mucosal barrier and may increase the risk of HIV infection and transmission [51].

When adult worms begin to produce eggs, the host's immune response shifts toward a $T_H2$ cell type of help. The sequestration of schistosome ova in tissue provokes a complex cellular and humoral immune response. Granulomata are formed, which are composed among other cell types of activated lymphocytes, macrophages, epithelioid cells, and Langerhans' cells, cells known to express the $CD4^+$ receptor [52]. It is likely that, after penetration through the friable and eroded epithelium of the cervix, the virus is rapidly bound by these $CD4^+$ receptor-bearing cells.

Recently, the first patient has been described in which cervical schistosomiasis, HIV, and human papilloma virus infection coexisted and in whom clinical and laboratory data suggested that genital schistosomiasis paved the way for the viral infections [53]. Corresponding to the findings in women, a study in Madagascar revealed that infection with *S haematobium* in men caused inflammation of the prostate and of the seminal vesicles [54]. This chronic inflammation might result in an increased viral shedding in the semen of individuals with dual infection.

## HIV and onchocerciasis

Onchocerciasis occurs in West Africa and in a few foci in Brazil, Venezuela, Guatemala, Mexico, and Yemen (see Tables 1–3). About 18 million people are estimated to be infected with *Onchocerca volvulus*, of whom 99% is in Africa. Parasite-vector associations are very specific with certain species of blackflies (*Simulium* spp) being responsible for the transmission in one focus, but not in others. From an immunologic point of view onchocerciasis is a spectral disease with a hyperergic form (Sowda) at one end and a hypoergic clinical picture (nodular onchocerciasis) at the other end of the spectrum. Before control was attempted through mass distribution of ivermectin, onchocerciasis was the leading cause of blindness in sub-Saharan Africa.

There is little information about interaction of HIV and onchocerciasis. No significant epidemiologic association or difference in microfilariae density was detected in a case-control study of 1910 patients with onchocerciasis and 276 controls [55]. The same authors did not find any difference in the efficacy of treatment with ivermectin or in the occurrence of side effects in those dually infected, even if CD4 cell counts were reduced. This is to be expected because killing of microfilariae by the drug ivermectin is known to be independent of cellular immunity.

Sentongo et al [56] showed a decreased cellular immune responsiveness of peripheral blood mononuclear cells of individuals with dual infections as opposed to those with only *O volvulus* infection. Similarly, the antibody response to *O volvulus* antigen was decreased in HIV-infected individuals with onchocerciasis as opposed to those without HIV infection [57]. The impact of these findings on transmission rates or disease progression is not known.

## HIV, lymphatic filariasis, and loiasis

Although lymphatic filariasis is widely distributed in the tropics, loiasis occurs in limited hot and humid areas of sub-Saharan Africa (see Tables 1–3). The causal agents of lymphatic filariasis are transmitted by various mosquito species and *Loa loa* by different *Chrysops* flies.

Human lymphatic filariasis is mainly caused by two species, *Wuchereria bancrofti* and *Brugia malayi*. These parasites are mutually exclusive in their geographic distribution. Most of the pathology in lymphatic filariasis is associated with the adult worms and their location in the lymphatic system with a spectrum of clinical manifestations seen in the endemic area. There are asymptomatic carriers with dozens or hundreds of microfilariae per milliliter of blood, and there are those with inflammatory reactions of the lymphatic vessels who later develop chronic lymphatic pathology. Recurrent bacterial infections seem to be an important cofactor in the development of filarial lymphedema and subsequent elephantiasis.

No data are available on the impact of HIV on filariasis or loiasis. Gopinath et al [58], however, recently showed that in vitro HIV replication was significantly increased in peripheral blood mononuclear cells from patients with untreated lymphatic filariasis. This finding might implicate a risk for faster HIV disease progression in coinfection with lymphatic filariae. No impact of HIV on loiasis has been reported.

**HIV and intestinal helminths**

In impoverished populations, intestinal helminths are prevalent in all age groups. Fifty percent to 80% of poor populations may be infected with worms causing ascariasis, trichuriasis, and hookworm disease. In endemic areas children can expect to be infected as soon as they crawl, and to remain so or to be regularly reinfected for the rest of their lives. During infection, all important nematodes undergo a phase of tissue migration. Typical worm burdens in areas where HIV infection is common produce a million eggs per day, accompanied by copious amounts of secretory and excretory products that exert an influence on the host's immune system.

There is no current evidence that immunosuppression by HIV facilitates or aggravates helminthic infections, with the possible exception of strongyloidiasis [59]. Helminths could, however, have an effect on the natural history of HIV on three levels: (1) increased susceptibility toward infection, (2) decreased protection against disease, and (3) faster disease progression.

Peripheral blood mononuclear cells of patients with helminthic infection are significantly more susceptible to infection with HIV than those of uninfected controls [60]. Furthermore, elevated levels of interleukin-4, a cytokine characteristic of the $T_H2$-type of immune response in helminthic infections, down-regulate $T_H1$ differentiation and function [61].

HIV replicates preferentially in $T_H2$- and $T_H0$-type clones, and $T_H2$ cells are usually abundant in individuals infected with helminths [62]. After HIV has spread to the systemic circulation its replication is limited by the fact that usually few activated lymphocytes and differentiated macrophages are present in the blood stream and that resting T cells and undifferentiated monocytes are not susceptible to HIV infection. In patients infected with intestinal helminthes, however, the number of activated T cells expressing HLA-DR and HIV coreceptors is elevated [63]. Further evidence for an influence of chronic helminthic infection on the natural history of HIV infection was observed in a field study in Ethiopia. Here, individuals with various helminthic infections had significantly higher HIV loads than those without helminths and, following antiparasitic treatment, the viral load decreased [64].

## References

[1] Harms G, Feldmeier H. HIV infection and tropical parasitic diseases: deleterious interactions in both directions? Trop Med Int Health 2002;7:479–88.
[2] Bloland PB, Wirima JJ, Steketee RW, et al. Maternal HIV infection and infant mortality in Malawi: evidence for increased mortality due to placental malaria infection. AIDS 1995;9: 721–6.
[3] Verhoeff FH, Brabin BJ, Hart CA, et al. Increased prevalence of malaria in HIV-infected pregnant women and its implications for malaria control. Trop Med Int Health 1999;4: 5–12.
[4] Ayisi JG, van Eijk AM, ter Kuile FO, et al. The effect of dual infection with HIV and malaria on pregnancy outcome in western Kenya. AIDS 2002;17:585–94.
[5] Brahmbhatt H, Kigozi G, Wabwire-Mangen F, et al. The effects of placental malaria on mother-to-child HIV transmission in Rakai, Uganda. AIDS 2003;17:2539–41.
[6] Mwapasa V, Rogerson SJ, Molyneux ME, et al. The effect of *Plasmodium falciparum* malaria on peripheral and placental HIV-1 RNA concentrations in pregnant Malawian women. AIDS 2004;18:1051–9.
[7] Whitworth J, Morgan D, Quigley M, et al. Effect of HIV-1 and increasing immunosuppression on malaria parasitaemia and clinical episodes in adults in rural Uganda: a cohort study. Lancet 2000;23:1051–6.
[8] French NJ, Nakiyingi J, Lugada E, et al. Increasing rates of malarial fever with deteriorating immune status in HIV-1-infected Ugandan adults. AIDS 2000;15:899–906.
[9] Grimwade K, French N, Mbatha DD, et al. HIV infection as a cofactor for severe falciparum malaria in adults living in a region of unstable malaria transmission in South Africa. AIDS 2004;18:547–54.
[10] Hoffman IE, Jere CS, Taylor TE, et al. The effect of *Plasmodium falciparum* malaria on HIV-1 RNA blood plasma concentration. AIDS 1999;13:487–94.
[11] Nathoo SL, Serghides L, Kain KC. Effect of HIV-1 antiretroviral drugs on cytoadherence and phagocytic clearance of *Plasmodium falciparum*-parasitised erythrocytes. Lancet 2003; 362:1039–41.
[12] Hunt H, Grau GE. Cytokines: accelerators and brakes in the pathogenesis of cerebral malaria. Trends Immunol 2003;24:491–9.
[13] World Health Organization. Leishmania/HIV co-infection, south-western Europe, 1990–1998. Wkly Epidemiol Rec 1999;74:365–75.
[14] Desjeux P, Alvar J. Leishmania/HIV co-infections: epidemiology in Europe. Ann Trop Med Parasitol 2003;97:3–15.
[15] Bernier R, Barbeau B, Trenblay MJ, et al. The lipophosphoglycan of *Leishmania donovani* up-regulates HIV-1 transcription in T cells through the nuclear factor kB elements. J Immunol 1998;160:2881–8.
[16] Alvar J, Canavate C, Gutierrez-Solar B, et al. Leishmania and human immunodeficiency virus co-infection: the first ten years. Clin Microbiol Rev 1997;10:298–319.
[17] Lopez-Velez R, Perez-Molina JA, Guerrero A, et al. Clinicoepidemiologic characteristics, prognostic factors, and survival analysis of patients co-infected with human immunodeficiency virus and leishmania in an area of Madrid, Spain. Am J Trop Med Hyg 1998;58: 436–43.

[18] Rosenthal E, Marty P, le Fichoux Y, et al. Clinical manifestation of visceral leishmaniasis associated with HIV-infection: a retrospective study of 91 French cases. Ann Trop Med Parasitol 2000;94:37–42.
[19] Pintado V, Martin-Rabadan P, Rivera ML, et al. Visceral leishmaniasis in HIV-infected and non-HIV-infected patients: a comparative study. Medicine 2001;80:54–73.
[20] Bossolasco S, Gaiera G, Olchini D, et al. Real-time PCR assay for clinical management of human immunodeficiency virus-infected patients with visceral leishmaniasis. J Clin Microbiol 2003;41:5080–4.
[21] Laguna F, Videla S, Jimenez-Mejias ME, et al. Amphotericin B lipid complex versus meglumine antimonite in the treatment of visceral leishmaniasis in patients infected with HIV: a randomised pilot study. J Antimicrob Chemother 2003;52:464–8.
[22] Delgado J, Macias J, Pineda JA, et al. High frequency of serious side effects from meglumine antimonite given without an upper limit dose for the treatment of visceral leishmaniasis in human immunodeficiency virus type-1-infected patients. Am J Trop Med Hyg 1999;61: 766–9.
[23] Tumbarello M, Tacconelli E, Bertagnolio S, et al. Highly active antiretroviral therapy decreases the incidence of visceral leishmaniasis in HIV-infected individuals. AIDS 2000;14: 2948–9.
[24] Lopez-Velez R. The impact of highly active antiretroviral therapy (HAART) on visceral leishmaniasis in Spanish patients co-infected with HIV. Ann Trop Med Parasitol 2003;97: 143–7.
[25] Villanueva JL, Alarcon A, Bernabeu-Wittel M, et al. Prospective evaluation and follow-up of European patients with visceral leishmaniasis and HIV-1 coinfection in the era of highly active antiretroviral therapy. Eur J Clin Microbiol Infect Dis 2000;19:798–801.
[26] Lopez-Velez R, Videal S, Marquez M, et al. Amphotericin B lipid complex versus treatment in the secondary prophylaxis of visceral leishmaniasis in HIV-infected patients. J Antimicrob Chemother 2004;53:540–3.
[27] Noireau F, Brun-Vezinet F, Larouze B, et al. Absence of relationship between human immunodeficiency virus 1 and sleeping sickness. Trans R Soc Trop Med Hyg 1987;81: 1000.
[28] Louis JP, Moulia-Pelat JP, Jannin J, et al. Absence of epidemiological inter-relations between HIV infection and African human trypanosomiasis in central Africa. Trop Med Parasitol 1991;42:155.
[29] Meda HA, Doua F, Laveissiere C, et al. Human immunodeficiency virus infection and human African trypanosomiasis: a case-control study in Cote d'Ivoire. Trans R Soc Trop Med Hyg 1995;89:639–43.
[30] Pepin J, Ethier L, Kazadi C, et al. The impact of immunodeficiency virus infection on the epidemiology and treatment of *Trypanosoma brucei gambiense* sleeping sickness in Nioko, Zaire. Am J Trop Med Hyg 1992;47:133–40.
[31] Blum J, Nkunku S, Burri C. Clinical description of encephalopathic syndromes and risk factors for their occurrence and outcome and outcome during melarsoprol treatment of human African trypanosomiasis. Trop Med Int Health 2001;6:390–400. Accessed May 23, 2004.
[32] World Health Organization 2003. http://www.who.int/ctd/chagas/burdens.htm.
[33] Perez-Ramirez L, Barnabe C, Sartori AM, et al. Clinical analysis and parasite genetic diversity in human immunodeficiency virus/Chagas disease coinfection in Brazil. Am J Trop Med Hyg 1999;61:198–206.
[34] Sartori AM, Neto JE, Visone Nunes EL, et al. Parasitemia in chronic Chagas' disease: comparison between human immunodeficiency virus (HIV)-positive and HIV-negative patients. J Infect Dis 2002;186:872–5.
[35] Ferreira MS, Nishioka SA, Sivestre MT, et al. Reactivation of Chagas' disease in patients with AIDS: a report of three new cases and a review of the literature. Clin Infect Dis 1997;25: 1397–400.

[36] Pacheco RS, Ferreira MS, Machado MI, et al. Chagas' disease and HIV co-infection: genotypic characterisation of the Trypanosoma cruzi strain. Mem Inst Oswaldo Cruz 1998; 93:165–9.

[37] Ferreira MS, Nishioka SA, Rocha A, et al. Acute fatal *Trypanosoma cruzi* meningoencephalitis in a human immunodeficiency virus-positive hemo-philiac patient. Am J Trop Med Hyg 1991;45:723–7.

[38] Cohen JE, Tsai EC, Ginsberg HJ, et al. Pseudotumoral chagasic meningoencephalitis as the first manifestation of AIDS. Surg Neurol 1998;49:324–7.

[39] Di Lorenzo GA, Pagano MA, Taratuto AL, et al. Chagasic granulomatous encephalitis in immunosuppressed patients. J Neuroimaging 1996;6:94–7.

[40] Sartori AM, Caiaffa-Filho HH, Bezerra RC, et al. Exacerbation of HIV viral load simultaneous with asymptomatic reactivation of chronic Chagas' disease. Am J Trop Med Hyg 2002;67:521–3.

[41] World Health Organization 2004. http://www.who.int/tdr/dw/schisto2004.htm. Accessed May 23, 2004.

[42] Karanja DM, Hightower AW, Colley DG, et al. Resistance to reinfection with *Schistosoma mansoni* in occupationally exposed adults and effect of HIV-1 co-infection on susceptibility to schistosomiasis: a longitudinal study. Lancet 2002;360:592–6.

[43] Mwinzi PN, Karanja DM, Colley DG, et al. Cellular immune responses of schistosomiasis patients are altered by human immunodeficiency virus type 1 coinfection. J Infect Dis 2001; 184:488–96.

[44] Karanja DM, Boyer AE, Strand M, et al. Studies on schistosomiasis in western Kenya. II. Efficacy of praziquantel for treatment of schistosomiasis in persons coinfected with HIV-1. Am J Trop Med Hyg 1998;59:307–11.

[45] Mwanakasale V, Vounatsou P, Sukwa TY, et al. Interactions between *Schistosoma haematobium* and human immunodeficiency virus type 1: the effects of coinfection on treatment outcomes in rural Zambia. Am J Trop Med Hyg 2003;69:420–8.

[46] Feldmeier H, Krantz I, Poggensee G. Female genital schistosomiasis as a risk factor for the transmission of HIV. Int J STD AIDS 1994;5:368–72.

[47] Feldmeier H, Poggensee G, Krantz I, Helling-Giese G. Female genital schistosomiasis: new challenge from a gender perspective. Trop Geograph Med 1995;47:2–15.

[48] Poggensee G, Feldmeier H, Krantz I. Schistosomiasis of the female genital tract: public health aspects. Parasitol Today 1999;15:378–81.

[49] Poggensee G, Kiwelu I, Wege V, et al. Female genital schistosomiasis of the lower reproductive tract: prevalence and schistosome-related morbidity. J Infect Dis 2000;181: 1210–3.

[50] Attili VR, Hira SK, Dube MK. Schistosomal genital granuloma: a report of 10 cases. Br J Venerol Dis 1983;59:269–72.

[51] Mabey D. Interaction between HIV infection and other sexually transmitted diseases. Trop Med Int Health 2000;5:32–6.

[52] Helling-Giese G, Sjaastad A, Poggensee G, et al. Female genital schistosomiasis (FGS): relationship between gynecological and histopathological findings. Acta Trop 1996;62: 257–67.

[53] Mosunjac MB, Tadros T, Beach R, et al. Cervical schistosomiasis, human papilloma virus (HPV), and human immunodeficiency virus (HIV): a dangerous coexistence or coincidence? Gynecol Oncol 2003;90:211–4.

[54] Leutscher P, Ramarokoto CE, Reimert CM, et al. Genital schistosomiasis in males: a community-based study from Madagascar. Lancet 2000;355:117–8.

[55] Fischer P, Kipp W, Kabwa P, et al. Onchocerciasis and HIV in Western Uganda: prevalences and treatment with ivermectin. Am J Trop Med Hyg 1995;53:171–8.

[56] Sentongo E, Rubaale T, Buettner DW, et al. T cell responses in coinfection with *Onchocerca volvulus* and the human immunodeficiency virus type 1. Parasite Immunol 1998;20:431–9.

[57] Tawill SA, Gallin M, Erttmenn KD, et al. Impaired antibody responses and loss of reactivity to *Onchocerca volvulus* antigens by HIV-seronegative onchocerciasis patients. Trans R Soc Trop Med Hyg 1996;90:85–9.
[58] Gopinath R, Ostrowski M, Justement SJ, et al. Filarial infections increase susceptibility to human immunodeficiency virus infection in peripheral blood mononuclear cells in vitro. J Infect Dis 2000;182:1804–8.
[59] Fincham JE, Markus MB, Adams VJ. Could control of soil-transmitted helminthic infection influence the HIV/AIDS pandemic? Acta Trop 2003;86:315–33.
[60] Shapira Nahor O, Kalinkovich A, Weisman Z, et al. Increased susceptibility to HIV-1 infection of peripheral blood mononuclear cells from chronically immuno-activated individuals. AIDS 1998;12:1731–3.
[61] Bentwich Z, Kalinkovich A, Weisman Z. Immune activation is a dominant factor in the pathogenesis of African AIDS. Immunol Today 1995;16:187–91.
[62] Bentwich Z, Kalinkovich A, Weisman Z, et al. Immune activation in the context of HIV infection. Clin Exp Immunol 1998;111:1–2.
[63] Kalinkovich A, Weisman Z, Greenberg J, et al. Decreased CD4 and increased CD8 counts with T cell activation is associated with chronic helminth infection. Clin Exp Immunol 1998;114:414–21.
[64] Bentwich Z, Maartens G, Torten D, et al. Concurrent infections and HIV pathogenesis. AIDS 2000;14:2071–81.

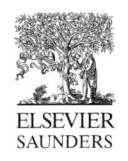

# Update in Traveler's Diarrhea

David R. Shlim, MD

*Jackson Hole Travel and Tropical Medicine, PO Box 40, Kelly, WY 83011, USA*

It has been 50 years since the concept of traveler's diarrhea (TD) was first introduced in studies of travelers to Mexico by Dr. Benjamin Kean. Before World War II, infectious diarrhea was well known, but mainly associated with poverty and war. There was not enough leisure worldwide travel to draw attention to the risks of TD in casual travelers.

After World War II, the advent of increasing prosperity coupled with expanding commercial air travel allowed ordinary people to take trips to more exotic destinations. Mexico became a popular destination for Americans, and Kean became interested in the phenomenon of diarrhea associated with travel.

At the time that he began to focus on travelers, the etiology and risk factors for TD were unknown. Although assumed to be infectious, cultures for *Salmonella* and *Shigella* species (the only bacterial intestinal pathogens outside of *Vibrio cholerae* that were known at the time) were almost always negative [1]. A subsequent search for protozoal pathogens was likewise unrevealing [1]. This led to hypotheses that TD was caused by changes in climate, diet, and stress associated with travel. An elegant study comparing tourists who had traveled to Hawaii with tourists who had traveled to Mexico proved that the risk of TD in Mexico was three times higher than of travelers in Hawaii [1].

Evidence that TD was probably caused by as yet unknown bacterial pathogens stemmed from proving the protective effect of using poorly absorbed antibiotics as prophylaxis in travelers to Mexico [2]. If antibiotics could prevent TD, then the suspicion was that bacterial pathogens must be involved.

A major breakthrough came in the early 1970s with the discovery of toxin-producing strains of *Escherichia coli*, subsequently dubbed enterotoxigenic *E coli* (ETEC) [3]. ETEC proved to be the cause of nearly half the TD cases in travelers to Mexico. With the additional finding of

*E-mail address:* drshlim@wyom.net

*Campylobacter* species as a cause of TD in 1978, the understanding of TD took a further leap. Viral pathogens were also discovered in the decade of the 1970s, but these added only a few percentage points each to the overall etiology of TD.

Etiologic studies have now been done in Mexico, Asia, Africa, and South America. These studies confirm the bacterial etiology of TD, but none of the studies found a pathogen in greater than 60% to 80% of subjects [4]. In the group of patients without a proved pathogen present, antibiotics shorten the illness of a significant percentage, suggesting the presence of an undetected bacterial pathogen or pathogens. The effort begun 50 years ago to confirm the etiology of TD is not complete, and continues to this day.

Once the bacterial etiology of TD was confirmed, the use of antibiotics to shorten the illness slowly began to take hold. The adoption of antibiotics was slow because there was a widely held belief that TD was a benign, self-limited illness that did not require treatment. Finding that some people with *Salmonella* had a prolonged excretion rate of that organism after antibiotic treatment (even though they were then found to be clinically well) also fueled the reluctance to treat. Even when treatment was considered, there was an absence of controlled clinical trials to determine if treatment was indeed effective, and which antibiotics should be used.

Early use of ampicillin and tetracyclines as treatment for TD was unsupported by clinical trials. Cotrimoxazole began to be used in the early 1980s, and studies in Mexico confirmed its efficacy against a broad range of bacterial diarrheal pathogens. It was ineffective against *Campylobacter*, however, and by the mid-1980s in Asia cotrimoxazole had begun to encounter enough bacterial resistance from other organisms that its empiric use was hampered.

Nalidixic acid, the precursor of today's modern fluoroquinolones, was first used against TD in Asia, with great efficacy. It was generally well-tolerated, and liquid preparations were available for pediatric use. As the fluoroquinolones came into use, nalidixic acid was supplanted by norfloxacin and ciprofloxacin, and later generations of fluoroquinolones. These drugs were effective against nearly 100% of bacterial enteric pathogens. They were so effective that the length of treatment gradually shortened from 5 to 7 days to 1 day, and in some cases a single dose [5,6].

Although the seriousness of TD was often dismissed by physicians, travelers continued to live in fear of severe episodes, or having key parts of their trip ruined by cramps and the need to stay proximate to a toilet. This concern led to studies to see if taking antibiotics prophylactically was a practical way to prevent TD.

The first of these prophylaxis studies were done in the 1970s using doxycycline, 100 mg per day. The use of doxycycline reduced the risk of TD by 59% to 86% [7–9]. Studies with cotrimoxazole showed 79% to 94% protective efficacy, and later studies with ciprofloxacin showed an 80% to

100% reduction in TD [9]. Despite the demonstrated efficacy, the use of daily antibiotic prophylaxis against TD never became widespread. Physicians were concerned about the side effects of antibiotics when used in a large population of well people [10]. There were also concerns about how to treat someone who had already become ill using the primary treatment antibiotic. Because early treatment of TD with 1 day's course of antibiotic usually shortens the illness to less than 1 day, the feelings remained that travelers should carry presumptive treatment, but not take daily antibiotic prophylaxis.

## Prevention of traveler's diarrhea through personal hygiene precautions

From a traveler's point of view, not getting TD at all is the most favorable outcome. Despite the increase in interest in travel medicine over the past 15 years, the rates of TD in all destinations have not dropped below the levels first detected in the 1950s. Early studies found that 33% of travelers to Mexico reported TD in the first 1 to 2 weeks of travel [1]. Since then, rates in Mexico are at least that high, and rates in other destinations range from 8% to 90% [11].

In the meantime, doctors and nurses continue to promote the view that avoiding tap water that has not been boiled, or foods that have not been peeled or cooked, prevents TD. Only seven studies have directly addressed this question in the past 50 years, and six of seven found no correlation with personal hygiene measures and the rate of TD. These studies demonstrate a remarkable consistency in not finding a connection between personal hygiene choices and the rate of diarrheal illness:

- "Drinking bottled liquids, and avoiding salads, raw vegetables, and unpeeled fruits failed to prevent illness" (Mexico 1973) [12].
- "Illness was not associated with consumption of water or iced beverages. Illness was similarly not associated with consumption of vendor food, salads containing raw vegetables, other raw vegetables, or unpeeled fruits" (Mexico 1976) [13].
- "Thus, diarrhea seemed to occur more frequently the more a person tried to elude it!" (worldwide 1983) [14].
- "No significant differences between those who did and did not observe the rules were observed in children below the age of 15 years" (worldwide 1991) [15].
- "The incidence of TD was not associated with the presence or absence of any specific dietary errors or the number of them committed. The rate of TD among people who reported no errors was 33%" (Morocco 1995) [16].
- "Our study failed to confirm as risk factors certain foods widely believed to be associated with TD, such as leafy vegetables, unpeeled fruits, untreated water, and ice" (Nepal 1996) [17].

The seventh study showed a correlation between the number of dietary mistakes and the risk of getting diarrhea in the first 5 days of travel [18]. This study has been widely cited as the basis for dietary precautions in TD. The study has some limitations, however, that should prevent it from carrying the entire burden of proof that dietary caution prevents TD. The study design included handing out 2240 questionnaires to departing Swiss travelers to a wide variety of destinations. The questionnaires were meant to encourage participants to record what they ate at each meal for 3 days, and then to report whether they had TD within the first 5 days of travel. The travelers were completely unsupervised, and only 688 (31%) of the questionnaires were returned. This huge drop out rate makes it difficult to evaluate the validity of the questionnaires that were returned, as the authors of the study acknowledge.

The question as to whether dietary precautions prevent TD has been difficult to distinguish from the question of whether travelers are able to follow the precautions adequately. Three studies have shown that 95% to 98% of travelers made dietary "mistakes" during a typical holiday. The same studies have shown, however, that there is no direct correlation between the number of such mistakes and the risk of getting TD [12,14,19].

At this point it is worth acknowledging the evidence that personal hygiene precautions are sensible, even if they are not completely adequate to protect the traveler against TD. Bacterial enteric pathogens have been cultured from food items in open markets, and from street stands selling meals [20]. Water is known to be contaminated in most developing countries. Avoiding certain types of food and water makes sense. Why then do TD rates not change in the face of even careful travelers' efforts?

Virtually all tourists must take their meals in restaurants. There have been several studies that have shown that eating in a restaurant, compared with eating at one's own home or apartment, is an independent risk factor for developing TD, not related to the types of food eaten in the restaurant [21,22]. The risks of preparing a large volume of food for clients have been well known for decades. Restaurants in developed countries must be licensed to handle food, and willing to undergo periodic inspections of their food handling procedures. If violations are found, the restaurant can be shut down.

These types of licensing and inspection procedures have not been instituted in most developing countries. Food handlers may never receive training in hygienic practices. Further limitations may include lack of an adequate supply of water or electricity, resulting in poor handwashing and counter cleaning procedures, and intermittent refrigeration. Thawing meat can be placed in refrigerators above already prepared but uncovered casseroles or lasagnas, allowing raw meat juices to contaminate them. An inspection survey that was conducted in Kathmandu in 1995 to 1996 documented the 10 most common hygienic errors in tourist-oriented restaurants (Table 1) [CIWEC Clinic Travel Medicine Center, unpublished data].

Given the frequency and magnitude of restaurant hygiene violations in many developing countries, the efforts that travelers make to select clean foods may be sabotaged. For example, a cucumber may be peeled and sliced on a cutting board that has just been used to cut up raw chicken. The cucumber ordinarily is considered an acceptable choice, because it is peeled. Some travelers have promoted the idea of only eating foods that have reached an internal temperature of 165°F, and even use a thermometer to confirm their choices. This may not prove acceptable or practical, however, for most travelers.

Whether increased food precautions and fewer mistakes decrease the rate of TD is not known. What is known is that the rate of TD has not been demonstrated to decrease in the last 50 years, despite efforts to educate travelers in personal food precautions. It may be that only gradual improvements in food handling in developing countries will eventually change this situation.

Table 1
The 10 most common hygiene errors in a survey of restaurants in Kathmandu, Nepal

| | |
|---|---|
| 1. Cross-contamination | Raw meat and vegetables cut on same cutting board with same knife |
| 2. Employee hygiene | Soap not available at all sinks, including bathrooms and kitchen sinks; employees not washing hands after handling raw meats |
| 3. Hazardous foods unrefrigerated and uncovered all day | Lasagna, quiche, refried beans, white sauce are not subsequently heated to a high enough temperature |
| 4. Tap-water contamination | Blenders for fruit and yoghurt drinks or milkshakes and fruit presses are rinsed with tap water between use |
| 5. Iodine solutions are not strong enough | Vegetables are not soaked long enough or in deep enough containers to disinfect their surface |
| 6. Auxilliary foods and sauces not refrigerated or covered | Yogurt, milk, mayonnaise, and butter |
| 7. Improper food storage in refrigerator | Meats, raw and cooked, not covered and stacked on top of each other; uncovered and thawing raw meats dripping onto uncovered vegetables, noodles, beans, and so forth |
| 8. Inadequate refrigeration capacity | Refrigerators too old and small for the volume of food stored; refrigerator not cold enough; foods stored outside of refrigerator because of lack of space; interrupted electricity supply for hours at a time |
| 9. Sanitizing solutions not being used | Cutting boards, knives, counters, and tables |
| 10. Dish and utensil contamination | Employees handling clean glasses by rim, and silverware by the heads; clean, wet dishes stacked before drying; dirty towels used to dry clean dishes |

## Prevention of traveler's diarrhea through nonantibiotic methods

The use of antibiotics to prevent TD is effective, but not embraced by travel health professionals. Nonantibiotic methods have been used to try to reduce the risk of TD. Among these methods are bismuth subsalicylate and *Lactobacillus*.

Bismuth subsalicylate, sold as Pepto-Bismol in the United States, is perhaps an underused tool to prevent TD. Two studies have demonstrated up to 62% protective efficacy over a 7-day period [23,24]. The dose is two tablets four times per day. This dosage provides 800 mg of salicylate per day. Travelers who have reasons to avoid salicylates, such as those taking anticoagulants (blood-thinning medications), should avoid bismuth subsalicylate. Additional limitations to the use of bismuth subsalicylate are the amount of medication that needs to be brought along, and the occurrence of both black tongue and black stools caused by the medication.

There are many strains of *Lactobacillus* that have been used to try to prevent TD. Some strains work better than others, affording protection in the 15% to 30% range [25]. One study has been done among travelers who took *Lactobacillus GG,* an acid-resistant strain, which demonstrated 63% reduction in TD [26].

## Etiology of traveler's diarrhea

Studies on the etiology of TD depend on the efforts that are made by the laboratory involved. Given the enormous number of bacteria in normal stool, pathogens are discovered by using selective media and other techniques to isolate the organisms that are sought. Protozoa are looked for microscopically, and increasingly by antigen tests and polymerase chain reaction. Viruses can be observed with electron microscopy, but the specific type of virus is usually proved by antigen detection assays. Even with all of these efforts, all studies of travelers with TD fail to find a known pathogen in 20% to 50% of cases. Given the history of TD, with new organisms discovered through the decade of the 1970s, it is likely that more bacterial organisms will be found in this currently unknown category. Indeed, a putative pathogen has emerged in the last few years.

Enteroaggregative *E coli* (EAEC) are *E coli* with the propensity to form a distinctive cascading adherence pattern when grown on Hep-2 cells, and that do not secrete heat-stable or heat-labile enterotoxin [27]. Several studies have shown that this is actually a group of organisms that differ with respect to their virulence properties [28]. A prospective study in Mexico in 2002 looked at stool colonization by EAEC and ETEC over a 4-week period [24]. Fourteen subjects developed diarrhea within the first 2 weeks of the study, of which 12 had EAEC present. Half of those infected with EAEC, however, had another known pathogen present (five had ETEC present, and one had

*Salmonella*). During the course of the study, 20 of 40 subjects had asymptomatic EAEC infection.

A subsequent attempt was made to determine whether the symptomatic infections with EAEC in this same group of students could be predicted by the presence of known virulence factors in the symptomatic cases. The study showed no correlation, however, between virulence factor-positive EAEC and clinical illness [29].

A study of intestinal markers of inflammation in TD in two geographic regions of the world, Mexico and India, found that EAEC was often present without signs of inflammation. Inflammatory markers, such as lactoferrin, were more commonly found in the travelers in India rather than Mexico. This study was taken as further evidence that not all EAEC strains are pathogenic [30]. A study of travelers in three major destinations (Guadalajara, Mexico; Goa, India; and Ocho Rios, Jamaica) found that EAEC was present in 33%, 19%, and 26%, respectively, of travelers who presented with TD [31]. Only 90 (14%) of 636 of patients with diarrhea, however, had EAEC as the only pathogen. Mixed infections were again common.

EAEC seems to be a potentially important contributor to the etiology of TD in some parts of the world, but its exact significance will not be known until clinicians can diagnose its presence in the stool more easily, and evaluate whether that particular strain is pathogenic or not [32]. So far, the strains seem to be sensitive to the usual antibiotics that are used in TD. Of concern is the fact that EAEC strains are associated with persistent diarrhea in children in developing countries [33] and may be a cause of AIDS-related chronic diarrhea [34].

**Diagnosis of traveler's diarrhea**

TD is a clinical syndrome defined by a change in bowel habits and accompanying symptoms. The etiology is caused by a number of pathogenic organisms, including bacteria, protozoa, and viruses, and preformed toxins. The diagnosis of the etiology of TD is complex, encompassing microscopic examination of the stool, before and after concentration; culturing for pathogenic bacteria; and performing antigen-antibody testing on stool. In the context of travel, laboratories that are considered reliable are rarely available, and in any case, obtaining the results takes several days. The treatment of TD is usually empiric unless the problem is particularly severe or persistent.

A clinical definition of bacterial diarrhea is: "the sudden onset of relatively uncomfortable diarrhea." Sudden onset means the person can remember the time of day their illness began. Relatively uncomfortable refers to any combination of cramps, urgency, watery stools, up to and including fever, vomiting, and bloody stools.

Protozoal diarrhea, in contrast, usually presents as the more gradual onset of not-so-severe diarrhea. Patients can rarely recall the exact day their illness began, and often tolerate their symptoms for 1 to 2 weeks before seeking medical care [35]. In Nepal, protozoa account for 10% to 15% of the etiology of TD, depending on the season [30,36,37].

Stool examination is still a very useful tool in making a diagnosis during an episode of TD. The presence of fecal leukocytes is highly associated with a bacterial pathogen. The absence of fecal leukocytes, however, does not mean that a bacterial pathogen is not present. Half the bacterial pathogens isolated at the CIWEC Clinic in Kathmandu were in stools that did not show fecal leukocytes [unpublished data].

Specific antigen tests exist for *Giardia lamblia*, *Cryptosporidium*, and *E histolytica–E dispar*. These seem to compare favorably with stool examinations as a diagnostic tool. It is important to remember, however, that one only finds what one is looking for with these tests: if one orders a test for *Giardia* alone, and the patient has *Cryptosporidium* or *E histolytica*, one will not accidentally discover the true diagnosis. Stool examination, in skilled hands, still provides this opportunity.

**Treatment of traveler's diarrhea**

The decade of the 1990s may be viewed as a golden age in TD therapeutics. For a period of time, all bacterial enteric pathogens were susceptible to one class of antibiotics, the fluoroquinolones, which could be given for as short a course as 1 day [5]. Resistance to ciprofloxacin, the most commonly used fluoroquinolone was first detected in the early 1990s among *Campylobacter* infections in Thailand. In vitro *Campylobacter* resistance increased steadily in Thailand from 0% in 1987 to 96% in 1997. *Campylobacter* resistance also has increased in other areas. A study at the CIWEC Clinic Travel Medicine Center in Nepal from 2001 to 2003 found that 70% of *Campylobacter* isolates were resistant to ciprofloxacin (Prativa Pandey, MD, personal communication, 2004). The licensing of the use of fluoroquinolones in chicken feed in developed countries has coincided with increasing detection of resistant *Campylobacter* in the United States, Spain, and The Netherlands [38].

Fortunately, however, most other bacterial enteric pathogens have not yet become resistant to fluoroquinolones. ETEC studies from 1999 to 2002 show 0% to 1% resistance rates in five different studies [39]. *Shigella boydii* and *Shigella flexneri* also have shown little resistance so far. The more severe *Shigella dystenteriae* has demonstrated 60% resistance in India in 1998 [40], but remains susceptible to ciprofloxacin in most of the world.

The impact of high level *Campylobacter* resistance on the empiric treatment of TD can be calculated. In Nepal, where *Campylobacter* accounts for 28% of bacterial infections, a 70% resistance rate means that empiric treatment with ciprofloxacin of all suspected bacterial diarrheal infections theoretically fails in 20% of cases. This figure should be tempered with the knowledge that in vitro resistance of *Campylobacter* to ciprofloxacin does not always predict clinical failure. In Mexico, where *Campylobacter* constitutes only 1% to 5% of the etiology of TD in travelers, the impact of high-level resistance is tiny.

Where *Campylobacter* resistance has proved problematic, azithromycin has been used as a replacement for fluoroquinolones [41]. Azithromycin has also proved useful against other bacterial enteric pathogens. In a head-to-head comparison study, azithromycin, 1000 mg as a single dose, was compared with levofloxacin, 500 mg as a single dose, in the treatment of TD in Guadalajara, Mexico [42]. Cure rates and side effects were comparable between the two drugs. Drug sensitivity testing was not performed. Resistance to azithromycin seems to be developing, although results have been mixed. One study in 1994 in Bangkok showed 15% resistance of *Campylobacter* to azithromycin [43], but a subsequent study in 1995 showed no azithromycin resistance among *Campylobacter* isolates [41].

One new drug on the horizon that may contribute to treating or preventing TD is rifaximin, a virtually nonabsorbed antibiotic. Rifaximin has been licensed in some European countries for up to 15 years, but was not used in a systematic way to treat TD. The drug received Food and Drug Administration approval on May 26, 2004, for adults over the age of 12 years.

Several trials have been performed using rifaximin to treat TD in various geographic locations. Three hundred eighty travelers were studied in Guatemala, Mexico, and Kenya. Rifaximin, 200 mg three times a day for 3 days, was compared with rifaximin, 400 mg three times a day for 3 days, and placebo for 3 days in a double-blind study. Both dosing regimens shortened the time to the last unformed stool from 60 hours in the placebo group to 33 hours in the treatment groups ($P = .0001$) [44]. Rifaximin was compared with ciprofloxacin in a study in Mexico and Jamaica. One hundred eighty-seven people were randomized to receive either rifaximin, 400 mg twice a day for 3 days, or ciprofloxacin, 500 mg twice a day for 3 days. Clinical improvement and side-effects were comparable in both groups [45]. Because rifaximin is not absorbed from the intestinal tract, it should be safe to use in both children and pregnant women, although one review urged caution in pregnancy [46]. The drug may not be effective against invasive organisms, such as *Shigella* or *Campylobacter* [46]. Because of those limitations in treatment, the drug may prove to have greater value as a daily prophylaxis against TD. Studies testing rifaximin prophylaxis against TD have been performed, but not yet published.

Patients with TD often feel weak and orthostatic. They should always be encouraged to maintain adequate hydration to compensate for the magnitude of fluid losses commensurate with their particular illness. Particular care should be exercised when the patient has prolonged vomiting and diarrhea.

## Vaccines against traveler's diarrhea pathogens

The sheer burden of diarrheal disease around the world, and the mortality among infants in developing countries, has fueled the interest in vaccines to prevent the most severe diarrheal diseases. Injectable cholera vaccine dates to the early 1880s. An oral rotavirus vaccine was approved in the United States in August 1998, but was withdrawn from the American market in October 1999 because of concerns about intussusception following immunization. Live attenuated *Shigella* vaccines were first developed in the 1960s, but were later discontinued. An oral cholera vaccine containing whole-cell killed cholera bacteria with the B-subunit of cholera toxin has been licensed in a number of countries, but not the United States. This vaccine provides some limited protection against ETEC infection in travelers, but the duration of protection is short [47].

Vaccines against ETEC and *Campylobacter* are also being pursued. *Campylobacter* has emerged as a prominent and severe pathogen, particularly resistant to many antibiotics, but vaccine testing has been hampered by concerns that a vaccine might induce Guillain-Barré syndrome, a problem that has been associated with *Campylobacter* infections.

The overall problem in producing commercially viable vaccines against bacterial enteric pathogens is the fact that each bacterium has multiple serotypes, and there are several major bacteria to protect against. Vaccines that are produced individually are expensive to test, and are likely to be costly to the traveler. If efficacy were in the 50% to 60% range, and the bacteria accounted for only 20% of TD in a given area, the vaccine could deliver only 10% to 12% protection against the overall risk of TD. This is a hard sell for many travelers. Vaccines against enteric bacterial pathogens, however, hold out the promise of potentially reducing the severity of first-time TD attacks in travelers. This could allow travelers to have less fear of the consequences of their first episodes of TD, which occasionally result in all night bouts of vomiting, fever, abdominal cramps, and frequent diarrhea.

## Summary

TD has not proved as preventable as hoped, despite knowing that it is transmitted mainly through food. Travelers have little ability to select restaurants based on the kitchen hygiene. The rates of TD in travelers to developing countries have not changed in the past 50 years, either because the dietary precautions they are taught are not effective or they cannot be adhered to in the course of a pleasurable vacation.

Nonantibiotic prophylaxis with bismuth subsalicylate has the potential to prevent 40% to 60% of TD episodes in short-term travelers, and is probably underused. Antibiotic prophylaxis can prevent up to 90% of infections, but is not routinely recommended.

Empiric treatment of TD has been the best approach to dealing with this problem, but its usefulness is being undermined by growing antibiotic resistance in many parts of the world. Fluoroquinolones are still the most useful agents where *Campylobacter* is not a predominant pathogen. Rifaximin may prove to be a useful addition to the options for treatment and prophylaxis. If used for treatment, it may require a backup antibiotic in areas where *Campylobacter* and *Shigella* are prominent pathogens.

## References

[1] Kean BH. The diarrhea of travelers to Mexico: summary of five-year study. Ann Intern Med 1963;59:605–14.

[2] Kean BH, Schaffner W, Brennan RW, et al. The diarrhea of travelers: V. Prophylaxis with phthalylsulfathiazole and neomycin sulphate. JAMA 1962;180:367–71.

[3] Gorbach SL, Kean BH, Evans DG, et al. Travelers' diarrhea and toxigenic *Escherichia coli*. N Engl J Med 1975;292:933–6.

[4] Ostrosky-Zeichner L, Ericsson CD. Travelers' diarrhea. In: Zuckerman JN, editor. Principles and practice of travel medicine. Chichester: John Wiley & Sons; 2001. p. 154.

[5] Salam I, Katelaris P, Leigh-Smith S, et al. Randomised trial of single-dose ciprofloxacin for travellers' diarrhoea. Lancet 1994;344:1537–9.

[6] Petruccelli BP, Murphy GS, Sanchez JL, et al. Treatment of traveler's diarrhea with ciprofloxacin and loperamide. J Infect Dis 1992;165:557–60.

[7] Sack DA, Kaminsky DC, Sack RB, et al. Prophylactic doxycycline for travelers' diarrhea: results of a prospective double-blind study of Peace Corps volunteers in Kenya. N Engl J Med 1978;298:758–63.

[8] Sack RD, Froelich JL, Zulkh AW, et al. Prophylactic doxycycline for travelers' diarrhea: results of a prospective double-blind study of Peace Corps volunteers in Morocco. Gastroenterology 1979;76:1368–73.

[9] Rendi-Wagner P, Kollaritsch H. Drug prophylaxis for travelers' diarrhea. Clin Infect Dis 2002;34:628–33.

[10] Gorbach SL, Edelman R, editors. Travelers' diarrhea: National Institutes of Health Consensus Conference, Rev Infect Dis 1986;8(Suppl 2):S227–33.

[11] Steffen R, Sack RB. Epidemiology. In: Ericsson CD, DuPont HL, Steffen R, editors. Travelers' diarrhea. Hamilton, Ontario: BC Decker; 2003. p. 113.

[12] Loewenstein MS, Balows A, Gangarosa EJ. Turista at an international congress in Mexico. Lancet 1973;1:529–31.

[13] Merson MH, Morris GK, Sack DA, et al. Travelers' diarrhea in Mexico. N Engl J Med 1976; 294:1299–305.

[14] Steffen R, van der Linde F, Gyr K, et al. Epidemiology of diarrhea in travelers. JAMA 1983; 249:1176–80.

[15] Pitzinger B, Steffen R, Tschopp A. Incidence and clinical features of traveler's diarrhea in infants and children. Pediatr Infect Dis J 1991;719–23.

[16] Mattila L, Siitonen A, Kyronseppa H, et al. Risk behavior for travelers' diarrhea among Finnish travelers. J Travel Med 1995;2:77–84.

[17] Hoge CW, Shlim DR, Echeverria P, et al. Epidemiology of diarrhea among expatriate residents living in a highly endemic environment. JAMA 1996;275:533–8.

[18] Kozicki M, Steffen R, Schar M. Boil it, cook it, peel it or forget it: does this rule prevent travellers' diarrhoea? Int J Epidemiol 1985;14:169–72.

[19] Steffen R, Collard F, Tornieporth N. Epidemiology, etiology, and impact of traveler's diarrhea in Jamaica. JAMA 1999;281:811–7.

[20] Rasrinaul L, Suthienkul O, Echeverria PD, et al. Foods as a source of enteropathogens causing childhood diarrhea in Thailand. Am J Trop Med Hyg 1988;39:97–102.

[21] Tjoa WS, DuPont HL, Sullivan P, et al. Location of food consumption and travelers' diarrhea. Am J Epidemiol 1977;106:61–6.
[22] Ericsson CD, Pickering K, Sullivan P, et al. The role of location of food consumption in the prevention of travelers' diarrhea in Mexico. Gastroenterology 1980;79:812–6.
[23] Steffen R, DuPont HL, Heusser R, et al. Prevention of travelers' diarrhea by the tablet form of bismuth subsalicylate. Antimicrob Agents Chemother 1986;29:625–7.
[24] Steffen R. Worldwide efficacy of bismuth subsalicylate in the treatment of travelers' diarrhea. Rev Infect Dis 1990;6:153–7.
[25] Marteau PR, de Vrese M, Cellier CJ, et al. Protection from gastrointestinal diseases with the use of probiotics. Am J Clin Nutr 2001;73:430S–6S.
[26] Hilton E. *Lactobacillus GG* in prevention of travelers' diarrhea. J Travel Med 1997;4:41–3.
[27] Nataro J, Steiner T, Guerrant R. Enteroaggregative *Escherichia coli*. Emerg Infect Dis 1998;6:829–31.
[28] Adachi JA, Ericsson CD, Jiang ZD, et al. Natural history of enteroaggregative and enterotoxigenic *Escherichia coli* infection among US travelers to Guadalajara, Mexico. J Infect Dis 2002;185:1681–3.
[29] Huang DB, Jiang ZD, DuPont HL. Association of virulence factor-positive and -negative enteroaggregative *Escherichia coli* and occurrence of clinical illness in travelers from the United States to Mexico. Am J Trop Med Hyg 2003;69:506–8.
[30] Greenberg DE, Jiang ZD, Steffen R, et al. Markers of inflammation in bacterial diarrhea among travelers, with a focus on enteroaggregative *Escherichia coli* pathogenicity. J Infect Dis 2002;185:944–9.
[31] Adachi JA, Jiang ZD, Mathewson JJ, et al. Enteroaggregative *Escherichia coli* as a major etiologic agent in traveler's diarrhea in 3 regions of the world. Clin Infect Dis 2001;32:1706–9.
[32] Wanke CA. To know *Escherichia coli* is to know bacterial diarrheal disease. Clin Infect Dis 2001;32:1710–2.
[33] Bhan MK, Raj P, Levine MM, et al. Enteroaggregative *Escherichia coli* associated with persistent diarrhea in a cohort of rural children in India. J Infect Dis 1989;159:1061–4.
[34] Wanke CA, Gerrior J, Blais V, et al. Successful treatment of diarrhea disease associated with enteroaggregative *Escherichia coli* in adults with human immunodeficiency virus. J Infect Dis 1998;178:1369–72.
[35] Taylor DN, Houston R, Shlim DR, et al. Etiology of diarrhea among travelers and foreign residents in Nepal. JAMA 1988;260:1245–8.
[36] Hoge CW, Shlim DR, Echeverria P, et al. Epidemiology of diarrhea among expatriate residents living in a highly endemic environment. JAMA 1996;275:533–8.
[37] Shlim DR, Hoge CW, Rajah R, et al. Persistent high risk of diarrhea among foreigners in Nepal during the first two years of residence. Clin Infect Dis 1999;29:613–6.
[38] Smith KE, Besser JM, Hedberg CW, et al. Quinolone-resistant *Campylobacter jejuni* infections in Minnesota, 1992–1998. N Engl J Med 1999;340:1525–32.
[39] Vila J, Levy SB. Antimicrobial resistance. In: Ericsson CD, DuPont HL, Steffen R, editors. Travelers' diarrhea. Hamilton, Ontario: BC Decker; 2003. p. 61.
[40] Dutta S, Sinha T, Dutta P. Serotypes and antimicrobial susceptibility patterns of *Shigella* species isolated from children in Calcutta, India. Eur J Clin Microb Infect Dis 1998;17:298–9.
[41] Kuschner RA, Trofa AF, Thomas RJ, et al. Use of azithromycin for the treatment of *Campylobacter* enteritis in travelers to Thailand, an area where ciprofloxacin resistance is prevalent. Clin Infect Dis 1995;21:536–41.
[42] Adachi JA, Ericsson CD, Jiang ZD, et al. Azithromycin found to be comparable to levofloxacin for the treatment of US travelers with acute diarrhea acquired in Mexico. Clin Infect Dis 2003;37:1165–71.
[43] Hoge CW, Gambel JM, Srijan A, et al. Trends in antibiotic resistance among diarrheal pathogens isolated in Thailand over 15 years. Clin Infect Dis 1988;26:341–5.

[44] Steffen R, Sack DA, Riopel L, et al. Therapy of travelers' diarrhea with rifaximin on various continents. Am J Gastroenterol 2003;98:1073–8.
[45] DuPont HL, Jiang ZD, Ericsson CD, et al. Rifaximin versus ciprofloxacin for the treatment of traveler's diarrhea: a randomized, double-blind clinical trial. Clin Infect Dis 2001;33: 1807–15.
[46] Anonymous. Rifaximin (Xifaxan) for travelers' diarrhea. The Medical Letter 2004;46:74–5.
[47] Peltola H, Siitonen A, Kyronseppa H. Prevention of travellers' diarrhoea by oral B-subunit/whole-cell cholera vaccine. Lancet 1991;338:1285–9.

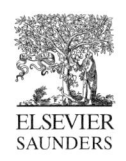

# Yellow Fever and Japanese Encephalitis Vaccines: Indications and Complications

Anthony A. Marfin, MD, MPH[a,*],
Rachel S. Barwick Eidex, PhD[b],
Phyllis E. Kozarsky, MD[b,c], Martin S. Cetron, MD[b,c]

[a]*Division of Vector-Borne Infectious Diseases, National Center for Infectious Diseases, Centers for Disease Control and Prevention, Fort Collins, CO 80522, USA*
[b]*Division of Global Migration and Quarantine, National Center for Infectious Diseases, Centers for Disease Control and Prevention, Atlanta, GA 30333, USA*
[c]*Department of Medicine, Emory University School of Medicine, Atlanta, GA, USA*

Appropriate administration of yellow fever (YF) or Japanese encephalitis (JE) vaccines to travelers requires an assessment of the traveler's risk for infection with these vector-borne flaviviruses during their travels and the presence of risk factors for adverse events following immunization. JE and YF vaccines have been more frequently associated with serious adverse events following immunization since the early 1980s and the late 1990s, respectively. This article describes the adverse events, the magnitude of their risk, and associated risk factors.

## Yellow fever

YF is a viral hemorrhagic fever caused by YF virus, a flavivirus. It only occurs in Africa and South America where an estimated 200,000 cases occur each year [1]. During urban human outbreaks, virus is spread by *Aedes aegypti*, a mosquito found in urban settings throughout the world. In contrast, YF viral transmission in rural areas involves tree-hole breeding mosquitoes [2]. After a 3- to 6-day viral incubation, fever, headache, photophobia, lumbosacral pain, epigastric pain, anorexia, and vomiting abruptly begin. Estimates vary but 15% or more of infected persons develop moderate to severe illness including overwhelming systemic disease. Severe

---

* Corresponding author. C/O PATH, 1455 NW Leary Way, Seattle, WA 98107.
 *E-mail address:* Aam0@cdc.gov (A.A. Marfin).

systemic disease is characterized by liver and renal failure and hemorrhage caused by thrombocytopenia and an acquired coagulopathy. Because there is no specific treatment, supportive care is the only treatment; the case fatality rate of severe systemic illness is about 20%, although it may be as high as 50% in some outbreaks.

Vaccination and eradication of *Ae aegypti* are the only effective strategies to reduce YF morbidity and mortality in affected areas. Since 1937, yellow fever vaccine (YEL) has been widely used in outbreaks and by military and civilian travelers to endemic areas. The Centers for Disease Control and Prevention (CDC) and the Advisory Committee on Immunization Practices recommend vaccination for travelers at risk for YF age 9 months and older going to specific areas in Africa and South America (Fig. 1) [3,4]. Over 125 countries legally require vaccination of international travelers for entry. Some countries require vaccination of all entering travelers, whereas others only require vaccination of travelers coming from YF-endemic areas. Generally, countries that have competent mosquito vectors require

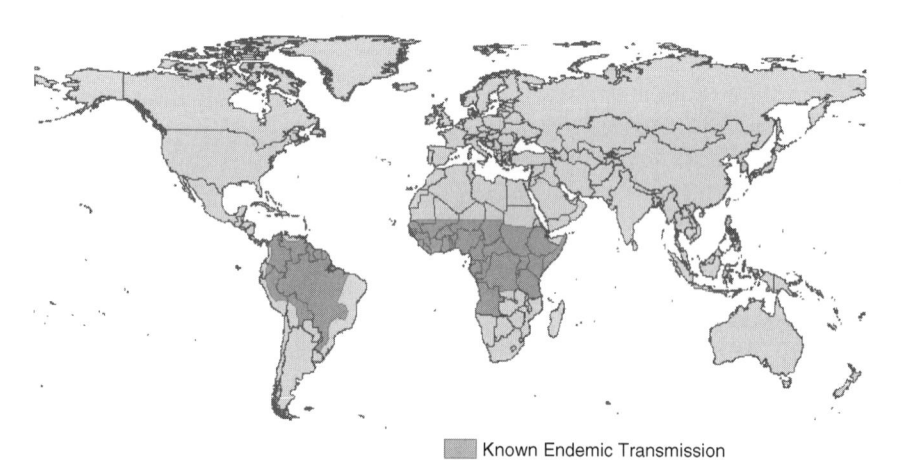

Fig. 1. Countries and regions with endemic yellow fever virus transmission. Shading is based on recent reports of human yellow fever infections or on the continued presence of ecologic factors associated with yellow fever virus transmission in areas with historical reports of human yellow fever infections. The map should be used only as a general guide to areas of risk of exposure to yellow fever. Some regions (eg, western Paraguay) are excluded from the endemic zone despite being bordered by areas of known yellow fever transmission and having ecologic zones that seem conducive to yellow fever transmission. These omissions likely reflect the absence of surveillance data rather than absence of transmission. Because areas of risk fluctuate at the borders of the endemic zone during periods of epizootic and epidemic activity, travelers are advised to seek updated information, particularly those who visit areas at the fringe of the endemic zone. The Centers for Disease Control and Prevention, tropical and travel medicine professionals, and local (in-country) public health departments are sources of additional information about geographic risk areas. (*Adapted from* the Centers for Disease Control and Prevention. Health information for international travelers, 2005–2006 [Yellow Book]. A frequently updated version of Yellow Book can be found at http://www.cdc.gov/travel/yb/index.htm and may be used to determine a person's actual need for yellow fever immunization).

vaccination to prevent an asymptomatic and viremic traveler from infecting local mosquitoes and establishing domestic transmission. The United States is a notable exception and has no vaccine entry requirement.

In the 1930s, *Ae aegypti* was present throughout the Caribbean and Central and South America. By 1970, control campaigns eradicated this vector from all large South American cities and greatly reduced the geographic range of *Ae aegypti*. Since 1970, *Ae aegypti* has re-established itself in areas that it previously occupied and spread across South America [5]. In Africa, *Ae aegypti* eradication never occurred and YF epidemics regularly occur in urban and rural settings [6,7].

The number of travelers going to YF-endemic areas is increasing; an estimated 500,000 to 1,000,000 unvaccinated American travelers enter such areas annually. In contrast, only about 200,000 American civilians receive YEL annually. As the number of unvaccinated travelers to YF-endemic areas has increased, there has been an increase in the reported number of imported YF cases into the United States and Europe [8–12]. In 1996 there was a report of an imported case of YF in an American traveler, the first American case in 72 years [12]. Since 1996, there have been two more American cases [9,10]. All three cases occurred in unvaccinated travelers and were fatal.

## Yellow fever vaccine

The need for YF vaccination remains. Although YEL has been considered one of the safest vaccines, recent reports of YEL-associated adverse events have raised concerns about vaccine safety [2,13]. YEL is a live, attenuated vaccine made with the 17D YF virus strain. Three distinct but related lineages (17D-204, 17DD, and 17D-213) have been developed; these three strains share 99.9% nucleic acid sequence homology [2,14,15]. The 17D-204 vaccine is manufactured in the United States, Europe, and Australia, and used in these countries and New Zealand; the 17DD vaccine is manufactured and used in South America; and the 17D-213 vaccine is manufactured in Germany.

## Adverse events

### General adverse events

Reactions to YEL are typically mild. After vaccination, vaccinees often report mild headaches, myalgia, low-grade fevers, or other minor symptoms for 5 to 10 days. In clinical trials, where symptoms are actively elicited, up to 25% of vaccinees report mild adverse events and up to 1% of vaccinees curtail regular activities [16,17]. Following primary vaccination, vaccine strain viremia occurs frequently among healthy persons but is usually waning or absent after the first week [2,18]. Viremia is generally not detectable in persons receiving repeat doses of YEL.

Immediate hypersensitivity reactions, characterized by rash, urticaria, or asthma, occur among persons with histories of allergies to egg or other substances; this is estimated to occur in 1 out of 131,000 vaccinations [19]. Gelatin, used as a stabilizer in YEL, has been implicated as a cause of allergic reactions to other vaccines and may play a role in reactions to YEL [17,20–22].

*Yellow fever vaccine–associated neurologic disease*

Before 1945, YEL-associated encephalitis among children was the most commonly reported serious adverse event following immunization. After standardization of the 17D seed lot system, such events decreased to one case per 8 million doses administered [2]. From 1945 to 2001, 23 YEL-associated encephalitis cases were reported worldwide; of these, 16 occurred among children aged 9 months or less and 7 among persons aged 3 to 76 years. In 1965, the first American case involved a 3-year-old child who died with encephalitis; this was the only fatal case among the 23 encephalitis cases. A second American case of neurologic disease involved a 76-year-old traveler who also developed severe systemic disease with hepatic and renal involvement [23].

Unlike these 23 earlier cases, most recently reported YEL-associated encephalitis cases occurred among adults. Since 2001, four Americans with encephalitis (aged 16, 36, 41, and 71 years) were reported to the Vaccine Adverse Event Reporting System (VAERS). All had illness onset 4 to 23 days following 17D-204 vaccination [24]. A retrospective review of 1995 to 2002 VAERS data identified four additional persons with Guillain-Barré syndrome, and since 2002 three cases of persons with demyelinating disease after vaccination were reported to VAERS. All 11 persons were hospitalized; none died. All developed illness after their first YEL vaccination but the time to illness onset was variable (4–23 days after vaccination). Of the encephalitis cases in which cerebrospinal fluid samples were tested, most had cerebrospinal fluid pleocytosis and all contained YF virus–specific IgM antibody. YEL-associated neurologic disease has also been recently reported from outside of the United States. In 2002, a 53-year-old man with a previously unrecognized HIV infection who developed encephalitis following vaccination and died was reported from Thailand [25]. In addition, four other international cases were reported to vaccine manufacturers from 1991 through 2001; these included two cases of encephalitis, one case of Guillain-Barré syndrome, and one case of bulbar palsy [26].

*Yellow fever vaccine–associated viscerotropic disease*

In 2001, a syndrome of fever and multiorgan system failure was first described among recipients of 17D-204 and 17DD vaccines [23,27,28]. During 1996 to 2003, nine American citizens (mean age: 67 years; range: 22–79 years) became ill 2 to 5 days after receiving 17D-204 [23,24]. All nine persons required intensive care after developing fever, hypotension, respiratory failure, elevated hepatocellular enzymes and bilirubin, lymphocytopenia, and thrombocytopenia; seven died. Vaccine-type virus was isolated from the blood of two patients 7 and 8 days after vaccination [23]. A third isolate came from cerebrospinal fluid obtained when the patient developed encephalitis. In three fatal cases, YF viral antigen was identified using immunohistochemistry. In two cases, antigen was found in multiple tissues (lung, lymph node, spleen, heart, liver, and muscle) and, in the third, antigen was only found in the liver. Flavivirus-like particles consistent with YF virus were identified by electron microscopy from tissue in one of these cases.

In addition to these American cases, two Brazilian citizens (aged 5 and 22 years) became ill 3 to 4 days after receiving 17DD vaccine in 1999 and 2000 [28], and an Australian citizen (aged 56 years) became similarly ill after receiving a 17D-204 vaccination in 2001 [24]. All died from 8 to 11 days following vaccination. In these cases, histopathologic changes similar to severe YF including midzonal necrosis, microvesicular fatty change, and Councilman's bodies were noted in the liver. YF antigen was identified in areas of midzonal necrosis from two recipients using immunohistochemistry. In the third patient, flavivirus-like particles were identified by electron microscopy in areas of midzonal necrosis. Vaccine strain virus was isolated from blood and autopsy material (ie, brain, liver, kidney, spleen, lung, skeletal muscle, or skin) from all three. Because the recovered viruses retained their vaccine-type phenotype in animals and did not have genomic changes previously associated with a reversion to virulence, Brazilian authorities assumed that these adverse events following immunization resulted from undefined host factors [29].

Since these initial reports, three more cases of severe adverse events after YF vaccination have been reported in the medical literature [30–32]. All were hospitalized with fever, renal abnormalities, and elevated hepatocellular enzymes; all recovered from their illness. Although YEL strain viremia infrequently occurs more than 1 week after vaccination [2,18], virus was isolated from the blood of one person 13 days after vaccination [32].

Most recently, in 2004, three more international cases of possible YEL-associated viscerotropic disease and fulminant hepatic failure were reported to the CDC through October. These include a 44-year-old Colombian man, a 61-year-old American man living in China, and a 26-year-old Spanish woman with illness onsets 6, 4, and 7 days after vaccination, respectively. The Colombian man and Spanish woman died 11 and 8 days after vaccination, respectively. In the case of the Colombian man, real-time, quantitative reverse transcriptase polymerase chain reaction detected 17DD vaccine strain sequences in a serum sampled 10 days after vaccination. No wild-type South American YF virus RNA sequences were found and no virus was isolated (B.W. Johnson, CDC, personal communication, 2004). The other two cases are under investigation.

## Risk factors for adverse events following immunization

*Age-associated risk*

Accurately measuring vaccine-associated viscerotropic and neurologic disease incidence is difficult because adequate prospective data are unavailable. Although VAERS solicits reports of adverse events after vaccination, it is a passive surveillance system that likely underestimates the true number of events and may have biased reporting [33]. In addition, the true number of YEL doses given to American civilians within each age group is unknown. Despite these limitations, using the number of cases reported to VAERS, the total vaccine doses sold in the United States and the age distribution of travelers receiving YEL at travel clinics, the authors estimated the reporting rate of these adverse events. Aventis Pasteur, the sole American YEL manufacturer, provided the annual number of single-dose vials purchased by civilian health care providers from 1990 through 2003. Because American health care providers previously reported minimal YEL wastage, it was assumed that the number of doses sold was a good estimate of administered doses [34]. In 1998, a survey was performed in 13 American clinics supporting the activities of GeoSentinel, an international network of travel-tropical medicine clinics established by the International Society of Travel Medicine and the CDC. To estimate the proportion of vaccine recipients by age group, these clinics reviewed and reported 12 months of YEL administration [34,35]. YEL-associated adverse events among American citizens reported to VAERS from 1990 through 2003 were categorized as viscerotropic or neurologic disease and classified by age group. Reporting rates for YEL-associated viscerotropic disease and neurologic disease in the United States were calculated by dividing the events reported by an estimate of the number of YEL vaccinations in each age group.

The American reporting rate of YEL-associated neurologic disease was estimated to be four cases per million distributed civilian doses. For viscerotropic disease, it was estimated to be three cases per million. A similar incidence has recently been reported in the United Kingdom [26].

For vaccinees aged 60 years and older, there were 17 cases of YEL-associated neurologic disease per million distributed civilian doses. This was more than seven times higher than the rate among younger persons, which was 2.3 cases per million. This increased age-related risk was more pronounced for YEL-associated viscerotropic disease. For vaccinees aged 60 and older, there were 20.5 cases of YEL-associated viscerotropic disease per million distributed civilian doses. This was more than 20 times higher than the rate among younger persons, which was one case per million. The rate of either YEL-associated syndrome among persons aged 60 to 69 years and 70 years or older was 35 cases and 41 cases per million distributed civilian doses, respectively.

*Thymus disease*

Only 25 cases of YEL-associated viscerotropic disease have been identified worldwide as of October 2004; thus, identifying risk factors for this adverse event remains challenging. Surprisingly, four (16%) had a history of thymic tumor and thymectomy, both uncommon conditions, suggesting that thymus disease is another independent risk factor for YEL-AVD. One fatal case, a 67-year-old woman, was vaccinated with YEL approximately 2 years after a thymectomy for a malignant thymoma. A second fatal case was a 44-year-old Colombian man who had a thymectomy 2 years before vaccination to remove a benign thymoma. A third case was a 70-year-old man with a history of myasthenia gravis and thymoma who was vaccinated approximately 20 years after a thymectomy. A fourth case was a 50-year-old man who had a thymectomy to remove a benign thymoma 8 years before vaccination. These latter two cases survived. Thymus tumors have been associated with significant abnormalities of the humoral and cellular immune systems, although the mechanisms are not well-understood [36–38]. The package insert for YF-Vax was updated in 2003 to include thymoma as a potential contraindication.

**Yellow fever: conclusion**

Physicians need to balance carefully the risks and benefits of YEL and only administer vaccine to persons truly at risk for YF viral infection. Currently, in the United States there is underuse of YEL among travelers who need protection from infection and inappropriate vaccination of persons traveling to areas that do not have a significant risk of YF. Both practices may be caused by a misinterpretation of the vaccine requirements for country entry or an inadequate review of the traveler's itinerary. In addition, there is an emergence of new high-risk populations for serious YEL-associated adverse events that includes persons aged 60 years and older and persons with thymoma or history of thymectomy.

To improve the quality of these travelers' risk assessments, information concerning known or probable infected areas is available from the World Health Organization (http://www.who.int), the Pan American Health Organization (http://www.paho.org), and the CDC (http://www.cdc.gov/travel).

**Japanese encephalitis**

JE virus, a mosquito-borne flavivirus, is the leading cause of viral encephalitis in Asian children, where as many as 50,000 cases may be reported annually [39,40]. Although less than 1% of infected persons develop encephalitis [41], the severity of illness, case fatality rate up to 25%, and occurrence of neuropsychiatric sequelae in 50% of survivors are strong arguments for travelers to consider JE vaccination when traveling to endemic areas.

In JE endemic areas, infection is common. Seroprevalence studies show that most persons have developed JE-specific antibody by the time they are young adults [42,43]. Before establishing vaccination programs, the annual incidence of encephalitis was as high as 10 to 20 per 100,000 in endemic countries. Because as many as 250 people may be infected and asymptomatic for every one case of JE, the actual infection rate may be as high as 5% per year in these areas. Older residents are protected from illness because of their acquired immunity following natural infection but travelers from nonendemic countries do not have this immunity unless they are immunized.

Two transmission patterns are present in Asia (Fig. 2). One pattern is seasonal transmission that may result in large epidemics in more temperate northern regions (eg, Japan, People's Republic of China, Taiwan, Korea, northern Vietnam, northern Thailand, northern India, and Nepal). The second pattern is year-around transmission and occurs in tropical southern regions (eg, southern Vietnam, southern Thailand, southern India, Indonesia, Malaysia, Philippines, and Sri Lanka). Year-around transmission can cause epidemics but it is more generally characterized by endemic or sporadic transmission [43]. JE virus is primarily transmitted

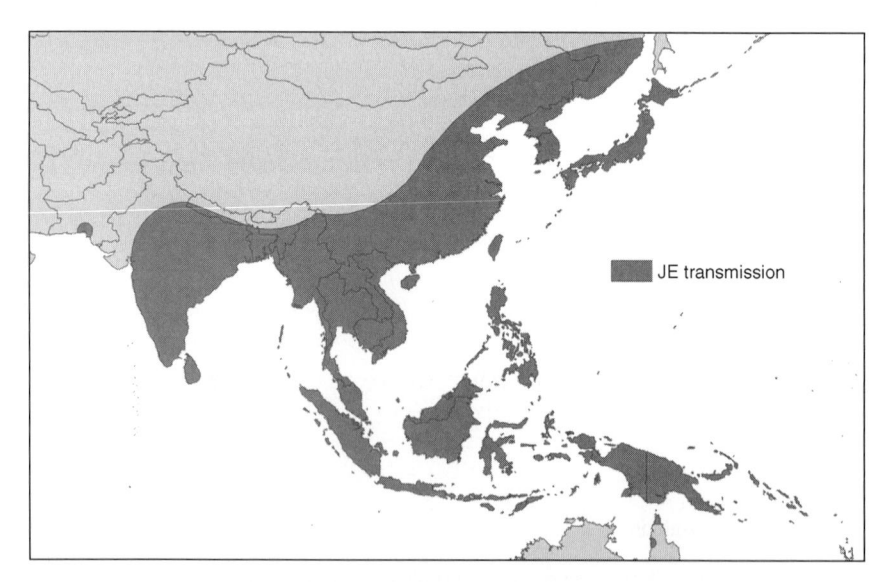

Fig. 2. Countries and regions with endemic Japanese encephalitis virus transmission. Shading is based on recent reports of Japanese encephalitis or on the continued presence of ecologic factors associated with Japanese encephalitis transmission in a country with a history of Japanese encephalitis transmission (*Modified from* Centers for Disease Control and Prevention at http://www.cdc.gov/ncidod/dvbid/jencephalitis/map.htm. Accessed October 29, 2004).

in an enzootic cycle between *Culex* mosquitoes (eg, *C tritaeniorhyncus, C vishnui, C pseudovishnui*) and amplifying vertebrate hosts (eg, domestic pigs, ardeid birds [egrets, herons]). In contrast to YF virus where humans may be critical to virus transmission as the amplifying host, humans play no role in the maintenance or amplification of JE virus in the transmission cycle. Consequently, in areas where JE vaccine coverage or natural immunity is high and human cases do not occur, JE virus may still be transmitted in an enzootic cycle.

Vector mosquito species are prolific in rural areas of Asia where they breed in flooded fields associated with rice production. In these areas, JE mosquito infection rates may be as high as 3%. The abundance of vector mosquitoes fluctuates with rainfall, but in many tropical locations irrigation patterns have now become a more important factor affecting vector abundance. The conditions specific to rural settings in Asia (ie, large populations of pigs, wading birds, rice production) greatly increase the risk of JE virus infection in unvaccinated persons. Because of the potential for year-round transmission in rural areas, the ineffectiveness of vector control, and the high morbidity and mortality of symptomatic disease, JE vaccination has been considered the primary prevention method in endemic areas.

JE viral incubation is 5 to 15 days. The earliest symptoms are the abrupt onset of fever, headache, abdominal pain, nausea, and vomiting. Over the course of several days, less than 1% of infected persons develop encephalopathy including agitated delirium, unsteady gait, and abnormal motor movements before progressing to somnolence and coma. The most frequently reported clinical syndrome is acute encephalitis, especially among hospitalized persons, but it is likely that milder neurologic syndromes (eg, aseptic meningitis, febrile headache) occur. Recent studies have drawn attention to cases of acute flaccid paralysis without signs of encephalitis, initially misdiagnosed as poliomyelitis cases [44,45]. Most clinical accounts are derived from case series of children living in endemic areas; the degree to which their clinical course is modified by previous exposure to other flaviviruses or by their young age is not known. As a result, generalizing clinical findings to older travelers from nonendemic countries should be done with caution.

Supportive care remains the most important treatment. Although there is no known specific antiviral treatment for JE virus or other closely related flaviviruses, this supportive care and the use of modalities to reduce intracerebral pressure (eg, mannitol) or seizures (eg, phenobarbital) when present may reduce morbidity and mortality. In controlled trials, dexamethasone and interferon alfa-2a did not improve clinical outcome [42,45,46].

## Japanese encephalitis vaccines

Since the mid-1970s, more than 500 million doses of JE vaccine (JEV) have been administered in the People's Republic of China, Japan, Korea, and Taiwan and disease incidence has been reduced to near-elimination levels [47]. Three types of JEV have been widely used [48]: (1) an inactivated mouse brain–derived vaccine; (2) an inactivated primary hamster kidney cell–derived vaccine; and (3) a live, attenuated vaccine (SA14-14-2). Only inactivated mouse brain–derived vaccine is available internationally for travelers from nonendemic countries. This is a formalin-inactivated vaccine prepared by purifying JE virus from the brains of mice inoculated intracerebrally with JE virus. Although the vaccine undergoes two major purification steps including ultracentrifugation, complete removal of mouse proteins is not possible. Each 1-mL dose of vaccine contains less than 50 ng of mouse serum proteins and no detectable murine myelin basic protein [49]. It is this potential contamination that elicits concern for allergic reactions and other adverse events following immunization. Other constituents include gelatin from bovine and porcine sources, formaldehyde, and thimerosal. Except for a 1989 change in the strain used to produce vaccine for Japan's domestic market, there have been no changes in the manufacturing process.

The efficacy of the inactivated, mouse brain–derived JE vaccine has been demonstrated in a placebo-controlled, randomized clinical trial in Thai children [39]. In a trial of more than 40,000 children, JE incidence among persons receiving two vaccine doses was 5 cases per 100,000 compared with 51 cases per 100,000 among persons who were not vaccinated. No serious side effects were reported following both the first or second dose, and the rates of lesser side effects (eg, headache, sore arm, rash, local swelling) were less than 1% and similar to the rates among placebo recipients.

The vaccine efficacy, low rate of side effects, and high morbidity and mortality among children with severe disease should make incorporation of this vaccine into national children's vaccination programs for children living in endemic areas a relatively easy decision. The greatest impediments to vaccine use in these settings have been the high cost of the mouse brain–derived vaccine, the cost and logistics of delivery imposed by a two-dose regimen, and the need for a boosting dose.

Since 1992, the inactivated, mouse brain–derived vaccine has been licensed in the United States. It is recommended that travelers and other persons who do not reside in areas endemic for JE virus receive three vaccine doses rather than the two doses recommended for persons living in endemic countries [49]. Because travelers, in general, do not have background flaviviral antibody, the additional dose is intended to improve the antibody response.

Because travelers do not share the same lifelong risk of infection and may not have the same high rates of morbidity and mortality, indications for the use of the vaccine are less clear. In addition, since the early 1980s, the risk of serious adverse events among western travelers and military personnel have been more frequently reported and made the risk-benefit analysis much more complex [50].

## Adverse events

### General adverse events

More than 500 million doses of the inactivated mouse brain–derived JE vaccine have been given in Asia since the late 1950s and have been associated with a low-to-moderate frequency of local and mild systemic adverse effects in Asian residents and travelers [40,51]. Tenderness, redness, swelling, and other local effects at the injection site were reported in about 20% of vaccinees. Fever, headache, malaise, rash, and other systemic effects (eg, chills, dizziness, myalgia, nausea, vomiting, and abdominal pain) were reported in approximately 10% of JEV recipients.

### Serious allergic adverse events

In early studies of an earlier preparation of the current inactivated vaccine, more serious adverse events following vaccination were seen. In a large study of more than 53,000 American military personnel vaccinated in 1947, 19 developed allergic reactions including urticaria and angioedema, a rate of 3.5 allergic events per 10,000 vaccinees [52].

From the late 1980s through the mid-1990s, a new pattern of serious allergic adverse events emerged. Adverse events following immunization with JE vaccine including angioedema and urticaria were first reported from Europe, North America, and Australia [49,50]. Of concern was the fact that many of these reactions were delayed by days and sometimes weeks after vaccination and the rate of allergic adverse events was increased when compared with the earlier studies performed in American military personnel. The reactions have been characterized by urticaria, often in a generalized distribution, or angioedema of the extremities, face (especially of the lips), and oropharynx. Although no cases of anaphylaxis were specifically noted, respiratory distress was reported in three vaccinees and collapse caused by hypotension or other causes leading to hospitalization was noted in several other cases. Most reactions were treated successfully with antihistamines or oral steroids; however, some patients were hospitalized for parenteral steroid therapy.

An important feature of these reactions has been the interval between vaccination and onset of symptoms. Roughly half of the reactions after the first immunization dose occurred 12 hours after administration (88% of reactions occurred within 3 days). The interval between administration of a second dose and onset of allergic symptoms generally was longer (median 3 days after administration; ranging up to 2 weeks). Reactions have occurred after a second or third dose, when preceding doses were received uneventfully.

Throughout the 1990s, several prospective, cohort studies were performed to determine the risk of allergic reactions following immunization with the inactivated mouse brain–derived vaccine [50]. For example, during a 7-month period from 1991 to 1992, 35,253 US Navy personnel and their dependents were vaccinated with the inactivated mouse brain–derived vaccine; 220 developed allergic symptoms [49]. Overall, the rate of mildly to moderately severe adverse events (including urticaria, angioedema, generalized itching, or wheezing) was 62 per 10,000 vaccinees. Of 35,253 vaccinees, nine were hospitalized (2.6 per 10,000 vaccinees) for refractory urticaria to receive intravenous steroids but none were considered life-threatening reactions. One death occurred in a 21-year-old man with a recurrent history of hypersensitivity reactions including a previous episode of anaphylaxis; the cause of death could not be established at autopsy. The rate of adverse events was greater following the first and second doses. The adverse event rate per 10,000 vaccinees was 27, 31, and 12 after the first, second, or third dose, respectively. A case-control study was conducted as part of this immunization campaign. Persons developing these reactions were nine times more likely to have had a past history of urticaria or angioedema after hymenoptera envenomation; following use of medications (eg, nonsteroidal anti-inflammatory drugs, sulfonamides, opioids); following physical triggers (eg, dermatographism, cold); or a history of chronic idiopathic urticaria. An increased risk for allergic adverse events among persons with an allergic predisposition was also noted in a Danish case-control study reported in 2000 [53]. The specific vaccine constituents responsible for these adverse reactions have not been identified.

*Serious neurologic adverse events*

The small amount of murine neural tissue in the vaccine has always raised concerns about the possibility of vaccine-related neurologic side effects. Surveillance of JEV-related neurologic complications in Japan during the years 1965 to 1973 identified cases of neurologic illness, such as encephalitis, seizures, and peripheral neuropathy, occurred at a rate of 1 to 2.3 per million vaccinees [49]. Very rarely, deaths occurred with vaccine-associated encephalitis. Despite decades of vaccine use, the first nine cases of postvaccination acute disseminated encephalomyelitis were reported in Japan in the 1990s [54,55]. In addition, in the late 1990s, a case of acute disseminated myelitis developed in a Japanese adolescent 2 weeks after receiving the inactivated vaccine [50]. In all 10 of these reported cases, symptom onset occurred within 1 month of vaccination and diagnostic white matter lesions were demonstrated with MRI; in some, increased levels of the myelin basic protein were demonstrated. Because of the presumed immunologic basis for these processes, all were treated with intravenous corticosteroids. A slightly different process was described when a 4-year-old Japanese girl developed acute transverse myelitis 2 weeks following vaccination with the inactivated vaccine. MRI showed diffuse swelling of the cervical and lumbar cord. Although the pathologic process was unknown, a cellular autoimmune mechanism against JE vaccine components was suspected and the child was treated with intravenous corticosteroids. No prospective studies to determine the rates for these events have been performed.

From 1983 through 1996, 384,000 doses of inactivated vaccine were administered to Danish travelers; 10 adult travelers were reported to have moderate to severe neurologic symptoms within weeks of their vaccination. All symptoms involved the central nervous system including encephalitis, seizures, gait disturbances, parkinsonism, development of white matter lesions, and myelitis [56]. Although causality was not established, this resulted in a rate of serious neurologic adverse event of 26 events per million vaccinations, roughly 10 times higher than previously reported rates from Japan in the 1960s and 1970s.

Based on postmarketing surveillance data from Japan and the United States in the late 1990s, the reported rates for all adverse events following the administration of inactivated mouse brain–derived JE vaccine doses was 2.8 in Japan and 15 in the United States per 100,000 [57]. In Japan, 17 neurologic disorders were reported, an estimated rate of two events per 1,000,000 doses. This rate was similar to the rates reported in the mid-1970s in Japan. In the United States, no serious neurologic adverse events were reported. The rates for allergic adverse events were 0.8 and 6.3 per 100,000 doses in Japan and the United States, respectively. Although VAERS data are passively collected, they suggest that hypersensitivity reactions with a delayed onset continue to occur among recipients of the inactivated JEV and that conservative recommendations limiting its use to travelers at high risk of infection with JE are appropriate.

### Traveler's risk

After the deaths of two American citizens who developed JE while staying in Beijing in the early 1980s, the use of this inactivated JEV was extended to travelers and military personnel from North America and Western Europe visiting JE-endemic areas.

Five factors should be considered when determining the appropriateness of JE vaccination for western travelers to an Asian country: (1) enzootic virus activity may be widespread in the absence of human disease, (2) the rate of JE viral illness is low among travelers, (3) JE viral encephalitis has high mortality and high rates of permanent disability in survivors, (4) there is no virus-specific treatment that can change the outcome of illness, and (5) there have been increasing concerns over the safety of the vaccine over the past 15 to 20 years [43].

Assessing an unvaccinated traveler's risk of infection and progression to illness is difficult. Like West Nile and St. Louis encephalitis viruses in North America, JE virus is a zoonotic virus that circulates between vertebrate amplifying hosts and zoophilic mosquito species. In countries where introduction of national immunization programs has reduced human disease incidence to near-elimination levels, JE virus may still circulate in animal populations [58]. In countries where national immunization programs have not been established, poor JE disease surveillance and lack of diagnostic testing likely result in an underestimate of JE incidence. Human JE incidence in such countries may not be a good gauge for traveler's risk.

The rate of disease among travelers from the United States, Canada, and Western Europe may be used to assess risk. Unfortunately, systematically collected data for travel-associated JE illnesses are not available. From 1978 through 1992, only 24 travel-related cases of JE were reported to the CDC. They included 11 American residents, of whom eight cases were military personnel or their dependents; only one case was a tourist. No cases were reported to the CDC from 1993 through 2003. In 2004, one unvaccinated American college student traveling in rural Thailand developed a nonfatal case of JE viral encephalitis and required mechanical ventilation and intensive care (Mira Leslie, personal communication, 2004). Despite the limitations of these data, the incidence among travelers seems low and is estimated to be far less than one in a million American travelers to endemic areas [49]. This estimate is likely to be low because persons making short trips or trips to urban centers where risk is low have been included in the denominator and because JE viral illness is likely to be underreported.

Unvaccinated western travelers or military personnel living in rural areas should have the same risk for JE as unvaccinated residents. As a result, risk can be extrapolated from incidence rates in the resident population. Assuming an incidence rate of 10 per 10,000 and a 5-month transmission period, the estimated risk for JE during the transmission season is 0.5 to 2 per 10,000 per week. In studies of unvaccinated military personnel with intense exposure in endemic areas from 1945 through 1991, the rate of JE was estimated to be up to 2.1 per 10,000 per week and comparable with the incidence among unvaccinated children in these same areas [41,49].

Because travelers' exposure to infected mosquitoes is often lower than residents of affected areas, the decision to use JEV must balance the risk of infection; the risk of developing illness after infection; the availability and use of personal protection (eg, insect repellents, protective clothing, well-screened or air-conditioned sleeping quarters, and avoidance of outdoor activity when vector mosquitoes are feeding); and the side effects of vaccination. The risk of being bitten by a JE-infected mosquito is rarely known. In general, this risk increases when travelers have longer stays during periods of epidemic virus transmission. The risk of becoming infected decreases when travelers are properly vaccinated and when the traveler has decreased exposure to infected mosquitoes through the use of personal protections that reduce nocturnal feeding by *Culex* mosquitoes. The risk for JE infection and illness is believed to be low for westerners visiting Asia but the risk of infection is highly variable and dependent on the destination of travel, the activities of the traveler, and the season of travel.

## Vaccine recommendations for travelers

Vaccine has been recommended for persons 1 year of age and older spending a month or longer in epidemic or endemic areas during the transmission season, especially with travel to rural areas [49]. Local JE incidence, the conditions of housing, nature of activities, duration of stay, and the potential for unexpected travel to high-risk areas are factors that must be considered when making the decision to vaccinate. Depending on the circumstances, vaccine should be considered for persons spending less than 30 days when their activities place them at particularly high risk for exposure (eg, outdoor activities in rural area). In all instances, regardless of their JE vaccination status, travelers are still advised to take personal precautions to reduce exposure to mosquito bites.

In endemic countries that use the inactivated mouse brain–derived vaccine, a two-dose regimen is recommended [49]. Two doses are effective in this setting because pre-existing immunity to related flaviviruses and subsequent flaviviral infections contribute to a robust and durable immune response. Based on studies performed in western military personnel and travelers [49,51], three doses of the inactivated mouse brain–derived vaccine given over a 30-day period (given on Days 0, 7, and 30) are recommended for residents of nonendemic countries. In persons from nonendemic countries who only received two doses, neutralizing antibody titers greater than or equal to 8 was found in only 77% of recipients. In addition, antibody levels declined substantially in most vaccines within 6 months of the second dose. Because the full duration of protection is not known, boosters are recommended every 3 years or when JE virus–specific neutralizing antibody is no longer present.

Little is known about risk factors for developing serious neurologic illness [42]. Like West Nile and St. Louis encephalitis viruses, two closely related viruses, advanced age may be a risk factor for developing symptomatic illness after infection among travelers. In addition, conditions that lower the integrity of the blood-brain barrier may increase the probability of developing JE. Infection acquired during pregnancy carries the potential for intrauterine infection and fetal death. These factors should be considered when advising elderly persons and pregnant women who plan visits to JE-endemic countries.

Adverse reactions to JEV manifesting as generalized urticaria or angioedema may occur within minutes following vaccination. Persons with a past history of urticaria or angioedema after hymenoptera envenomation, following use of medications (eg, nonsteroidal anti-inflammatory drugs, sulfonamides, opioids), or following physical triggers (eg, dermatographism, cold) or a history of chronic idiopathic urticaria may have a greater risk of developing reactions to JEV. This history should be considered when weighing risks and benefits of the vaccine for an individual patient. When patients with such a history are offered vaccine, they should be alerted to their increased risk for reaction and monitored appropriately. There are no data supporting the efficacy of prophylactic antihistamines or steroids in preventing JEV-related allergic reactions.

**Japanese encephalitis: conclusions**

The decision to use JEV in travelers should balance the risk of becoming infected and ill, the risk of adverse events following immunization, and the availability and acceptability of repellents and other alternative measures to reduce risk of infection. Risk of infection should be interpreted cautiously because risk can vary within areas and from year to year and available data are often incomplete.

**Acknowledgments**

The authors thank Ms. Jodi Udd of PATH, Seattle, Washington, for the maps of yellow fever and Japanese encephalitis transmission that were derived from maps on the websites of the US Centers for Disease Control and Prevention.

**References**

[1] WHO. District guidelines for yellow fever surveillance. Yellow fever technical consensus meeting. Geneva, March 2–3, 1998. WHO/EPI/GEN/98.08, 1–25. Geneva, Switzerland: WHO; 1998.
[2] Monath TP. Yellow fever. In: Plotkin SA, Orenstein WA, editors. Vaccines. Philadelphia: WB Saunders; 2004. p. 1095–176.
[3] Centers for Disease Control and Prevention. Health information for international travel 2003–2004. Atlanta (GA): US Department of Health and Human Services; 2003.
[4] Cetron MS, Marfin AA, Julian KG, et al. Yellow fever vaccine. Recommendations of the Advisory Committee on Immunization Practices (ACIP), 2002. MMWR Recomm Rep 2002;51:1–11.
[5] Gubler DJ. The changing epidemiology of yellow fever and dengue, 1900 to 2003: full circle? Comp Immunol Microbiol Infect Dis 2004;27:319–30.
[6] Monath TP. Facing up to re-emergence of urban yellow fever. Lancet 1999;353:1541.
[7] Nasidi A, Monath TP, DeCock K, et al. Urban yellow fever epidemic in western Nigeria, 1987. Trans R Soc Trop Med Hyg 1989;83:401–6.
[8] Barros ML, Boecken G. Jungle yellow fever in the central Amazon. Lancet 1996;348:969–70.
[9] Centers for Disease Control and Prevention. Fatal yellow fever in a traveler returning from Amazonas, Brazil, 2002. MMWR Morb Mortal Wkly Rep 2002;51:324–5.
[10] Fatal yellow fever in a traveler returning from Venezuela, 1999. MMWR Morb Mortal Wkly Rep 2000;49:303–5.
[11] Colebunders R, Mariage JL, Coche JC, et al. A Belgian traveler who acquired yellow fever in the Gambia. Clin Infect Dis 2002;35:e113–6.
[12] McFarland JM, Baddour LM, Nelson JE, et al. Imported yellow fever in a United States citizen. Clin Infect Dis 1997;25:1143–7.

[13] Barrett AD. Yellow fever vaccines. Biologicals 1997;25:17–25.
[14] Smithburn KC, Durieux C, Koerber R, et al. Yellow fever vaccination. WHO Monograph Series, Number 30. Geneva, Switzerland: World Health Organization; 1956.
[15] Pugachev KV, Ocran SW, Guirakhoo F, et al. Heterogeneous nature of the genome of the ARILVAX yellow fever 17D vaccine revealed by consensus sequencing. Vaccine 2002;20: 996–9.
[16] Lang J, Zuckerman J, Clarke P, et al. Comparison of the immunogenicity and safety of two 17D yellow fever vaccines. Am J Trop Med Hyg 1999;60:1045–50.
[17] Monath TP, Nichols R, Archambault WT, et al. Comparative safety and immunogenicity of two yellow fever 17D vaccines (ARILVAX and YF-VAX) in a phase III multicenter, double-blind clinical trial. Am J Trop Med Hyg 2002;66:533–41.
[18] Reinhardt B, Jaspert R, Niedrig M, et al. Development of viremia and humoral and cellular parameters of immune activation after vaccination with yellow fever virus strain 17D: a model of human flavivirus infection. J Med Virol 1998;56:159–67.
[19] Kelso JM, Mootrey GT, Tsai TF. Anaphylaxis from yellow fever vaccine. J Allergy Clin Immunol 1999;103:698–701.
[20] Kelso JM, Jones RT, Yunginger JW. Anaphylaxis to measles, mumps, and rubella vaccine mediated by IgE to gelatin. J Allergy Clin Immunol 1993;91:867–72.
[21] Sakaguchi M, Inouye S. Two patterns of systemic immediate-type reactions to Japanese encephalitis vaccines. Vaccine 1998;16:68–9.
[22] Miyazawa H, Saitoh S, Kumagai T, et al. Specific IgG to gelatin in children with systemic immediate- and nonimmediate-type reactions to measles, mumps and rubella vaccines. Vaccine 1999;17:2176–80.
[23] Martin M, Tsai TF, Cropp B, et al. Fever and multisystem organ failure associated with 17D-204 yellow fever vaccination: a report of four cases. Lancet 2001;358:98–104.
[24] Centers for Disease Control and Prevention. Adverse events associated with 17D-derived yellow fever vaccination—United States, 2001–2002. MMWR Morb Mortal Wkly Rep 2002;51:989–93.
[25] Kengsakul K, Sathirapongsasuti K, Punyagupta S. Fatal myeloencephalitis following yellow fever vaccination in a case with HIV infection. J Med Assoc Thai 2002;85:131–4.
[26] Kitchener S. Viscerotropic and neurotropic disease following vaccination with the 17D yellow fever vaccine, ARILVAX. Vaccine 2004;22:2103–5.
[27] Chan RC, Penney DJ, Little D, et al. Hepatitis and death following vaccination with 17D-204 yellow fever vaccine. Lancet 2001;358:121–2.
[28] Vasconcelos PF, Luna EJ, Galler R, et al. Serious adverse events associated with yellow fever 17DD vaccine in Brazil: a report of two cases. Lancet 2001;358:91–7.
[29] Galler R, Pugachev KV, Santos CL, et al. Phenotypic and molecular analyses of yellow fever 17DD vaccine viruses associated with serious adverse events in Brazil. Virology 2001;290: 309–19.
[30] Adhiyaman V, Oke A, Cefai C, et al. Effects of yellow fever vaccination. Lancet 2001;358: 1907–8.
[31] Troillet N, Laurencet F. Effects of yellow fever vaccination. Lancet 2001;358:1908–9.
[32] Werfel U, Popp W. Effects of yellow fever vaccination. Lancet 2001;358:1909.
[33] Rosenthal S, Chen R. The reporting sensitivities of two passive surveillance systems for vaccine adverse events. Am J Public Health 1995;85:1706–9.
[34] Martin M, Weld LH, Tsai TF, et al. Advanced age a risk factor for illness temporally associated with yellow fever vaccination. Emerg Infect Dis 2001;7:945–51.
[35] Freedman DO, Kozarsky PE, Weld LH, et al. GeoSentinel: the global emerging infections sentinel network of the International Society of Travel Medicine. J Travel Med 1999;6:94–8.
[36] Goldstein AL, Badamchian M. Thymosins: chemistry and biological properties in health and disease. Expert Opin Biol Ther 2004;4:559–73.
[37] Linton PJ, Dorshkind K. Age-related changes in lymphocyte development and function. Nat Immunol 2004;5:133–9.

[38] Kelleher P, Misbah SA. What is Good's syndrome? Immunological abnormalities in patients with thymoma. J Clin Pathol 2003;56:12–6.
[39] Hoke CH, Nisalak A, Sangawhipa N, et al. Protection against Japanese encephalitis by inactivated vaccines. N Engl J Med 1988;319:608–14.
[40] Gajanana A, Thenmozhi V, Samuel PP, et al. A community-based study of subclinical flavivirus infections in children in an area of Tamil Nadu, India, where Japanese encephalitis is endemic. Bull World Health Organ 1995;73:237–44.
[41] Halstead SB, Tsai TF. Japanese encephalitis vaccines. In: Plotkin SA, Orenstein WA, editors. Vaccines. Philadelphia: WB Saunders; 2004. p. 919–58.
[42] Solomon T. Flavivirus encephalitis. N Engl J Med 2004;351:370–80.
[43] Shlim DR, Solomon T. Japanese encephalitis vaccine for travelers: exploring the limits of risk. Clin Infect Dis 2002;35:183–8.
[44] Misra UK, Kalita J. Anterior horn cells are also involved in Japanese encephalitis. Acta Neurol Scand 1997;96:114–7.
[45] Solomon T, Kneen R, Dung NM, et al. Poliomyelitis-like illness due to Japanese encephalitis virus. Lancet 1998;351:1094–7.
[46] Hoke CH Jr, Vaughn DW, Nisalak A, et al. Effect of high-dose dexamethasone on the outcome of acute encephalitis due to Japanese encephalitis virus. J Infect Dis 1992;165: 631–7.
[47] Vaughn DW, Hoke CH Jr. The epidemiology of Japanese encephalitis: prospects for prevention. Epidemiol Rev 1992;14:197–221.
[48] Solomon T. Vaccines against Japanese encephalitis. In: Jong EC, Zuckerman JN, editors. Travelers' vaccines. Hamilton, Ontario, Canada: BC Decker; 2004. p. 219.
[49] Tsai TF. Inactivated Japanese encephalitis virus vaccine. Recommendations of the Advisory Committee on Immunization Practices (ACIP). MMWR Recomm Rep 1993;42:1–15.
[50] Plesner AM. Allergic reactions to Japanese encephalitis vaccine. Immunol Allergy Clin North Am 2003;23:665–97.
[51] Poland JD, Cropp CB, Craven RB, et al. Evaluation of the potency and safety of inactivated Japanese encephalitis vaccine in US inhabitants. J Infect Dis 1990;161:878–82.
[52] Sabin AB. Epidemic encephalitis in military personnel. JAMA 1947;133:281–93.
[53] Plesner A, Ronne T, Wachmann H. Case-control study of allergic reactions to Japanese encephalitis vaccine. Vaccine 2000;18:1830–6.
[54] Ohtaki E, Murakami Y, Komori H, et al. Acute disseminated encephalomyelitis after Japanese B encephalitis vaccination. Pediatr Neurol 1992;8:137–9.
[55] Ohtaki E, Matsuishi T, Hirano Y, et al. Acute disseminated encephalomyelitis after treatment with Japanese B encephalitis vaccine (Nakayama-Yoken and Beijing strains). J Neurol Neurosurg Psychiatry 1995;59:316–7.
[56] Plesner AM, Arlien-Soborg P, Herning M. Neurological complications to vaccination against Japanese encephalitis. Eur J Neurol 1998;5:479–85.
[57] Takahashi H, Pool V, Tsail TF, et al. Adverse events after Japanese encephalitis vaccination: review of post-marketing surveillance data from Japan and the United States. The VAERS Working Group. Vaccine 2000;18:2963–9.
[58] Konishi E, Shoda M, Kondo T. Prevalence of antibody to Japanese encephalitis virus nonstructural 1 protein among racehorses in Japan: indication of natural infection and need for continuous vaccination. Vaccine 2004;22:1097–103.

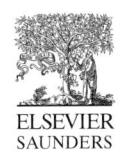

# A Travel Medicine Guide to Arthropods of Medical Importance

Richard J. Pollack, PhD[a],*,
Leonard C. Marcus, VMD, MD[b,c,d]

[a]Laboratory of Public Health Entomology, Department of Immunology and Infectious Diseases, Harvard School of Public Health, 665 Huntington Avenue, Boston, MA 02115, USA
[b]Travelers' Health & Immunization Services, 148 Highland Avenue, Newton, MA 02465, USA
[c]Department of Environmental and Population Health, Tufts University School of Veterinary Medicine, North Grafton, MA, USA
[d]Department of Medicine, University of Massachusetts School of Medicine, Worcester, MA, USA

Arthropod-transmitted diseases cause enormous morbidity, mortality, and economic losses worldwide. Global surveillance data on many of these diseases are reviewed elsewhere in this issue. Although residents of North America seem most concerned about encounters with hematophagous arthropods and vector-borne agents while traveling abroad, they are also at risk in their own neighborhoods and during journeys throughout their own continent. For example, 9862 human cases of disease caused by West Nile virus were reported in the United States during 2003, 2866 of which were neuroinvasive [1]. Lyme disease cases numbered 23,763 during 2002 [2]. In contrast, of the 1337 cases of malaria reported in 2002, all but five were acquired abroad [3]. Although autochthonous cases of leishmaniasis are rare in the United States, the Centers for Disease Control and Prevention dispenses sodium stibogluconate to treat an average of 30 to 40 imported cases annually.

Those who travel for business and pleasure may put themselves at particular risk by their choices of destination, season of travel, accommodations, and activities. Military personnel constitute a special class of traveler, and because they often cannot exercise avoidance, they face particularly elevated risks of vector-borne disease. More than 350 American

---

* Corresponding author.
*E-mail address:* rpollack@hsph.harvard.edu (R.J. Pollack).

troops have acquired leishmaniasis while serving in Iraq from May 2002 to January 2004 [4].

This article describes clinically relevant aspects of the biology, ecology, and epidemiology of the main kinds of arthropods that directly injure people or transmit infections. Guidance is offered to clinicians so they might better educate and advise travelers how to protect themselves, and evaluate and manage complaints by travelers on their return.

## Arthropods as the cause of direct injury or as vectors

Arthropods can cause diverse problems for the traveler. At one end of the spectrum, they may cause distress simply by making their presence known. The characteristic whine produced by the beating wings of certain mosquitoes, for example, causes some people to panic and lose sleep, even if none land and feed. At the opposite extreme are situations in which insects and ticks transmit pathogenic agents that result in considerable illness and death. Between these extremes are various arthropods that infest, feed on, or otherwise harass travelers. The interval of contact may be fleeting (as the bite of a mosquito), more prolonged (as bot fly larvae developing in the skin), or chronic (as from a resident and perpetuating population of scabies mites or lice on the body).

Several reference works are available to guide the clinician in serving the traveler. Background information on vector-borne diseases and statistics on case reports are provided by Internet sites maintained by the Centers for Disease Control and Prevention [5]. Descriptions of the vectors and vector-borne pathogens are detailed in infectious disease and medical entomology texts [6,7], and in printed and online image atlases [8,9].

## Pathogen transmission

Transmission of a vector-borne agent, in general, requires the presence of an arthropod that is competent (ie, it must be physiologically able to acquire, maintain, and transmit a suitable quantum of the infectious agent). To serve as a suitable vector, it must also satisfy requirements of vectorial capacity. As such, it must survive long enough for the pathogen to develop or multiply within it, be abundant where and when the reservoir hosts are abundant, and focus it's feeding on hosts that are effective reservoirs [10]. An arthropod that has ingested pathogens from its host is considered infected. If the arthropod is not a competent vector, the pathogens fail to survive, develop, or multiply, or otherwise fail to be transmitted to a new host. A vector becomes infectious solely after the pathogens have developed or multiplied and journeyed to their relevant point of egress from the vector (eg, the saliva for Lyme disease spirochetes and malarial sporozoites, the hindgut for louse-borne typhus rickettsiae).

Generally, people acquire vector-borne pathogens while being fed on by the vector. Most often, the pathogenic agents are within the vector's saliva injected directly into the skin. In this manner, people become inoculated with agents as diverse as the sporozoites of malaria, the virions of arboviruses, and the bacterial agent of Lyme disease. The infectious particles are either mainlined directly into blood vessels or deposited into perivascular tissue in the skin. Infectious larvae, such as the nematode agents of lymphatic filariasis and onchocerciasis, forcibly escape from the mouthparts of their feeding mosquito and black fly hosts, respectively. A droplet of insect hemolymph on the skin protects these tiny worms for a fleeting moment until they enter the wound left by the insect's mouthparts, or they become stranded and die. The metacyclic trypomastigotes of American trypanosomiasis, in contrast, are passed not in the saliva, but in the feces of their triatomine vectors. The host is infected when these protozoa are scratched or rubbed into the wound or mucus membranes. Similarly, the agents of louse-borne typhus and louse-borne relapsing fever are passed in the feces of their body louse vectors. These kinds of agents must develop or proliferate within the vector's tissues, and in these cases the arthropod vector serves to effect biologic transmission.

Various pathogens may contaminate the mouthparts, gut, or body of an insect or tick, whether or not these arthropods engage in hematophagy. Microbes carried in this manner may then be passed on without any development or proliferation in the vector, a process termed "mechanical" transmission. Certain other agents rely on other mechanisms for transmission (eg, ingestion of the infected vector by the vertebrate host), but these are beyond the limited scope of this article.

**Modes of encounter**

Arthropods approach and molest people to find shelter and sustenance, or to deposit the eggs that give rise to their progeny. They locate hosts mainly by detecting body heat, and by following olfactory cues (carbon dioxide; lactic acid; and for certain African *Anopheles,* a particular constituent of foot odor), and visual cues (size, shape, color, pattern, and movement). Even where and when vector-borne pathogens are transmitted intensely, relatively few potential vectors are infected, and even fewer are infectious (terms defined previously).

They feed on blood mainly to nourish themselves and to acquire proteins needed for egg development. The agents they transmit to vertebrate hosts can also burden the vector or enhance the likelihood of their transmission. The malaria parasite may compel the infected mosquito to probe more extensively, the plague bacillus causes the flea to regurgitate, and filariae may reduce the flight range and longevity of their fly vectors.

The chance of encountering a potential vector is a function of geography, season, and the specific activities in which the traveler engages. Whatever the chances of this encounter, because a relatively small proportion of potential vectors in any site are likely to be infected, the risk of acquiring vector-borne disease from any single encounter is further reduced. The aggregate chance of infection, however, rises with each new contact. Generally, a single bite from an infectious vector is sufficient to transmit viral, bacterial, or protozoan infections and, because these pathogens multiply in the human host, one bite can produce disease. One mosquito bite can lead to malaria, one sand fly bite to leishmaniasis, and one tick bite to a case of tick-borne encephalitis or Lyme disease.

The vectors of filariasis inoculate the vertebrate host with motile larvae, each of which matures into one adult worm nearly a year later. Each mated female worm may produce many thousands of tiny motile microfilariae daily that then course through the host's skin or blood to await carriage by another vector. Generally, a person in a filariasis endemic region must suffer thousands of bites during a period of several years to acquire enough infective bites to cause demonstrable infection and clinical disease. The short-term traveler very rarely suffers clinical filariasis. An exception is loiasis where one adult worm can cause symptoms.

The brief moment during which flies (including mosquitoes) bite is sufficient to infect the new host. In comparison, ticks feed more slowly. Whereas the argasid (soft) ticks may complete their feeding in a matter of minutes, the ixodid (hard) ticks remain attached and feed for 3 or more days. Several kinds of pathogenic agents (eg, the spirochete of Lyme disease) do not appear in the tick's saliva until the tick has been feeding for about 2 days. Early recognition and removal of the feeding tick in such cases may preclude transmission before it becomes infectious.

Within North America, visitors can encounter an impressive array of potential vectors and vector-borne agents. Mosquitoes and ticks provide the most prominent threats to residents and travelers, alike. The *Culex* mosquitoes that serve as the main vectors of West Nile virus exploit the foul water within the ubiquitous storm water catch basins lining urban and suburban streets, and in clogged roof gutters, rain-filled trash barrels and toys, and in disused swimming pools. Although *Culex* mosquitoes tend to feed preferentially on birds, people serve as occasional hosts for these and other kinds of mosquitoes. The efficiency and intensity of West Nile virus transmission is evidenced by the rapid coast-to-coast spread of this epidemic. Prevalence of infection within mosquito and bird populations, and risk for people rises through the summer, peaking in late summer and into early autumn. Other mosquito-borne arboviruses, such as the agents of eastern equine and St. Louis encephalitis, follow a similar seasonal pattern, but are more restricted in their geographic ranges.

Deer ticks and the agents they vector (particularly those causing Lyme disease and human babesiosis) were, until recently, restricted to a few defined foci in New England, the upper Midwest, and California. The burgeoning deer population throughout the eastern United States now supports dense deer tick populations, and consequently, enhances risk of these deer tick–transmitted infections in suburban and rural areas. Risk to people is seasonal, and corresponds to the host-seeking activities of the nymphal ticks in late spring through early summer, and of the adult ticks in late autumn and in the springtime.

Visits abroad provide the traveler with diverse and often unfamiliar risks. Close relatives of American deer ticks occur throughout much of Europe and Asia, where they transmit agents causing Lyme disease and tick-borne encephalitis. Mosquitoes become of particular concern in regions endemic for malaria and dengue. Occasional autochthonous cases of malaria occur in the United States, mainly through the actions of imported infected vectors (airport malaria) or local transmission by indigenous vectors that acquired infection from a returning traveler [11]. Although the phlebotomine sand flies of the tropics and subtropics are diminutive and often go unnoticed, the leishmanial infections they can transmit often lead to disfiguring or significant illness.

Any kind of arthropod, whether a vector or not, can survive and flourish only within particular ecologic constraints. Whereas most insects and ticks tolerate an impressive range in temperature, humidity, and day length conditions, other kinds are restricted by narrow tolerances. Human head lice, for instance, thrive only when ambient conditions match those within an inch or so of the human scalp. Reduced daylight hours (such as during the approach of autumn) cause certain temperate *Culex* mosquitoes to enter physiologic diapause (a resting stage, similar to hibernation). When reared under such short day length conditions, the adults feed on sugars rather than blood, and seek shelter in which they may survive through the winter. Increasing daylight hours in the spring or warming temperatures stimulate these mosquitoes to seek blood meals and their ovaries to produce eggs. Such an innate timing mechanism may also restrict these mosquitoes to certain latitudes.

Just as the ambient temperature constrains the distribution of a vector, it may also limit the geographic range of the pathogen. The *Anopheles* mosquito vectors of malaria may survive and prosper at ambient temperatures at or below 20°C, but such low temperatures dramatically extend the extrinsic incubation period of the malarial agent within the vector. Few mosquitoes survive long enough to transmit sporozoites to a new host. At temperatures below 15°C and 18°C, *Plasmodium vivax* and *P falciparum*, respectively, fail to develop within the vector. The presence of the vector does not necessarily connote risk for certain vector-borne diseases. These temperature considerations limit the distribution of such infections as a function of latitude and altitude.

As with temperature, rainfall and other climatic conditions profoundly influence the seasonal abundance of many kinds of vectors and the transmission intensity of vector-borne disease. Ground depressions inundated by seasonal rains or run-off from snowmelt may give rise to prodigious populations of mosquitoes. The main malaria vectors in portions of sub-Saharan Africa may be scarce, and transmission of malaria virtually nonexistent, until after the rains have begun each year. Elsewhere, the main and ancillary vectors maintain transmission throughout the year.

The frequency of vector-host contact depends on the extent to which their activity overlaps. Each kind of mosquito exhibits its own characteristic daily pattern of host seeking. *Culex* and *Anopheles* mosquitoes, in general, seek hosts at night, whereas many *Aedes* attack at midday. Others time their meals at hours near dawn and dusk. Night-active mosquitoes may readily take blood meals from sleeping human hosts. Although certain *Anopheles* feed almost exclusively on hosts while outdoors, others readily enter dwellings in search of their meals. Other outdoor biters, such as black flies and tsetse flies, may accidentally enter a dwelling, but once inside they pursue escape rather than any available hosts. Soft (argasid) ticks, bed bugs, and certain mites remain close to their host's nest and await the predictable, often nightly, return of their meals. Bedrooms, thereby, serve as foci for these pests.

The work environment and quality of the accommodations profoundly influence the kinds of vectors encountered, and the frequency of such contact. Travelers staying within well-constructed and air-conditioned urban hotels and offices face minimal risks of encountering such pests while inside. They lose these protections, however, when outside such privileged confines. Those staying in less stellar surroundings face increased risks. Accommodations lacking window screens in malarious regions are best avoided, or the traveler should take care to use a bed net properly (preferably one that has been treated with an insecticide) and to take malarial prophylaxis. Even with screens and nets, the indoor environment may not be free of mosquito risk. Populations of the yellow fever mosquito, *Aedes aegypti,* can perpetuate without venturing outdoors. Their aquatic immature stages develop in water jugs and vases, and the adults of this mosquito feed and rest indoors. Primitive accommodations pose even greater risks. Thatched roofs in the American tropics and subtropics offer harborage for the cone-nosed or kissing bugs (triatomines) that transmit American trypanosomiasis.

Arthropods of public health importance may actively seek out a host for the few seconds needed to acquire a meal of blood or to lay their eggs, may passively lay in wait for the host to approach them, or may take up residence on or in the host's body. In the latter case, the arthropods are provided with unlimited food, security, and a likely means of contacting additional hosts. The following discussion briefly illustrates the ecology of the more prominent arthropods that may burden the traveler.

## Chronic and obligate parasites of human beings

People serve as the sole source of food and shelter for a few kinds of parasitic arthropods. Some of these cause chronic infestations, and the etiologic agents may accompany the traveler home. Most prominent of these are the scabies-inducing *Sarcoptes* mites and the three kinds of human-lice. *Sarcoptes scabiei* is a colorless, ovoid mite less than 1 mm long that excavates sinuous burrows in the stratum corneum. Adult females occasionally emerge from these burrows and crawl over the surface of the skin. Infestations are most prevalent in the tropics, and crowding promotes outbreaks. Transmission mainly depends on direct contact between hosts. Because these mites succumb in about 2 days when isolated from a human host, fomite transmission (eg, through contaminated clothing or bedding) is rarely important. Infestations are generally asymptomatic for a month or more, until cell-mediated and humoral immune hypersensitivity responses to the mite's saliva and feces cause inflammatory skin lesions. Pruritus, particularly when affecting one or more close contacts, raises suspicion of scabies. Definitive diagnosis should rest on discovery of the mites or their eggs extracted from their burrows (most often found in the web spaces between the fingers) or in skin scrapings or by epidermal shave biopsy. A single application of permethrin is usually sufficient to eliminate living mites, but persisting mite antigens may continue to provoke allergic reactions for many months.

Human beings are also the sole hosts for head lice (*Pediculus capitis*), body lice (*Pediculus humanus*), and pubic lice (*Pthirus pubis*). These wingless insects feed only on blood and infest the surface of the skin and hair; they are incapable of burrowing. Head lice infest children more often than adults. Transmission likely occurs by direct head-to-head contact with an infested person; fomites are relatively unimportant. Body lice, in contrast, mainly infest the indigent, and sequester in the seams of clothing worn for extended intervals. Body lice are transmitted mainly by direct contact, and by shared bedding and clothing. Pubic lice mainly infest sexually promiscuous people, and are primarily transmitted venereally. They are concentrated on the hair of the pubis, and occasionally also on hair ornamenting the face and axillae and on eyelashes. Infestations of head lice are generally asymptomatic, but transient pruritus may occur from allergic reactions to their saliva. Bites of body lice and pubic lice tend to cause more intense pruritus and an erythematous maculopapular rash. Body lice, but not head lice or pubic lice, may serve as vectors for louse-borne typhus, louse-borne relapsing fever, and trench fever. Body lice and these pathogenic agents are most frequently encountered in areas of civil strife, in prisons where inmates do not bathe or change clothes frequently, and in homeless shelters. Few business or leisure travelers are likely to encounter body lice or their pathogens. Diagnoses and treatment of louse infestations should rest on demonstrating a live louse, and not on the finding of their presumptive eggs. Lice and their eggs may be removed from hair by mechanical means, but applications of pediculicides are often necessary to eliminate the infestations [12]. Pyrethrins and synthetic pyrethroids are generally efficacious for killing lice, but they tend not to affect the eggs. Malathion formulations seem effective for killing louse eggs and lice that are resistant to pyrethroids. Body lice can be eliminated in most cases simply by bathing and changing to well-laundered clothes. Lice are usually host specific, so lice of lower animals very rarely, if ever, bite people.

**Parasites staying for limited, but extended, intervals**

An array of arthropods that are obligate parasites for part of their development may occasionally attack people. Whereas most kinds of fleas attack only briefly, the chigoe flea, *Tunga penetrans*, can infest travelers who walk barefoot or in sandals in rural sites in Africa, Latin America, and India. The fertilized female penetrates the stratum corneum of the skin, and beneath the margins of toenails, and causes an enlarging furuncular lesion as the flea swells to the size of a pea. Although the lesion is generally self-limiting, it is painful and may cause sloughing of skin. The developing flea should be removed as soon as possible by means of a sterile needle.

Many kinds of hard (ixodid) ticks readily feed on people. These ticks tend to quest passively and await a passing host to sweep them off of vegetation. A host's warmth and exhaled carbon dioxide stimulates other ticks to approach from a short distance. These ticks imbed their harpoon-like mouthparts into the skin and remain in place and feed for several days. Once engorged, they drop off and wander away. Hiking in woods or through high grass enhances contact with these ticks, some of which may transmit agents of Lyme disease, human babesiosis, Rocky Mountain spotted fever, and various kinds of tick-borne encephalitis viruses. Some level of protection is afforded by pretreatment of clothing with permethrin. Hikers should inspect their bodies each day to locate and remove attached ticks before they transmit pathogens. Fine-tipped forceps are most suitable to grasp and withdraw the ticks by the base of their mouthparts.

Larvae of several kinds of flies invade wounds or intact tissue to produce myiasis (maggot infestation), usually in skin, but sometimes in body orifices, intestine, eye, or other organs. In Central and South America, the human bot fly *(Dermatobia hominis)* attaches her eggs to the body of a mosquito or other flying insect that serves as a vehicle to carry them to a large mammal. Heat from the mammal causes larvae to hatch, drop from their transport host, and penetrate the mammal's skin. The larvae mature in a boil-like lesion, and after about a month of development, they emerge and pupate away from the host. In parts of Africa, female tumbu flies, *Cordylobia anthropophaga*, deposit numerous eggs on urine- or sweat-contaminated clothing. Clothing that has been washed in a stream and dried in the open serve as attractive and suitable substrates. The eggs embryonate within 2 days and remain viable for about 2 weeks. Contact with warm, moist skin stimulates the larvae to emerge, penetrate skin, and form boils from which larvae emerge within 9 days. Travelers should ensure that their clothes are ironed if they have been traditionally laundered in endemic regions. In

North America, horse botflies, *Gasterophilus intestinalis*, deposit their eggs on the flanks of horses. A human rider's warm, moist, bare leg substitutes for the horse's tongue to stimulate larvae to hatch and penetrate skin. Larvae migrate through the skin, producing narrow raised pruritic tunnels. Covering the lesion with an occlusive ointment or gentle pressure is often sufficient to coax the air-breathing larvae to emerge. In other cases, surgical excision is required.

Larvae of about 20 kinds of trombiculid mites (chiggers) normally feed on reptiles, small mammals, and birds, but attack people, causing dermatitis and occasionally transmitting pathogens. These tiny (approximately 0.25 mm long) mites climb and cluster on grass tips and wait for a passing host. They tend to attach to skin around the waist or wherever clothing is constricting, and feed for several days on host tissues liquefied by their saliva. The harvest mite of Europe and the American chigger of North America cause seasonal risk in late summer through early autumn. Their bites cause intense itching and wheals and pustules within hours of feeding, but they do not serve as vectors. In parts of Asia, several kinds of chiggers transmit the rickettsial agent of scrub typhus, but the bites themselves are insignificant. Insect repellents on skin and clothing provide some protection from chigger attack.

**Nest parasites**

Various kinds of arthropods sequester in and around the nests of their vertebrate hosts, and patiently wait for their meals to return. Because people's homes (or hotels, hostels, dormitories) are, functionally, glorified nests, it should not be surprising to find these inhabited by parasitic arthropods. Chief among these are bedbugs, soft (argasid) ticks, and cone-nosed (triatomine) bugs, all of which feed exclusively on blood.

Bedbugs and their close relatives inhabit nests and roosts of birds and bats worldwide, and feed on these and other hosts. During the past few years, the cosmopolitan bedbugs have become increasingly recognized as a pest in hovels, homes, and high-class hotels throughout North America and Europe. These flattened, wingless bugs hide in cracks and crevices, often in the bed frame and mattress, and emerge at night to feed painlessly on their sleeping victims. They feed frequently when hosts are available, but can survive nearly a year between meals if necessary. Although not known to transmit infectious agents to people, the reactions to the saliva from these bugs can be exceedingly distressing. Infestations of bedbugs are sometimes apparent by detecting the blood spots voided by the fed bugs onto mattresses, linens, and even the walls, and by a peculiar odor characteristic of dense bug populations. To add insult to injury, bedbugs occasionally hide in luggage and accompany travelers home and establish a new infestation there. Pyrethroid insecticidal treatments to the sleeping quarters, particularly to the bed frame and mattress, can diminish their populations and associated bites. Eradication of bedbugs, however, often requires protracted and costly treatments to the premises.

The cone-nosed (triatomine) bugs of tropical and subtropical Central and South America burden people with more than their bites. As with bedbugs, cone-nosed bugs conceal themselves during the day (often in thatched roofs) and seek blood from almost any available warm-blooded host at night. Some triatomine bugs serve as vectors for the agent of American trypanosomiasis (Chagas disease), passing the infectious forms in their feces while feeding painlessly. Adults are winged and fly when disturbed or to establish new infestations. In heavily infested homes, residents may suffer dozens of bites each night, with individual adult bugs drawing up to 4 g of blood per meal. Applications of insecticidal fogs and residues to roof and walls of domiciles can reduce the population of the bugs and disease risk. Travelers in endemic regions are wise to select accommodations with solid (not thatched) ceilings or roofs, and with smooth walls without crevices.

Certain soft (argasid) ticks occasionally bite travelers staying in rodent-infested rustic cabins in the western United States. *Ornithodoros hermsii* ticks readily attack people at night. The brief (15–45 minute) episodes of blood feeding are generally unrecognized. These ticks may survive for a decade, with only an occasional meal needed for survival each year. These soft ticks pose occasional risk as vectors of the tick-borne relapsing fever spirochete that has sickened several people and proved fatal in a few cases [13].

Unlike lice, most fleas are not very host specific. Diverse fleas of rodents abound in and near the nests of their hosts, and readily bite people and their usual rodent hosts. In parts of the western United States and elsewhere in the world [14], rodents harbor the agent of plague. Backcountry trekkers to endemic areas should avoid camping near rodent burrows, and they may benefit from the use of insect repellents. In addition to plague, some rodent fleas can transmit murine typhus. Cat and dog fleas (*Ctenocephalides felis* and *C canis*, respectively) also readily bite people. *C felis* transmits *Bartonella henselae* to cats, and possibly to people. Eliminating cat and dog fleas depends on treating the animal hosts and premises, not the transient human host.

**Parasites of momentary duration**

Travelers are most aware of those arthropods that mount momentary attacks, such as mosquitoes, black flies, and tsetse flies. Less appreciated are the stealthy sand flies that pose risk of transmitting leishmaniasis. The habits, host preferences, and local abundance of each of these flies are functions of the region, season, and species composition. In general, protection from their bites outdoors is offered by covering exposed skin with clothing, and by use of insect repellents on skin and clothing. Clothing is most protective if it has a tight weave and is loose and baggy. Window screens, bed nets, and air conditioning can markedly reduce annoyance and risk from those biting insects that live or venture indoors. Although certain biting flies, such as the certatopogonids ("no-see-ums") and psychodids (sand flies) are small enough to pass through the mesh of standard window screens and mosquito nets, they may be blocked with fine mesh screens or with ones that have been treated with insecticides.

## Nonparasitic arthropods of medical significance

A broad array of arthropods may inflict damage simply in defensive mode, by accidental contact, or while foraging indiscriminately. Travelers virtually anywhere in North America or abroad may experience stings or bites from wasps, bees, ants, scorpions, spiders, and centipedes, but none of these serve as a vector. Similarly, urticating setae or blistering agents adorn some millipedes, beetles, and caterpillars. Travelers should exercise caution when handling arthropods unknown to them, reaching into dark recesses that might harbor a biting or stinging creature, or approaching nests of wasps and other social insects.

## Pretrip and post-trip considerations

Just as travel-minded clinicians evaluate and offer their patients relevant pretravel vaccinations, prophylactic treatments, and guidance, so too should they consider and prepare the traveler to deal with arthropods and vector-borne illnesses they might encounter. Travel agents are rarely prepared to offer appropriate guidance [15]. Discussions should focus on the travelers' destinations, choice of accommodations, and on the risks accompanying their planned activities (Table 1). Efficacious insect repellents should be packed or purchased at the destination and applied appropriately. Formulations based on DEET remain the best available repellents [16,17]. Clothing treatment with permethrin should be considered, and tick removal devices packed, for those likely to encounter ticks. Bed nets are commercially available; compactly packed; readily deployed; and can offer significant protection (especially if they are impregnated with insecticide) to travelers staying in endemic regions and where window screens or similar amenities may be absent.

Regardless of the precautions taken, certain unwanted guests, including bot flies, scabies mites, and lice, occasionally accompany the returning traveler home. Complaints of sensations elicited by these parasites may be suggestive of an active infestation or lingering reactions (sometimes for weeks afterward) of bites experienced while traveling. The clinician should

Table 1
Representative arthropods burdening travelers, and strategies to reduce risk of annoyance and disease

| Ecologic group | Representative taxa | Geography | Manner of contact | Representative disease risks | Protection methods[a] |
|---|---|---|---|---|---|
| Chronic, perpetuating parasitism | Scabies mite (*Sarcoptes scabiei*) | Worldwide | Direct contact with infested person, bedding, or clothing | Pruritus, disseminated cutaneous infestation in immunocompromised hosts | A, H |
| | Human body louse (*Pediculus humanus*) | Worldwide | Direct contact with infested person, bedding, or clothing | Pruritus, systemic disease: louse-borne typhus, louse-borne relapsing fever, trench fever | A, D, E, H, I |
| | Human head louse (*Pediculus capitis*) | Worldwide | Direct head-to-head contact with infested person | Pruritus | G, H |
| | Human pubic louse (*Pthirus pubis*) | Worldwide | Direct (usually promiscuous) contact with infested person, bedding, or clothing | Pruritus | A, G, H |
| Extended stay for feeding or development | Chigoe flea (*Tunga penetrans*) | Tropics and subtropics | Exposed feet in infested areas | Local irritation, secondary bacterial infection | A, B, F, G |
| | Hard (Ixodid) ticks (eg, deer ticks (*Ixodes*); dog or wood ticks (*Dermacentor*); *Amblyomma* | Worldwide | Ticks quest for hosts in high grass and brush-covered sites | Lyme disease, human babesiosis, ehrlichiosis (anaplasmosis), tick-borne encephalitis (*Ixodes*); Rocky Mountain Spotted Fever, tick paralysis (*Dermacentor*); African tick-bite fever (*Amblyomma*) | A, B, C, D, F, G |
| | Myiasis-inducing fly larvae (eg, *Cordylobia anthropophaga*, *Dermatobia hominis*, *Gasterophilus intestinalis*) | Mainly tropics and subtropics | Adult female fly oviposits on body of host (*Gasterophilus*), on sweat or urine stained clothing (*Cordylobia*), or on a 'carrier' arthropod (*Dermatobia*), | Furuncular, wound, creeping dermal injury | B, C, D, E, G, I |

| | | | | | |
|---|---|---|---|---|---|
| Nest-inhabiting parasites | Bed bugs and relatives (*Cimex spp*) | Worldwide | Nocturnal feeding, mainly near beds | Pruritus | A, E, F |
| | Kissing or cone-nose bugs (Triatomines) | Tropical and subtropical Americas | Nocturnal feeding; bugs hide in thatched roofs and cracked mud walls | Chagas disease (American trypanosomiasis) | A, D, E, F |
| | Soft (Argasid) ticks; diverse hematophagous mites | Worldwide | Proximity to nests and dens of mammals, birds, reptiles | Tick-borne relapsing fever (certain soft ticks); rickettsialpox and pruritus (certain hematophagous mites) | A, C, D, F |
| | Fleas (eg, cat fleas, dog fleas, fleas of rodents) | Worldwide | Proximity to infested dogs, cats, rodents, and residences and yards where they may have roamed within past several months | Pruritus, often around ankles; plague (rodent fleas in endemic areas) | A, C, D, F |
| Ephemeral visitors (brief contact and feeding) | Mosquitoes (eg, *Anopheles*, *Aedes*, *Culex*) | Worldwide | Depending on kind of mosquito, females seek hosts outdoors or inside shelters; some feed mainly at night, others during the day, or mainly around dawn and dusk | Malaria, arboviruses, filariases | A, B, C, D, E |
| | Black flies (*Simulium*) | Worldwide | Diurnal, outdoor feeding, mainly near rivers and streams | Onchocerciasis | A, B, C, D |
| | Sand flies (eg, *Lutzomyia*, *Phlebotomus*) | Tropics and subtropics | Mainly nocturnal | Leishmaniasis | A, B, C, D, E, F |

[a] Protection methods: A, Avoidance; B, Clothing barrier (long pants, long sleeves, socks, closed-toe shoes; baggy fabric or densely woven); C, Application of insect or tick repellents to body, clothing (DEET-containing repellents are most effective); D, Insecticide-impregnated clothing; E, Insecticide-treated nets (bed nets, screening); F, Area insecticide applications; G, Mechanical removal of parasite; H, Treatment of patient with appropriate antiparasitic agent; and I, Heat treating clothing.

make reasonable efforts to evaluate these cases fully, carefully considering the patient's destination and the activities he or she engaged in while away. Earnest attempts should be made to demonstrate an etiologic agent, and to submit any questionable specimen to an expert for evaluation. If neither the agent is discovered nor relief is offered by symptomatic or presumptive treatments, delusional parasitosis should be considered. Travelers who made use of accommodations infested with ticks, mites, bedbugs, or other vermin are advised to unpack and inspect their luggage and belongings carefully, and to launder their clothing immediately on their return. These steps may preempt the establishment of a new infestation.

## Summary

Guidance has been offered to clinicians so they might better educate and advise travelers how to protect themselves, and evaluate complaints by travelers once they have returned. Any biting arthropod may cause direct injury, and the bite of just one infectious vector can be enough to prove fatal to the unprotected. Travelers and travel medicine practitioners should familiarize themselves with the vectors and vector-borne agents likely to be encountered corresponding to the traveler's specific itinerary, accommodations, and planned activities, and devise a rational strategy to reduce risk.

## References

[1] Centers for Disease Control and Prevention. 2003 West Nile virus activity in the United States (reported as of May 21, 2004). Available at: http://www.cdc.gov/ncidod/dvbid/westnile/surv&controlCaseCount03_detailed.htm. Accessed June 6, 2004.
[2] Centers for Disease Control and Prevention. Notice to readers: final 2002 reports of notifiable diseases. MMWR Morb Mortal Wkly Rep 2003;52:741–50.
[3] Centers for Disease Control and Prevention. Malaria facts. Available at: http://www.cdc.gov/malaria/facts.htm. Accessed June 6, 2004.
[4] Centers for Disease Control and Prevention. Update: cutaneous leishmaniasis in US military personnel—Southwest/Central Asia, 2002–2004. MMWR Morb Mortal Wkly Rep 2004;53:264–5.
[5] Centers for Disease Control and Prevention. National Center for Infectious Diseases: travelers' health. Available at: http://www.cdc.gov/travel/. Accessed June 6, 2004.
[6] Spielman A, Wachtel M, Pollack RJ. Arthropods. In: Gorbach SL, Bartlett JG, Blacklow NR, editors. Infectious diseases. 3rd edition. Philadelphia: Lippincott Williams & Wilkins; 2004. p. 2401–14.
[7] Lane RP, Crosskey RW. Medical insects and arachnids. London: Chapman & Hall; 1993.
[8] Peters W. A colour atlas of arthropods in clinical medicine. London: Wolfe Publishing; 1992.
[9] Centers for Disease Control and Prevention. Public health image library. Available at: http://phil.cdc.gov/phil/. Accessed June 6, 2004.
[10] Telford SR III, Pollack RJ, Spielman A. Emerging vector-borne infections. Infect Dis Clin North Am 1991;5:7–17.
[11] Centers for Disease Control and Prevention. Multifocal autochthonous transmission of malaria—Florida, 2003. MMWR Annual Review of Entomology 2004;53:412–3.

[12] Burgess IF. Human lice and their control. Annu Rev Entomol 2004;49:457–81.
[13] Schwan TG, Policastro PF, Miller Z, et al. Tick-borne relapsing fever caused by *Borrelia hermsii*, Montana. Emerg Infect Dis 2003;9:1151–4.
[14] Centers for Disease Control and Prevention. NCID travelers' health: plague. Available at: http://www.cdc.gov/travel/diseases/plague.htm. Accessed June 6, 2004.
[15] Centers for Disease Control and Prevention. Fatal yellow fever in a traveler returning from Amazonas, Brazil, 2002. MMWR Morb Mortal Wkly Rep 2002;51:324–5.
[16] Fradin MS, Day JF. Comparative efficacy of insect repellents against mosquito bites. N Engl J Med 2002;347:13–8.
[17] Fradin MS. Mosquitoes and mosquito repellents: a clinician's guide. Ann Intern Med 1998; 128:931–40.

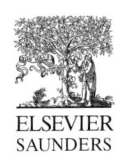

# New Strategies for the Prevention of Malaria in Travelers

Lin H. Chen, MD[a,b,]*, Jay S. Keystone, MD, MSc (CTM), FRCPC[c,d]

[a]*Department of Medicine, Harvard Medical School, Boston, MA, USA*
[b]*Division of Infectious Diseases, Mount Auburn Hospital, 330 Mount Auburn Street, Cambridge, MA 02238, USA*
[c]*Department of Medicine, University of Toronto, Toronto, Ontario, Canada*
[d]*Center for Travel and Tropical Medicine, Toronto General Hospital, 200 Elizabeth Street, 9ES-411A, Toronto, Ontario M5G 2C4, Canada*

Malaria causes significant morbidity and mortality in travelers. One barrier to effective prevention of malaria in travelers is poor adherence to recommended chemoprophylaxis, often the result of medication side effects; this problem is further complicated by spreading drug resistance. This article highlights some recent epidemiologic studies and laboratory techniques that assess travelers' malaria, reviews recent reports on personal protective measures, summarizes data on the use of atovaquone-proguanil and recommendations for the use of primaquine as primary prophylaxis, reviews the guidelines for standby treatment, and presents data on the development of a new antimalarial, tafenoquine.

## Epidemiology of malaria in travelers

Malaria causes at least 300 million clinical attacks and 2.7 million fatalities annually in developing countries [1,2]. It also causes significant morbidity and mortality among travelers. Approximately 25 to 30 million international travelers visit malaria-endemic countries each year, and 30,000 cases of malaria are estimated to occur among them [3,4]. The World Health Organization (WHO) European Region reported 13,000 cases of imported malaria in 1999, eight times the number reported in 1972, although

---

* Corresponding author. Division of Infectious Diseases, Mount Auburn Hospital, 330 Mount Auburn Street, Cambridge, MA 02238, USA.
 *E-mail address:* lchen@hms.harvard.edu (L.H. Chen).

underreporting is widely recognized [5]. Case fatality rates for falciparum malaria range from 0.7% to 3.6% in developed countries [3]. Factors contributing to the increased numbers of imported malaria cases include increased immigration by persons from malarious areas and their subsequent visits to friends and relatives in their home countries (VFRs); rising number of tourists visiting malaria-endemic countries; spread of drug resistance; poor adherence to chemoprophylaxis regimens; and environmental influences, such as irrigation for agricultural projects, that lead to increased risk in endemic countries and expansion of malaria-endemic regions [5].

Data on the risk of malaria to travelers are crucial in making pretravel recommendations. In the United States, 1540, 1402, 1383, and 1337 cases of malaria were reported to the Centers for Disease Control and Prevention (CDC) in 1999, 2000, 2001, and 2002, respectively; only 19% to 23% of imported civilian cases had taken recommended chemoprophylaxis [6–9]. The most frequent reason for travel was to visit friends and relatives (35.9%–45%), followed by tourism (10.2%–10.7%), and missionary work (9.2%–10.6%). Most cases were acquired in Africa (58.9%–72.1%, predominantly West Africa), followed by the Americas (11.3%–20.1%, predominantly Central America), and Asia (12.5%–17.9%, predominantly India) [6–9]. Short-term European travelers were found to contract malaria at an incidence rate of 12 per 1000 travelers per month to East Africa and 24 per 1000 travelers per month to West Africa, or 0.4 to 0.8 per 1000 persons per night in high transmission areas [10]. Peace Corps volunteers from the United States contracted falciparum malaria at a rate of 25 per 1000 persons per month in West Africa [11]. All data illustrate that travelers to Sub-Saharan Africa, especially West Africa, are at highest risk. An approximation of malaria risk in various areas of the world is presented in Table 1 [12].

**Surveillance strategies**

New strategies to assess the incidence and risk of malaria in travelers are being used by networks of travel clinics, namely GeoSentinel and TropNet Europe, which collect data on travel-related illnesses. An analysis of the GeoSentinel database that included 1140 cases of malaria reported from November 1997 to December 2002 confirmed that most were caused by *Plasmodium falciparum* (60%) and *Plasmodium vivax* (24%) [13]. The most frequently cited reasons for travel were to visit friends and relatives (35%) and tourism (26%); 75% of infections were acquired in Sub-Saharan Africa, but travel to Oceania also presented significant risk [13]. A TropNet Europe analysis of 1659 immigrants and European residents with imported falciparum malaria also indicated that those visiting friends and relatives in their home countries were the group most likely to acquire malaria and it occurred most frequently among travelers returning from West Africa [14].

Laboratory techniques have also been applied to assess malaria epidemiology in returning travelers. One such tool is the measurement of

Table 1
Malaria risk for 1 month of travel without chemoprophylaxis

| Region | Morbidity (per 100,000 travelers) | Mortality (assuming case fatality rate of 2%) | Malaria risk (extrapolated from morbidity data) |
|---|---|---|---|
| Solomons, PNG | 6000 | 30 | 1:17 |
| West Africa | 2400 | 43 | 1:40 |
| East Africa | 1500 | 27 | 1:70 |
| Indian subcontinent | 250 | 1.4 | 1:400 |
| Far East | 250 | <1.2 | 1:400 |
| South America | <50 | 0.14 | <1:2000 |
| Central America | <25 | 0.02 | <1:4000 |

*Data from* Steffen R, Jong EC. Travelers' and immigrants' health. In: Guerrant RL, Walker DH, Wyler PF, editors. Tropical infectious diseases: principles, pathogens and practice. Philadelphia: Churchill Livingstone; 1999. p. 108.

circumsporozoite antibodies. Circumsporozoite proteins are present on the surface of sporozoites, before their invasion of liver cells [15–17]. The presence of antibodies to circumsporozoite protein is consistent with transmission of sporozoites to the infected individual, but not necessarily with clinical disease. Studies using circumsporozoite antibodies have detected a malaria seroconversion of 4.9% and seroprevalence of 4.9% to 21% in returned travelers [15–17]. In addition to its use in epidemiologic surveillance, the technique has been applied to the evaluation of chemoprophylaxis efficacy, where the measurement of circumsporozoite antibodies serves as a marker for exposure to *P falciparum* [18].

## Existing chemoprophylaxis options and malaria drug resistance

Before the addition of atovaquone-proguanil for malaria chemoprophylaxis in 2000, available drugs recommended by the CDC for primary chemoprophylaxis of malaria included chloroquine, doxycycline, hydroxychloroquine, and mefloquine. Although the combination of chloroquine and proguanil was also recommended, proguanil was not available in the United States. Primaquine was recommended as a "terminal prophylaxis" to reduce the risk of relapse from hypnozoites of *P vivax* or *Plasmodium ovale*.

The drugs used for primary prophylaxis of malaria have uncommon but potentially significant side effects. Mefloquine, for example, is associated with adverse events in 25% to 50% of users, although most resolve spontaneously; severe neuropsychiatric events requiring hospitalization occur at an estimated rate of 1 per 10,000 [10]. Up to 4% of mefloquine users experience less severe adverse events that still lead to its discontinuation (Table 2) [10,19–21].

The emergence of *P falciparum* resistance (Table 3) [22,23] and occurrence of adverse events from existing drugs have necessitated a

Table 2
Tolerability of chemoprophylaxis drugs

| Medication | Mild-moderate AEs (%) | Severe AEs (%) | Moderate-severe neuropsychiatric AEs (%) | Moderate-severe skin AEs (%) | Withdrawal (%) |
|---|---|---|---|---|---|
| Chloroquine-proguanil | 45 | 11 | 30 | 8 | 5 |
| Mefloquine | 42 | 12 | 37 | 1 | 4 |
| Doxycycline | 33 | 6 | 24 | 3 | 3 |
| Atovaquone-proguanil | 32 | 7 | 20 | 2 | 2 |

*Abbreviation:* AEs, adverse events.

*Data from* Schlagenhauf P, Tschopp A, Johnson R, et al. Tolerability of malaria chemoprophylaxis in non-immune travelers to sub-Saharan Africa: multicentre, randomized, double blind, four-arm study. BMJ 2003;327:1078–83.

continuous search for additional chemoprophylaxis regimens. Chloroquine resistance was identified as early as 1957, proguanil resistance in 1949, mefloquine resistance in 1982, and atovaquone-proguanil resistance was recently documented in Africa [24,25]. Chloroquine-resistant *P falciparum* is widespread except for Central America, Mexico, Haiti, Dominican Republic, northern Argentina, and parts of the Middle East and China. Mefloquine resistance is present along the Thai-Cambodian and Thai-Myanmar borders.

Chloroquine-resistant *P vivax*, first recognized in 1989, has been reported in Papua New Guinea, Papua (Irian Jaya), Vanuatu, Thailand, Myanmar, Guyana, Somalia, and Latin America [26–29].

Recently, chloroquine-resistant *Plasmodium malariae* has been documented on the island of Sumatra, Indonesia [30]. A monkey malaria, *Plasmodium knowlesi*, has also been identified in humans in Borneo, but the parasite seems to be sensitive to chloroquine [31].

New techniques are available to assess resistance at a molecular level, and can contribute to the recommendations for malaria chemoprophylaxis in travelers. These techniques have been successful in identifying the mutations that confer drug resistance [22]. In one study, *P falciparum* isolates from Canadian travelers with imported malaria from 1994 to 2000 were analyzed for *pfcrt*, *dhfr*, and *dhps* polymorphisms. East African isolates were much more likely to have mutations in *pfmdr1* and *pfcrt*, consistent with chloroquine resistance [32].

## Atovaquone-proguanil

One recent addition to the options for malaria chemoprophylaxis is atovaquone-proguanil (Malarone), available in the United States since 2000, and supplied in a fixed-dose combination of 250 mg atovaquone and 100 mg proguanil for adults. Atovaquone inhibits mitochondrial electron transport at the cytochrome $b$-$c_1$ complex, collapses mitochondrial membrane

Table 3
Resistance of *Plasmodium falciparum* to chemoprophylaxis

| Medication | Mechanism of action | Resistance identified, year | Mechanism for resistance | Areas with resistance |
|---|---|---|---|---|
| Chloroquine | 4-Aminoquinoline, inhibits parasite's hemoglobin degradation in food vacuole leading to toxic heme accumulation and disruption of parasite membrane; acts on erythrocytic stage | 1957 | Decreased chloroquine uptake by parasite vacuole; associated with mutations in *pfmdr1*, *pfcg2*, and *pfcrt* genes | Widespread in Africa, Oceania, Asia, and South America |
| Atovaquone-proguanil | Atovaquone inhibits mitochondrial electron transport and collapses mitochondrial membrane potential; proguanil metabolite, cycloguanil, inhibits dihydrofolate reductase; acts on hepatic and erythrocytic stages | 1996 (resistance to proguanil was identified in 1949) | Mutations in cytochrome *b* gene; reduced drug affinity to dihydrofolate reductase; associated with mutations in *pfdhfr* | Africa |
| Doxycycline | Binds to ribosomal mRNA and inhibits protein synthesis; acts on erythrocytic stage and some hepatic stage activity | No data | Not identified | Not identified |
| Mefloquine | Competes with parasite protein for heme binding and forms complexes that disrupt parasite membrane; acts on erythrocytic stage | 1982 | Unclear, possibly similar to chloroquine or cross-resistance with other antimalarials | Border areas between Thailand, Cambodia, and Myanmar |
| Primaquine | 8-Aminoquinoline, acts on mitochondria by generation of toxic metabolites and oxidative stress; acts on hepatic and erythrocytic stages | No data | Chesson strain of *P vivax* is primaquine-tolerant; a higher dose is needed | Chesson strain of *P vivax* is present in tropical areas, especially Southeast Asia and Oceania; also noted in Somalia and Guyana |

*Data from* Refs. [22,23,33,34,43,44,51,98–104].

potential, and decreases pyrimidine synthesis and parasite replication [33,34]. Proguanil inhibits dihydrofolate reductase by its metabolite, cycloguanil, and also enhances atovaquone's effect on mitochondrial membrane potential [33]. The combination is synergistic, and has demonstrated causal prophylactic activity [33,35,36]. A causal prophylactic drug is effective against the hepatic stage of malaria infection, which occurs for about 7 days after exposure to parasites, and which occurs before the erythrocytic stage of infection. The chemoprophylaxis may be started 1 day before entering a malaria risk area, and only needs to be continued for 1 week after departure from the risk area. Protective efficacy against *P falciparum* has been shown to be 95% to 100% (Table 4) [18,21,36–42] and against *P vivax*, 84% [41].

Atovaquone-proguanil offers some advantages over other chemoprophylaxis regimens. Because it does not require advanced loading and prolonged dosing after travel, the dosing schedule is more convenient for some travelers. The side effect profile is often more acceptable than other chemoprophylactic drugs. In a comparison of tolerability of atovaquone-proguanil compared with mefloquine, doxycycline, and chloroquine-proguanil in nonimmune travelers seen in travel clinics in Switzerland, Germany, and Israel (N = 623), atovaquone-proguanil was less frequently associated with mild to moderate adverse events and moderate to severe neuropsychiatric events (see Table 2) [19]. One additional advantage is the pediatric formulation (62.5 mg atovaquone and 25 mg proguanil), which can be dosed by weight for children greater than 11 kg [37,40]. The only significant disadvantage to atovaquone-proguanil is the high cost of the drug compared with other prophylactic agents, particularly for prolonged travel in malarious areas. Cost is not usually an issue, however, for short trips of 2 weeks or less. Because of its convenience of administration, many practitioners recommend the drug for both chloroquine-sensitive and chloroquine-resistant areas.

The safety of atovaquone-proguanil during pregnancy has not been established. Although proguanil is believed to be safe during pregnancy, data are lacking regarding atovaquone. The drug should not be administered to pregnant women.

Resistance to atovaquone arises from mutations on the cytochrome $b$-$c_1$ gene [43]. A mutation in codon 268 of cytochrome $b$ was identified in a nonimmune traveler returning from Kenya with atovaquone-proguanil–resistant *P falciparum* [25]. Postmarketing surveillance of safety and efficacy of atovaquone-proguanil estimated that 1.28 million people had been prescribed atovaquone-proguanil as of April 2003, predominantly for malaria prophylaxis [44]. Forty-eight postmarketing prophylaxis failures and 15 falciparum malaria treatment failures were reported up to April 2003. Five cases of clinical failure were confirmed to have such a mutation in codon 268 of cytochrome $b$, with associated reduction in parasite binding affinity to atovaquone. The countries in which a confirmed failure has been

Table 4
Studies of atovaquone-proguanil for malaria prophylaxis

| Study site | Dates of study | Subjects | Age of subjects (y) | Number of subjects taking AP (total, N) | Protective efficacy (%) | Reference |
|---|---|---|---|---|---|---|
| Human challenge | Before 2001 | Nonimmune volunteers | 18–50 | 12 (16) | 100 | 36 |
| Gabon | January to June 1997 | Semi-immune children | 4–16 | 112 (212) | 100 | 37 |
| Kenya | April to August 1996 | Semi-immune residents | 18–65 | 54 daily dose, 54 double dose (162) | 100 | 39 |
| Zambia | Before 1999 | Semi-immune residents | 18–65 | 102 (213) | 95 | 38 |
| Gabon | January through June 2000 | Semi-immune children | 4–16 | 143 (255) | 97 | 40 |
| Papua, Indonesia | April through December 1999 | Nonimmune transmigrants | 12–65 | 148 (297) | 93 overall 96 Pf 84 Pv | 41 |
| 21 travel clinics in Europe, Canada, South Africa | April to October 1999 | Nonimmune travelers | ≥14 (and 50 kg) | 501 (1008) | 100 | 18 |
| 15 travel clinics in Europe, Canada, South Africa | April through September 1999 | Nonimmune travelers | ≥3 (and 11 kg) | 489 (966) | 100 | 21 |
| Eritrea | 1997–1999 | Nonimmune Danish soldiers | Not available | 186 (300) | 100 | 42 |

*Abbreviations:* AP, atovaquone-proguanil; Pf, *P. falciparum*; Pv, *P. vivax*.

documented include Nigeria, Mali, Cameroon, Ivory Coast, Kenya, and Gabon.

**Primaquine**

Until recently, malaria chemoprophylaxis has targeted the prevention of fatal falciparum malaria, but *P vivax* is a frequent cause of travel-related malaria and is not effectively prevented with the prevailing chemoprophylaxis strategy. The CDC recommendations include the use of primaquine for terminal prophylaxis to prevent *P vivax* malaria, but the guidelines are broad and adherence is difficult. Data in travelers illustrated that current chemoprophylaxis prevented primary attacks of *P falciparum* and *P vivax* but not relapses of *P vivax* or *P ovale*. In 1995 to 1996, groups of Israeli travelers returning from Ethiopia were found to have a high incidence (50%) of *P vivax* occurring 3 months after exposure despite recommended chemoprophylaxis [45]. More recently, analyses of malaria surveillance in civilian residents of Israel from 1994 to 1999 (N = 300) and the United States from 1992 to 1998 (N = 2822) showed that *P vivax* and *P falciparum* caused most malaria cases, and were comparable in incidence (44.6%–50.8% versus 43.5%–44%, respectively) [46]. Thirty-five percent to 45% of malaria cases occurred more than 2 months after return; *P vivax* and *P ovale* caused the overwhelming majority of late cases, and 62% to 81% of these patients had taken recommended chemoprophylaxis other than primaquine [46]. Most patients with *P falciparum* presented within 2 months, however, and did not use appropriate chemoprophylaxis. The authors concluded that in Sub-Saharan Africa where *P falciparum* is the predominant cause of malaria, blood-stage prophylaxis is adequate. They recommended liver stage (primaquine) prophylaxis during travel in the Horn of Africa (Ethiopia and Somalia), however, where *P vivax* causes significant malaria cases, and other areas with significant *P vivax* and *P ovale* infection.

Most available malaria prophylactic agents kill blood-stage parasites and are considered suppressive, whereas causal prophylactic agents kill parasites during the liver stage. Among the compounds synthesized in the search of drugs for malaria control in the 1940s was 6-methoxy-8-aminoquinoline, later called plasmochin, plasmoquine, or pamaquine [47]. The compound killed gametocytes and also prevented relapses of *P vivax* infection, but was too toxic; further research identified less toxic and more effective 8-aminoquinolines, and led to the discovery of primaquine [47]. Primaquine was evaluated in the 1950s for its activity as a radical cure for malaria in American troops returning from the Korean War. Primaquine has demonstrated activity against the liver stage of *P vivax* and *P falciparum*, blood stage of *P vivax*, hypnozoite of *P vivax and P ovale*, and gametocytes; however, it has only minor activity against the asexual blood stage of *P falciparum* [47–49]. It is effective against chloroquine-resistant strains of

*P falciparum* [50]. Its mechanism of action is not clearly known, but is speculated to be a disruption of the parasite mitochondrial membrane by generation of toxic metabolites [51]. A challenge study with sporozoites of the Chesson strain of *P vivax* in subjects taking primaquine, 30 mg daily 1 day before, the day of, and 6 days after challenge, achieved 100% protective efficacy [52].

Clinical trials have been conducted since 1992 in Indonesia [53–55], Kenya [56], Colombia [57], and in Israeli travelers (Table 5) [58]. Thirty milligrams of primaquine base (15 mg base = 26.5 mg salt) equivalent to two tablets daily showed a protective efficacy of 85% to 93% for *P falciparum* and *P vivax*, although an alternate-day regimen provided inadequate protection for *P falciparum* [53]. In Indonesian transmigrants to Papua, overall protective efficacy was 93%, 88% to 95% for *P falciparum*, and 90% to 92% for *P vivax* [54,55]. In Kenyan children, 15-mg daily dose showed a protective efficacy of 85% for *P falciparum* [56]. A study in Colombian soldiers showed 89% overall protective efficacy, 94% for *P falciparum* and 85% for *P vivax* [57]. Finally, a retrospective study of travelers who took rafting trips to *P vivax*–hyperendemic areas in Ethiopia (October 1995 through April 1998) showed that travelers who took primaquine for chemoprophylaxis had a lower incidence of malaria (5.7%) compared with those who took doxycycline (53%) or mefloquine (52%) [58].

Primaquine seems to have a good safety and tolerability profile. Gastrointestinal disturbances are the primary complaints, but are minimized when the drug is taken with food [59]. Primaquine at 30 mg base every other day was better tolerated than weekly chloroquine [53]. Headache, cough, and sore throat were less likely to occur in the primaquine group compared with placebo [55]. Methemoglobinemia was infrequent, in the range of 6%, symptoms were mild and without clinical consequence; the maximum level of methemoglobinemia recorded following the use of primaquine was 13%, but resolved within 2 weeks even with long-term use [59]. Glucose-6-phosphate dehydrogenase (G6PD) deficiency is the most dangerous contraindication, because life-threatening hemolysis can occur. A G6PD level must be determined before prescribing the medication. Primaquine should not be given during pregnancy.

In 2003, an expert panel convened by the CDC reviewed the recommendations on malaria prophylaxis in travelers, and new recommendations were made regarding primaquine. First, the CDC added primaquine as a second-line chemoprophylaxis agent, to be given as a daily dose of 30 mg base starting 1 to 2 days before entering a malaria risk area, continued through exposure, and for 1 week after departing a malaria risk area [60]. Second, primaquine had previously been recommended at a dose of 15 to 30 mg daily for 14 days to eradicate the hypnozoites of *P vivax* or *P ovale* in patients with these infections (radical cure). The review of primaquine's efficacy as a radical cure showed that the Chesson strain of *P vivax* did not

Table 5
Studies of primaquine for malaria prophylaxis

| Study site | Dates of study | Subjects | Age of subjects (y) | Number of subjects taking primaquine (total, N) | Dose | Protective efficacy (%) | Reference |
|---|---|---|---|---|---|---|---|
| Irian Jaya (Papua), Indonesia | November 1992 to January 1993 | Nonimmune transmigrants | 7–59 | 45 (99) | 0.5 mg base/kg every other day | 74% Pf 90% Pv | 53 |
| Kenya | April to July 1992 and 1993 | Semi-immune children | 9–14 | 32 (165) | 15 mg daily | 85% | 56 |
| Irian Jaya (Papua), Indonesia | July 1993 to August 1994 | Nonimmune transmigrants | >15 | 43 (126) | 0.5 mg base/kg daily | Overall 93% Pf 95% Pf 90% Pv | 54 |
| Colombia | April to September 1997 | Nonimmune soldiers | 18–42 | 122 (176) | 30 mg daily | Overall 89% Pf 94% Pf 85% Pv | 57 |
| Papua, Indonesia | April through December 1999 | Nonimmune transmigrants | 12–65 | 97 (385) | 30 mg daily | Overall 93% Pf 88% Pf 92% Pv | 55 |
| Israel | October 1995 through April 1998 | Nonimmune travelers who visited Ethiopia | 22–65 | 106 (158) | 15 mg daily <70 kg 30 mg daily >70 kg | Incidence of malaria = 5.7% (doxycycline group = 53%, mefloquine group = 52%) | 58 |

*Abbreviations:* Pf, *P falciparum*; Pv, *P vivax*.

respond to the lower doses of primaquine. As a result, the recommendation for radical cure has been changed to 30 mg of primaquine daily for 14 days. Finally, the recommendation for terminal prophylaxis has also been changed to the increased dose, primaquine 30 mg daily for 14 days after departure from malaria risk areas [60].

For malaria chemoprophylaxis it has been proposed that primaquine base in a dose of 0.5 mg/kg daily may be started on arrival and continued through 3 days after leaving a malaria risk area [59]. Primaquine may be an ideal regimen for short trips, thereby improving compliance. The shortened course, however, needs further assessment and approval. Evaluation is also needed in children less than 8 years of age.

Table 6 lists currently recommended drugs for chemoprophylaxis and terminal prophylaxis.

## Tafenoquine

Not yet available, tafenoquine was developed by Walter Reed Army Institute of Research in search for alternatives to primaquine. Originally called WR238605 or etaquine, it is a synthetic analogue of primaquine ([±]-8-[{4-amino-1-methylbutyl} amino]-2,6-dimethoxy-4-methyl-5-[3-trifluoromethylphenoxy] quinoline succinate) [47,61,62]. In comparison with primaquine, tafenoquine seems to have comparable or greater efficacy, lower toxicity, and longer half-life [47,62,63]. Tafenoquine has a long absorption phase and is slowly metabolized; it reaches peak concentration at 12 hours, and has an elimination half-life of 14 days [62]. Tafenoquine has been described to be more potent than primaquine as a blood schizonticide, possibly because of its accumulation inside the red blood cell and longer half-life [62].

Tafenoquine has been evaluated as a causal prophylactic against *P falciparum*, a radical curative agent against *P vivax*, and a blood schizonticide against multidrug-resistant asexual blood stages of *P falciparum* or chloroquine-resistant *P vivax* [47]. A human challenge model using 600 mg of tafenoquine in a single dose 1 day before challenge with *P falciparum* protected three of four subjects, resulting in a protective efficacy of 75% [61]. Clinical trials of tafenoquine for chemoprophylaxis in semi-immune residents in Kenya, Ghana, and Gabon have demonstrated protection (Table 7) [64–66]. A dose-ranging study for weekly prophylaxis with tafenoquine showed protective efficacies of 86% (200 mg), 87% (100 mg), and 84% (50 mg), comparable with the 86% protective efficacy from weekly mefloquine [65]. Although one trial found a loading dose of tafenoquine, 125 mg and 250 mg daily for 3 days, to have protective efficacies of 93% and 100% at 70 days in semi-immunes [66], another trial found a protective efficacy of only 68% at 13 weeks following a 3-day course of tafenoquine, 400 mg daily [64]. In the latter trial, tafenoquine continued

Table 6
Summary of recommended drugs for malaria chemoprophylaxis and terminal prophylaxis

| Parasite sensitivity | Medication | Adult dose | Pediatric dose | Comments and directions |
|---|---|---|---|---|
| Areas with chloroquine-sensitive *P falciparum* | Chloroquine phosphate | 300 mg base (500 mg salt) orally once per week | 5 mg/kg base (8.3 mg/kg salt) once per week | Start 1–2 wk before entering risk area and through 4 wk after departure from risk area |
| | Hydroxychloroquine sulfate | 310 mg base (400 mg salt) orally, once per week | 5 mg/kg base (6.5 mg/kg salt) orally, once per week, up to 310 mg base | An alternative to chloroquine for primary prophylaxis in areas with chloroquine-sensitive *P falciparum* |
| Areas with chloroquine-resistant *P falciparum* | Atovaquone-proguanil | 250 mg atovaquone and 100 mg proguanil in a combined adult tablet orally daily | 62.5 mg atovaquone and 25 mg proguanil in a combined pediatric tablet daily<br>11–20 kg: 1 tablet<br>21–30 kg: 2 tablets<br>31–40 kg: 3 tablets<br>≥40 kg: 1 adult tablet daily | Also recommended for primary prophylaxis in areas with mefloquine-resistant *P falciparum*<br>Start 1–2 d before entering risk area and through 1 wk after departure from risk area<br>Contraindicated in pregnant women |
| | Doxycycline | 100 mg orally daily | ≥8 years of age: 2 mg/kg up to 100 mg daily | Also recommended for primary prophylaxis in areas with mefloquine-resistant *P falciparum*<br>Start 1–2 d before entering risk area and through 4 wk after departure from risk area<br>Contraindicated in pregnant women and children <8 y old |

| | | | |
|---|---|---|---|
| Mefloquine | 228 mg base (250 mg salt) orally, once per week | ≤15 kg: 4.6 mg/kg base (5 mg/kg salt) orally, once per week<br>15–19 kg: ¼ tablet<br>20–30 kg: ½ tablet<br>31–45 kg: ¾ tablet<br>≥46 kg: 1 tablet | Start 1–2 wk before entering risk area and through 4 wk after departure from risk area<br>Consider starting 3–4 wk before travel to assess tolerability<br>Contraindicated in persons with seizures, major psychiatric disorders, recent depression or anxiety reactions, and cardiac conduction abnormalities associated with arrhythmia<br>Second-line option for primary prophylaxis |
| Primaquine prophylaxis | 30 mg base (52.6 mg salt) orally daily | 0.6 mg/kg base (1 mg/kg salt) up to adult dose | Must check G6PD level first; contraindicated in persons with G6PD deficiency<br>Contraindicated in pregnancy and lactation |
| Terminal prophylaxis to prevent relapse of *P vivax* and *P ovale* | Primaquine | 30 mg base (52.6 mg salt) orally daily for 14 d after departure from the malarious area | 0.6 mg/kg base (1 mg/kg salt) up to adult dose, daily for 14 d after departure from the malarious area | Must check G6PD level first; contraindicated in persons with G6PD deficiency<br>Contraindicated in pregnancy and lactation |

*Adapted from* Centers for Disease Control and Prevention. Malaria. In: Health information for international travel 2003–2004. Atlanta: US Department of Health and Human Services, Public Health Service; 2003. p. 99–116.

Table 7
Studies of tafenoquine for malaria prophylaxis

| Study site | Dates of study | Subjects | Age of subjects (y) | Dose | Number of subjects (total N) | Protective efficacy | Reference |
|---|---|---|---|---|---|---|---|
| WRAIR | Before 1998 | Nonimmune volunteers | 25 +/- 5 y | 600 mg ×1 | 4 (6) | 75% | 61 |
| Kenya | May through September 1997 | Semi-immune residents | 18–55 | 400 mg daily ×3<br>200 mg daily ×3 then weekly<br>400 mg daily ×3 then weekly | 54<br>53<br><br>57 (223) | 68% (at 13 wk)<br>86%<br><br>89% | 64 |
| Ghana | August 1998 | Semi-immune residents | 18–60 | 25 mg,<br>50 mg,<br>100 mg,<br>or 200 mg daily ×3 then weekly | 93<br>91<br>94<br>91 (508) | 32%<br>84%<br>87%<br>86% | 65 |
| Gabon | February to July 1999 | Semi-immune residents | 12–20 | 250 mg daily ×3<br>125 mg daily ×3<br>62.5 mg daily ×3<br>31.25 mg daily ×3 | 84<br>79<br>86<br>79 (410) | 100%<br>93%<br>80%<br>0 (at 77 days) | 66 |
| Thailand | August 1996-June 1997 | Patients infected with *P vivax* | 18–60 | 300 mg daily ×7<br>500 mg daily ×3, repeated in 1 week<br>500 mg ×1 | 15<br>11<br><br>9 (44) | Overall 91% decrease in malaria relapse, follow-up for 6 mo | 67 |
| Papua New Guinea | November 1998 to September 1999 | Australian Defense Force, used for terminal prophylaxis | Not reported | 400 mg daily ×3<br>200 mg bid ×3 | 292<br>86 (586) | Rate of *P vivax* occurring within 12 mo of exposure was 1.85%, compared with 2.8% in primaquine group | 68 |

weekly after the 3-day loading dose provided much improved protection of 86% (200 mg) and 89% (400 mg), respectively [64].

The studies for chemoprophylaxis showed that gastrointestinal disturbances were more common in the group taking tafenoquine, 400 mg weekly; dermatologic complaints, such as furunculosis and rash, were more prevalent in the tafenoquine group [64]. Musculoskeletal complaints and respiratory tract infections were also reported. Some subjects were found to have mild alanine transaminase elevations [65]. As with primaquine, tafenoquine can cause methemoglobinemia and serious hemolysis in G6PD-deficient individuals [64,67].

Studies that assessed tafenoquine as a radical cure, using 400 mg or 500 mg daily dosing for 3 days have demonstrated reduction of *P vivax* relapses by 91% compared with no radical cure and similar efficacy compared with primaquine [67,68]. Chesson strain parasites refractory to primaquine were also refractory, however, to tafenoquine [68]. Gastrointestinal disturbances, such as abdominal discomfort and diarrhea, were more frequent in subjects who took tafenoquine than in those who took primaquine or chloroquine alone [67,68]. Nonetheless, the shorter course should be more convenient as a radical cure and terminal prophylaxis.

It has been suggested that wide use of tafenoquine may contribute to reduction of transmission because of its gametocidal action. It should be remembered, however, that low drug levels may lead to development of drug resistance [69].

## Azithromycin

Another drug that has been tested for its antimalarial properties is azithromycin. Azithromycin concentrates in tissues and intracellularly, and has a long half-life of 2.4 days [70]. It may be used safely in children under 8 years of age and in pregnant women. In a challenge study where subjects were infected with chloroquine-resistant *P falciparum* on day 3 of azithromycin therapy, three out of four volunteers who took azithromycin daily for 7 days were protected, indicating a protective efficacy of 75% [70]. The mechanism of action of azithromycin as an antimalarial is unknown, but may be caused by the inhibition of parasite mitochondrial protein synthesis [70]. Although causal prophylaxis was suggested, the results of another study refuted the effect [71].

A field trial in Kenya showed daily azithromycin to have a protective efficacy of 82.7%, but weekly azithromycin only resulted in a protective efficacy of 64.2%, compared with 92.6% for doxycycline (Table 8) [72]. In nonimmune Indonesians in Irian Jaya, the protective efficacy of daily azithromycin was found to be only 71.6% for *P falciparum* and 98.9% for *P vivax* (compared with 96.3% and 98% for doxycycline, respectively) [73]. To achieve adequate malaria protection, azithromycin needs to be used in

Table 8
Studies of azithromycin for malaria prophylaxis

| Study site | Date of study | Subjects | Age of subjects (years) | Dose | Number of subjects taking azithromycin, (total, N) | Protective efficacy | Reference |
|---|---|---|---|---|---|---|---|
| WRAIR | Before 1994 | Nonimmune volunteers | 18–40 | 500 mg then 250 mg daily x7 | 4 (19) | 75% | 70 |
| WRAIR | Before 1994 | Nonimmune volunteers challenged on day 14 | 18–46 | 500 mg then 250 mg daily for 7 days or 28 days after challenge | 10 (24) | 40% (7-day group) 100% (28-day group) | 71 |
| Kenya | April to August 1995 | Semi-immune residents | 18–55 | 250 mg daily 1000 mg weekly | 55 53 (213) | 82.7% 64.2% | 72 |
| Indonesia | July 1996 to January 1997 | Nonimmune transmigrants | 18–55 | 750 mg then 250 mg daily | 148 (300) | 71.6% Pf 98.9% Pv | 73 |

*Abbreviations:* Pf, *P falciparum;* Pv, *P vivax.*

combination with other agents. In vitro tests have shown additive to synergistic effects against multidrug-resistant *P falciparum* when azithromycin was combined with chloroquine, quinine, tafenoquine, or primaquine, but possible antagonism when combined with dihydroartemisinin [74]. At present, azithromycin cannot be recommended for malaria chemoprophylaxis. Further studies of its efficacy in combination with other agents are warranted.

**Standby treatment**

Chemoprophylaxis guidelines have been developed to protect travelers at risk of acquiring malaria, and aim to prevent symptomatic malaria infections. This benefit must be balanced against the risk of adverse events resulting from prophylactic medications. It is especially worrisome for those visiting remote areas that despite chemoprophylaxis, malaria can still occur. Among travelers who stayed in endemic areas for up to 1 month, 22% of malaria infections were treated while abroad in the endemic country, often with suboptimal medical care [75]. It should be noted that recent studies have shown that malaria is not infrequently overdiagnosed among travelers visiting developing countries, particularly in West Africa [76,77].

Standby emergency treatment evolved as another way to approach the problem of malaria in travelers and as a means to reduce the risks of prophylactic medications in areas of the world where the transmission of malaria is low. Standby treatment is generally considered "an option for clearly defined situations while prophylaxis remains the safest choice for travelers to areas of high transmission" [78].

Since 1988, the WHO has recommended self-administration of standby treatment by certain travelers to remote malaria-endemic regions when fever and flulike symptoms occur and immediate medical attention is not available [75,79]. In 1990, the CDC recommended chloroquine and sulfadoxine-pyrimethamine (Fansidar) for standby emergency treatment while medical care is sought; mefloquine was not recommended for standby treatment because of side effects [80]. The current CDC and WHO guidelines emphasize the use of chemoprophylaxis for travel to malarious areas. Standby emergency treatment is not a replacement for appropriate chemoprophylaxis. Standby emergency treatment may be recommended, however, for specific situations: travelers who choose to take no prophylaxis; who choose a suboptimal drug regimen; who may fall ill in remote areas even while taking effective prophylaxis, and do not have ready access to medical care; and who may need to self-diagnose [60,75]. Furthermore, the WHO also states that travelers visiting remote areas with low-risk multidrug-resistant *P falciparum* for 1 week or more (South East Asia border areas) can consider standby treatment over chemoprophylaxis [79]. All guidelines stress that standby treatment of possible malaria is only a temporary measure, that prompt medical attention is absolutely necessary, and that standby treatment should not replace immediate medical evaluation [60]. Chemoprophylaxis remains the safest choice for malaria prevention.

The WHO includes additional indications for certain occupations, such as aircraft crews. In this group it has been suggested that chemoprophylaxis be reserved for high-risk destinations, whereas at other times aircrew might use personal protective measures, seek immediate medical care for fever, and take standby treatment if medical care is not available [79]. Before the initiation of standby treatment, a survey of Swiss airline crew in 1984 found poor adherence with chemoprophylaxis, where only 25% used chemoprophylaxis [81]. From 1985 to 1988, Swissair changed its emphasis to personal protective measures and standby treatment with sulfadoxine-pyrimethamine rather than chemoprophylaxis for crew to Asia and South America [81]. After the adoption of standby treatment, there was no significant increase of malaria cases; standby treatment was carried by 83%, personal protective measures used by 61% to 73% [81]. Standby treatment was used by 1% of the crew per year, and the number of antimalarial tablets prescribed decreased dramatically from 138,000 (1984) to 45,000 (1988) [81].

Extensive and detailed instructions need to be communicated when prescribing standby treatment. Travelers should take standby treatment promptly if they develop a fever, chills, or other influenza-like illness, and if professional medical care is not available within 24 hours. Specific directions should be given concerning symptom recognition, when and how treatment should be administered, the regimen and side effects, possible drug failure, and the need to seek medical evaluation as soon as possible [79]. The WHO also recommends that the instructions specifically include the following [79]:

1. If fever occurs 1 week or more after entering malaria risk area, obtain medical evaluation immediately;
2. If access to medical care is unavailable within 24 hours after fever onset, start standby treatment and seek medical care;
3. Complete standby treatment and resume chemoprophylaxis 1 week after first treatment dose; mefloquine should be resumed 1 week after last treatment dose of quinine;
4. Treat fever with antipyretics first to minimize vomiting; give second full dose if vomiting occurs within 30 minutes; give additional half dose if vomiting occurs within 30 to 60 minutes; and
5. Use a different drug for standby treatment of malaria from that used for prophylaxis.

The choice of drugs for standby treatment varies according to national and regional guidelines [60,79,82]. The CDC currently recommends atovaquone-proguanil for standby treatment for travelers not taking atovaquone-proguanil for prophylaxis (Table 9). Because of resistance and toxicity, a traveler who is taking chemoprophylaxis should be given

Table 9
Standby treatment of malaria

| Drug | Adult dose | Pediatric dose | Comments |
|---|---|---|---|
| Atovaquone-proguanil (Malarone) | 4 tablets (each dose contains 1000 mg atovaquone and 400 mg proguanil) orally as a single daily dose for 3 consecutive days | One dose daily for 3 consecutive days using adult-strength tablets:<br>11–20 kg: 1 tablet<br>21–30 kg: 2 tablets<br>31–40 kg: 3 tablets<br>41 kg or more: 4 tablets | Self-treatment to be used if professional medical care is not available within 24 hours.<br>Medical care should be sought immediately after treatment.<br>Contraindicated in persons with severe renal impairment (creatinine clearance <30 mL/min).<br>Not recommended for self-treatment in persons on atovaquone-proguanil prophylaxis. Not currently recommended for children <11 kg, pregnant women, and women breast-feeding infants weighing <11 kg. |

*Adapted from* CDC. Malaria. In: Health information for international travel 2003–2004. Atlanta: US Department of Health and Human Services, Public Health Service; 2003. p. 99–116.

a different drug for standby treatment [60,79,82]. If atovaquone-proguanil cannot be used, the CDC Malaria Epidemiology Branch (Malaria Hotline 770-488-7788) can provide consultation to health-care providers on other options for self-treatment [60]. The options for standby treatment recommended by the WHO include chloroquine, mefloquine, quinine, and quinine plus doxycycline [79]. The United Kingdom guidelines include the following options: chloroquine; atovaquone-proguanil; co-artemether (artemisinin plus lumefantrine); quinine plus doxycycline; and quinine [82]. Sulfadoxine-pyrimethamine has been removed as an option for standby treatment because of widespread resistance. Halofantrine has been explicitly excluded because of QT prolongation and arrhythmias [60,82].

Concerns have been raised regarding standby treatment because of its misuse by travelers. Following the 1988 recommendation for standby treatment by Swiss experts, an assessment suggested overuse because 4% of travelers to East Africa used standby treatment where the attack rate was only 0.2% to 1.5% [78]. Another study found that only 5% of those travelers with possible malaria symptoms used standby treatment, and two thirds of ill travelers failed to seek medical attention or use medication [83]. Standby therapy may lead to the delay in diagnosis of other important infections, as was the case of a returned traveler who used standby treatment for fever without relief, only to be diagnosed later with an appendicular abscess [84]. An additional concern is that some travelers may discontinue chemoprophylaxis in favor of standby treatment, leading to greater malaria risk [85]. Finally, in this same study, most ill travelers erred on the dose of standby treatment [85].

**Rapid diagnostics for malaria: dipstick tests**

In the consideration of standby treatment for malaria, some experts have advocated that travelers obtain parasitologic confirmation along with self-treatment [78]. Self-diagnosis using microscopic tests is usually not feasible for travelers, but a number of rapid diagnostic tests (dipsticks) have been developed for field diagnosis, and have possible applications for use by travelers.

These rapid diagnostic tests, ParaSight F, ICT Malaria (MalaQuick), and OptiMAL, are based on antigen-capture assays. ParaSight F detects histidine-rich protein II present in the plasma of persons infected with *P falciparum* [86,87]. The dipstick consists of a nitrocellulose-glass fiber strip that is embedded with antibodies for histidine-rich protein II and a dye that marks a positive reaction [87,88]. ICT Malaria test, detecting *P falciparum*–specific histidine-rich protein II and panmalarial antigens, has demonstrated a sensitivity of 86.2% to 95% and specificity of 76.9% to 97% for *P falciparum* but poor sensitivity (2.9%) for nonfalciparum malaria [88,89]. A study using the ParaSight F test showed 14% false-negative samples [87]. The OptiMAL test detects parasite lactate dehydrogenase, seems to have reasonable specificity (*P falciparum* = 97%, non–*P falciparum* = 96.9%), but lacks sensitivity (*P falciparum* = 42.6%, non–*P falciparum* = 47.1%,) [88].

The use of rapid diagnostic tests for travelers exposed to malaria has been debated. Most studies of self-diagnosis have shown that travelers have significant difficulty in performing these tests or in their interpretation [87,90,91]. The high false-negative rate is unacceptable and these tests are especially difficult to perform when a traveler is ill [87,91]. In addition, weather conditions can degrade dipsticks and reduce their sensitivity. Rapid diagnostic tests for malaria are currently not recommended for use by travelers [79].

**Personal protective measures**

Insect repellents, insecticide-impregnated clothing, and bed nets continue to be important and significant measures in the prevention of malaria transmission. A study of Colombian soldiers found the use of permethrin-impregnated clothing to reduce the occurrence of malaria from 14% in controls to 3% in permethrin-treated group, or 75% effective protection for a 1-month exposure [92]. A comparison of repellents (DEET, botanical, soybean oil, citronella, IR3535) found DEET, or N, N-diethyl-m-toluamide, to provide the longest period of protection; higher concentrations of DEET correlated with longer periods of protection, but only products up to 23.8% DEET were tested [93]. Ethanol seems to increase the dermal absorption of DEET; nonalcohol formulations may reduce toxicity from DEET [94].

Safety of DEET and in utero exposure has been examined. Although DEET crossed placenta, and was detected in 8% of cord blood, infants born to women who used approximately 20% DEET in the second and third trimesters of pregnancy did not have adverse effects when followed up to 12 months [95]. Recently, the Environmental Protection Agency and the American Academy of Pediatrics have approved the use of DEET for protection of infants older than 2 months of age [96]. Finally, a new repellent, picaridin, seems to hold promise as an alternative to DEET. Nighttime use of 19.2% picaridin provided more than 94.7% protection for at least 9 hours against mixed species of mosquitoes; by comparison, 35% DEET provided more than 95% protection for 7 hours [97].

## Summary

Malaria prevention has benefited from many diverse disciplines of research, including epidemiologic monitoring, development of laboratory techniques, assessment of insect repellents, or pharmaceutical innovations. Strategies in all these sectors have been explored in recent years, resulting in improved options to prevent travelers' malaria. The addition of atovaquone-proguanil for malaria chemoprophylaxis and the recommendation of primaquine as primary prophylaxis have been significant advances. Tafenoquine seems promising. Standby treatment recommendations have been refined. Many areas still need better strategies. Problematic areas include chemoprophylaxis for long-term travelers, expatriates, and pregnant women; optimal criteria for terminal prophylaxis; and the prevention of malaria in populations that are least likely to seek pretravel evaluations, such as those visiting friends and relatives in their home countries (VFRs). Finally, research in travel and tropical medicine should continue to focus on additional strategies to confront the ever-widening challenge of drug-resistant malaria.

## References

[1] WHO. World malaria situation in 1994. Part I: Population at risk. Wkly Epidemiol Rec 1997;72:269–74.
[2] Breman JG. The ears of the hippopotamus: manifestations, determinants, and estimates of the malaria burden. Am J Trop Med Hyg 2001;64(1–2 Suppl):1–11.
[3] Muentener P, Schlagenhauf P, Steffen R. Imported malaria (1985–95): trends and perspectives. Bull World Health Organ 1999;77:560–6.
[4] Kain KC, Keystone JS. Malaria in travelers: epidemiology, disease, and prevention. Infect Dis Clin North Am 1998;12:267–84.
[5] Sabatinelli G, Ejoy M, Joergensen P. Malaria in the WHO European Region (1971–1999). Euro Surveill 2001;6:61–5.
[6] Newman RD, Barber AM, Roberts J, et al. Malaria surveillance—United States, 1999. MMWR Morb Mortal Wkly Rep 2002;51(SS01):15–28.
[7] Causer LM, Newman RD, Barber AM, et al. Malaria surveillance—United States, 2000. MMWR Morb Mortal Wkly Rep 2002;51(SS05):9–23.

[8] Filler S, Causer LM, Newman RD, et al. Malaria surveillance—United States, 2001. MMWR Morb Mortal Wkly Rep 2003;52(SS05):1–14.
[9] Shah S, Filler S, Causer LM, et al. Malaria surveillance—United States, 2002. MMWR Morb Mortal Wkly Rep 2004;53(SS01):21–34.
[10] Steffen R, Fuchs E, Schildknecht J, et al. Mefloquine compared with other chemoprophylactic regimens in tourists visiting East Africa. Lancet 1993;341:1299–303.
[11] Lobel HO, Miani M, Eng T, et al. Long-term malaria prophylaxis with weekly mefloquine. Lancet 1993;341:848–51.
[12] Steffen R, Jong EC. Travelers' and immigrants' health. In: Guerrant RL, Walker DH, Wyler PF, editors. Tropical infectious diseases: principles, pathogens and practice. Philadelphia: Churchill Livingstone; 1999. p. 106–14.
[13] Leder K, Black J, O'Brien D, et al. Malaria in travelers: a review of the GeoSentinel Surveillance Network. Clin Infect Dis 2004;39:1104–12.
[14] Jelinek T, Schulte C, Behrens R, et al. Imported falciparum malaria in Europe: sentinel surveillance data from the European network on surveillance of imported infectious diseases. Clin Infect Dis 2002;34:572–6.
[15] Nothdurft HD, Jelinek T, Bluml A, et al. Seroconversion to circumsporozoite antigen of *Plasmodium falciparum* demonstrates a high risk of malaria transmission in travelers to East Africa. Clin Infect Dis 1999;28:641–2.
[16] Jelinek T, Bluml A, Loscher T, et al. Assessing the incidence of infection with *Plasmodium falciparum* among international travelers. Am J Trop Med Hyg 1998;59:35–7.
[17] Jelinek T, Loscher T, Nothdurft HD. High prevalence of antibodies against circumsporozoite antigen of *Plasmodium falciparum* without development of symptomatic malaria in travelers to sub-Saharan Africa. J Infect Dis 1996;174:1376–9.
[18] Høgh B, Clarke PD, Nothdurft HD, et al. Atovaquone-proguanil versus chloroquine-proguanil for malaria prophylaxis in non-immune travelers: a randomized, double-blind study. Lancet 2000;356:1888–94.
[19] Schlagenhauf P, Tschopp A, Johnson R, et al. Tolerability of malaria chemoprophylaxis in non-immune travelers to sub-Saharan Africa: multicentre, randomized, double blind, four-arm study. BMJ 2003;327:1078–83.
[20] Croft A, Garner P. Mefloquine to prevent malaria: a systematic review of trials. BMJ 1997;315:1412–6.
[21] Overbosch D, Schilthuis H, Bienzle U, et al. Atovaquone-proguanil versus mefloquine for malaria prophylaxis in nonimmune travelers: results from a randomized, double-blind study. Clin Infect Dis 2001;33:1015–21.
[22] Wongsrichanalai C, Pickard AL, Wernsdorfer WH, et al. Epidemiology of drug-resistant malaria. Lancet Infect Dis 2002;2:209–18.
[23] Le Bras J, Durand R. The mechanisms of resistance to antimalarial drugs in *Plasmodium falciparum*. Fundam Clin Pharmacol 2003;17:147–53.
[24] Färnert A, Lindberg J, Gil P, et al. Evidence of *Plasmodium falciparum* malaria resistant to atovaquone and proguanil hydrochloride: case reports. BMJ 2003;326:628–9.
[25] Schwartz E, Bujanover S, Kain KC. Genetic confirmation of atovaquone-proguanil-resistant *Plasmodium falciparum* malaria acquired by a nonimmune traveler to East Africa. Clin Infect Dis 2003;37:450–1.
[26] Kain KC, Shanks GD, Keystone JS. Malaria chemoprophylaxis in the age of drug resistance. I. Currently recommended drug regimens. Clin Infect Dis 2001;33:226–34.
[27] Rieckmann KH, Davis DR, Hutton DC. *Plasmodium vivax* resistance to chloroquine? Lancet 1989;2:1183–4.
[28] Whitby M, Wood G, Veenendaal JR, et al. Chloroquine-resistant *Plasmodium vivax*. Lancet 1989;2:1395.
[29] Baird JK, Basri H, Purnomo, et al. Resistance to chloroquine by *Plasmodium vivax* in Irian Jaya, Indonesia. Am J Trop Med Hyg 1991;44:547–52.

[30] Maguire JD, Sumawinata IW, Masbar S, et al. Chloroquine-resistant *Plasmodium malariae* in south Sumatra, Indonesia. Lancet 2002;360:58–60.
[31] Singh B, Kim Sung L, Matusop A, et al. A large focus of naturally acquired *Plasmodium knowlesi* infections in human beings. Lancet 2004;363:1017–24.
[32] Labbe AC, Patel S, Crandall I, et al. A molecular surveillance system for global patterns of drug resistance in imported malaria. Emerg Infect Dis 2003;9:33–6.
[33] Srivastava IK, Rottenberg H, Vaidya AB. Atovaquone, a broad spectrum antiparasitic drug, collapses mitochondrial membrane potential in a malarial parasite. J Biol Chem 1997; 272:3961–6.
[34] Srivastava IK, Vaidya AB. A mechanism for the synergistic action of atovaquone and proguanil. Antimicrob Agents Chemother 1999;43:1334–9.
[35] Shapiro TA, Ranasinha CD, Kumar N, et al. Prophylactic activity of atovaquone against *Plasmodium falciparum* in humans. Am J Trop Med Hyg 1999;60:831–6.
[36] Berman JD, Nielsen R, Chulay JD, et al. Causal prophylactic efficacy of atovaquone-proguanil (Malarone) in a human challenge model. Trans R Soc Trop Med Hyg 2001;95: 129–32.
[37] Lell B, Luckner D, Ndjave M, et al. Randomised placebo-controlled study of atovaquone plus proguanil for malaria prophylaxis in children. Lancet 1998;351:709–13.
[38] Sukwa TY, Mulenga M, Chisdaka N, et al. A randomized, double-blind, placebo-controlled field trial to determine the efficacy and safety of Malarone (atovaquone/proguanil) for the prophylaxis of malaria in Zambia. Am J Trop Med Hyg 1999;60: 521–5.
[39] Shanks GD, Gordon DM, Klotz FW, et al. Efficacy and safety of atovaquone/proguanil as suppressive prophylaxis for *Plasmodium falciparum* malaria. Clin Infect Dis 1998;27: 494–9.
[40] Faucher J-F, Binder R, Missinou MA, et al. Efficacy of atovaquone/proguanil for malaria prophylaxis in children and its effect on the immunogenicity of live oral typhoid and cholera vaccines. Clin Infect Dis 2002;35:1147–54.
[41] Ling J, Baird JK, Fryauff DJ, et al. Randomized, placebo-controlled trial of atovaquone/proguanil for the prevention of *Plasmodium falciparum* or *Plasmodium vivax* malaria among migrants to Papua, Indonesia. Clin Infect Dis 2002;35:825–33.
[42] Petersen E. The safety of atovaquone/proguanil in long-term malaria prophylaxis of nonimmune adults. J Travel Med 2003;10(Suppl 1):S13–5.
[43] Korsinczky M, Chen N, Kotecka B, et al. Mutations in *Plasmodium falciparum* cytochrome b that are associated with atovaquone resistance are located at a putative drug-binding site. Antimicrob Agents Chemother 2000;44:2100–8.
[44] De Boever EH, Hedgley C, Alam F, et al. Post-marketing surveillance of Malarone (atovaquone and proguanil hydrochloride): efficacy update [abstract 245]. Presented at the 52nd Annual Meeting of the ASTMH. Philadelphia, December 3–7, 2003.
[45] Schwartz E, Sidi Y. New aspects of malaria imported from Ethiopia. Clin Infect Dis 1998; 26:1089–91.
[46] Schwartz E, Parise M, Kozarsky P, et al. Delayed onset of malaria: implications for chemoprophylaxis in travelers. N Engl J Med 2003;349:1510–6.
[47] Peters W. The evolution of tafenoquine: antimalarial for a new millennium? J R Soc Med 1999;92:345–52.
[48] Pukrittayakamee S, Vanijononta S, Chantra A, et al. Blood stage antimalarial efficacy of primaquine in *Plasmodium vivax* malaria. J Infect Dis 1994;169:932–5.
[49] Arnold J, Alving AS, Hockwald RS, et al. The antimalarial action of primaquine against the blood and tissue stages of falciparum malaria (Panama P-F-6 strain). J Lab Clin Med 1955;46:391–7.
[50] Geary TG, Divo AA, Jenson JB. Activity of quinoline antimalarials against chloroquine-sensitive and -resistant strains of *Plasmodium falciparum* in vitro. Trans R Soc Trop Med Hyg 1987;81:499–503.

[51] Jong EC, Nothdurft HD. Current drugs for antimalarial chemoprophylaxis: a review of efficacy and safety. J Travel Med 2001;8(Suppl 3):S48–56.
[52] Arnold J, Alving AS, Hockwald RS, et al. The effect of continuous and intermittent primaquine therapy on the relapse rate of Chesson strain vivax malaria. J Lab Clin Med 1954;44:429–37.
[53] Baird JK, Fryauff DJ, Basri H, et al. Primaquine for prophylaxis against malaria among nonimmune transmigrants in Irian Jaya, Indonesia. Am J Trop Med Hyg 1995;52:479–84.
[54] Fryauff DJ, Baird JK, Basri H, et al. Randomized, placebo-controlled trial of primaquine for prophylaxis of falciparum and vivax malaria in Indonesia. Lancet 1995;346:1190–3.
[55] Baird JK, Lacy MD, Basri H, et al. Randomized, parallel placebo-controlled trial of primaquine for malaria prophylaxis in Papua, Indonesia. Clin Infect Dis 2001;33:1990–7.
[56] Weiss WR, Oloo AJ, Johnson A, et al. Daily primaquine is effective for prophylaxis against falciparum malaria in Kenya: comparison with mefloquine, doxycycline, and chloroquine plus proguanil. J Infect Dis 1995;171:1569–75.
[57] Soto J, Toledo J, Rodriquez M, et al. Primaquine prophylaxis against malaria in nonimmune Colombian soldiers: efficacy and toxicity. Ann Intern Med 1998;129:241–4.
[58] Schwartz E, Regev-Yochay G. Primaquine as prophylaxis for malaria for nonimmune travelers: a comparison with mefloquine and doxycycline. Clin Infect Dis 1999;29:1502–6.
[59] Baird JK, Frauff DJ, Hoffman SL. Primaquine for prevention of malaria in travelers. Clin Infect Dis 2003;37:1659–67.
[60] CDC. Malaria. In: Health information for international travel 2003–2004. Atlanta: US Department of Health and Human Services, Public Health Service; 2003. p. 99–116.
[61] Brueckner RP, Coster T, Wesche DL, et al. Prophylaxis of *Plasmodium falciparum* infection in a human challenge model with WR 238605, a new 8-aminoquinoline antimalarial. Antimicrob Agents Chemother 1998;42:1293–4.
[62] Brueckner RP, Lasseter KC, Lin ET, et al. First-time-in-humans safety and pharmacokinetics of WR 238605, a new antimalarial. Am J Trop Med Hyg 1998;58:645–9.
[63] Shanks GD, Kain KC, Keystone JS. Malaria chemoprophylaxis in the age of drug resistance. II. Drugs that may be available in the future. Clin Infect Dis 2001;33:381–5.
[64] Shanks GD, Oloo AJ, Aleman GM, et al. A new primaquine analogue, tafenoquine (WR 238605), for prophylaxis against *Plasmodium falciparum* malaria. Clin Infect Dis 2001;33:1968–74.
[65] Hale BR, Owusu-Agyei S, Fryauff DJ, et al. A randomized, double-blind, placebo-controlled, dose-ranging trial of tafenoquine for weekly prophylaxis against *Plasmodium falciparum*. Clin Infect Dis 2003;36:541–9.
[66] Lell B, Faucher JF, Missinou MA, et al. Malaria chemoprophylaxis with tafenoquine: a randomized study. Lancet 2000;355:2041–5.
[67] Walsh DS, Looareesuwan S, Wilairatana P, et al. Randomized dose-ranging study of the safety and efficacy of WR 238605 (Tafenoquine) in the prevention of relapse of *Plasmodium vivax* malaria in Thailand. J Infect Dis 1999;180:1282–7.
[68] Nasveld P, Kitchener S, Edstein M, et al. Comparison of tafenoquine (WR238605) and primaquine in the post-exposure (terminal) prophylaxis of vivax malaria in Australian Defense Force Personnel. Trans R Soc Trop Med Hyg 2002;96:683–4.
[69] Kun JFJ, Lehman LG, Lell B, et al. Low-dose treatment with sulfadoxine-pyrimethamine combinations selects for drug-resistant *Plasmodium falciparum* strains. Antimicrob Agents Chemother 1999;43:2205–8.
[70] Kuschner RA, Heppner DG, Andersen SL, et al. Azithromycin prophylaxis against a chloroquine-resistant strain of *Plasmodium falciparum*. Lancet 1994;343:1396–7.
[71] Andersen SL, Berman J, Kuschner R, et al. Prophylaxis of *Plasmodium falciparum* malaria with azithromycin administered to volunteers. Ann Intern Med 1995;123:771–3.
[72] Andersen SL, Oloo AJ, Gordon DM, et al. Successful double-blinded, randomized, placebo-controlled field trial of azithromycin and doxycycline as prophylaxis for malaria in Western Kenya. Clin Infect Dis 1998;26:146–50.

[73] Taylor WR, Richie TL, Fryauff DJ, et al. Malaria prophylaxis using azithromycin: a double-blind, placebo-controlled trial in Irian Jaya, Indonesia. Clin Infect Dis 1999;28: 74–81.
[74] Ohrt C, Willingmyre GD, Lee P, et al. Assessment of azithromycin in combination with other antimalarial drugs against *Plasmodium falciparum* in vitro. Antimicrob Agents Chemother 2002;46:2518–24.
[75] WHO. Development of recommendations for the protection of short-stay travelers to malaria-endemic areas: memorandum from two WHO meetings. Bull World Health Organ 1988;66:177–96.
[76] Holtz TH, Onikpo F, Lama M, et al. Malaria microscopy in eight secondary health care facilities in Oueme, Cameroon [abstract 546]. Presented at the American Society of Tropical Medicine and Hygiene. Atlanta, November 11–15, 2001, p. 332.
[77] Silvers MJ, Purnomo, Tracy LA, et al. Assessing and improving accuracy of malaria slide reading for clinical trials [abstract 248]. Presented at the American Society of Tropical Medicine and Hygiene. Atlanta, November 11–15, 2001. p. 222.
[78] Schlagenhauf P, Steffen R. Stand-by treatment of malaria in travelers: a review. J Trop Med Hyg 1994;97:151–60.
[79] WHO. Stand-by emergency treatment. In: International travel and health. Available at: http://www.who.int/ith/chapter07_03.html. Accessed March 29, 2004.
[80] CDC. Recommendations for the prevention of malaria among travelers. MMWR Morb Mortal Wkly Rep 1990;39(RR-3):1–10.
[81] Steffen R, Holdener F, Wyss RK, et al. Malaria prophylaxis and self-therapy in airline crews. Aviat Space Environ Med 1990;6:942–5.
[82] Bradley DJ, Bannister B. Guidelines for malaria prevention in travelers from the United Kingdom for 2003. Commun Dis Public Health 2003;6:180–99.
[83] Schlagenhauf P, Steffen R, Tschopp A, et al. Behavioural aspects of travelers in their use of malaria presumptive treatment. Bull World Health Organ 1995;73:215–21.
[84] Lampe AS, Bakker RB, Smith SJ. Dangers of antimalarial standby treatment. Eur J Clin Microbiol Infect Dis 1994;13:322.
[85] Nothdurft HD, Jelinek T, Pechel SM, et al. Stand-by treatment of suspected malaria in travelers. Trop Med Parasitol 1995;46:161–3.
[86] Parra ME, Evans SB, Taylor DW. Identification of *Plasmodium falciparum* histidine rich protein-2 in the plasma of humans with malaria. J Clin Microbiol 1991;29:162–234.
[87] Trachsler M, Schlagenjhauf P, Steffen R. Feasibility of a rapid dipstick antigen-capture assay for self-testing of travellers' malaria. Trop Med Int Health 1999;4:442–7.
[88] Mason DP, Kawamoto F, Lin K, et al. A comparison of two rapid field immunochromatographic tests to expert microscopy in the diagnosis of malaria. Acta Trop 2002;82:51–9.
[89] Whitty CJM, Armstrong M, Behrens RH. Self-testing for falciparum malaria with antigen-capture cards by travelers with symptoms of malaria. Am J Trop Med Hyg 2000; 63:295–7.
[90] Jelinek T, Amsler L, Grobusch MP, et al. Self-use of rapid tests for malaria diagnosis by tourist. Lancet 1999;354:1609.
[91] Funk M, Schlagenhauf P, Tschopp A, et al. MalaQuick versus ParaSight F as a diagnostic aid in travellers' malaria. Trans R Soc Med Hyg 1999;93:268–72.
[92] Soto J, Medina F, Dember N, et al. Efficacy of permethrin-impregnated uniforms in the prevention of malaria and leishmaniasis in Colombian soldiers. Clin Infect Dis 1995;21: 599–602.
[93] Fradin MS, Day JF. Comparative efficacy of insect repellents against mosquito bites. N Engl J Med 2002;347:13–8.
[94] Fradin MS. Mosquitoes and mosquito repellents: a clinician's guide. Ann Intern Med 1998; 128:931–40.
[95] McGready R. Safety of the insect repellent N, N-diethyl-m-toluamide (DEET) in pregnancy. Am J Trop Med Hyg 2001;65:285–9.

[96] American Academy of Pediatrics. Follow safety precautions when using DEET on children. Available at: www.aap.org/family/wnv-jun03.htm. Accessed May 25, 2004.
[97] Frances SP, Van Dung N, Beebe NW, et al. Field evaluation of repellent formulations against daytime and nighttime biting mosquitoes in a tropical rainforest in northern Australia. J Med Entomol 2002;39:541–4.
[98] Goldberg DE, Slater AF, Beavis R, et al. Hemoglobin degradation in the human malaria pathogen *Plasmodium falciparum*: a catabolic pathway initiated by a specific aspartate protease. J Exp Med 1991;173:961–9.
[99] Slater AF, Cerami A. Inhibition by chloroquine of a novel haem polymerase enzyme activity in malaria trophozoites. Nature 1992;355:167–9.
[100] Schlesinger PH, Krogstad DJ, Herwaldt BL. Antimalarial agents: mechanisms of action. Antimicrob Agents Chemother 1988;32:793–8.
[101] Joshi N, Miller DQ. Doxycycline revisited. Arch Intern Med 1997;157:1421–6.
[102] Warhurst DC. Antimalarial interaction with ferriprotoporphyrin IX monomer and its relationship to the activity of the blood schizonticides. Ann Trop Med Parasitol 1987;81: 65–7.
[103] Khan B, Omar S, Kanyara JN, et al. Antifolate drug resistance and point mutations in *Plasmodium falciparum* in Kenya. Trans R Soc Trop Med Hyg 1997;91:456–60.
[104] Mockenhaupt FP. Mefloquine resistance in *Plasmodium falciparum*. Parasitol Today 1995; 11:248–53.

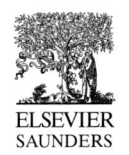

# Management of Severe Malaria: Interventions and Controversies

Geoffrey Pasvol, MA, MB, ChB, D Phil, FRCP, FRCPE[a,b,*]

[a]Department of Infection and Tropical Medicine, Lister Unit, Northwick Park Hospital, Harrow HA1 3UJ, United Kingdom
[b]Wellcome Centre for Clinical Tropical Medicine, Imperial College London, Room 233, Wright Fleming Institute, St. Mary's Campus, Norfolk Place, London W2 1PG, United Kingdom

The number of malarial infections acquired by international travelers from industrialized countries remains tiny compared with the annual global clinical caseload of nearly 500 million and 1 to 3 million deaths, mainly among young children in Africa. There are thought to be about 25,000 cases of malaria annually in travelers, only about half of which are reported and about 150 (<1%) are fatal [1]. About 1000 occur in the United States annually. In the United Kingdom alone well over 2000 cases are notified each year and there are around 10 to 20 deaths. Numbers are growing because of increasing international travel, increasing risk of transmission in areas where malaria control has declined, and the increasing prevalence of drug-resistant strains of parasites. The principles of prevention of imported malaria remain the avoidance of infective mosquito bites and appropriate chemoprophylaxis in the 30 million or so travelers who visit malarial-endemic regions each year [2]. The traveling population must be educated to seek advice before departure and also if they develop feverish symptoms within a few months or more of returning from a malarious area.

## Epidemiology of malaria in travelers

Of the four species of malarial parasites that commonly cause infections in man *Plasmodium falciparum* is responsible for virtually all the deaths. The other species, *Plasmodium vivax*, *Plasmodium ovale*, and *Plasmodium*

---

* Department of Infection and Tropical Medicine, Lister Unit, Northwick Park Hospital, Harrow HA1 3UJ, United Kingdom.
  *E-mail address:* g.pasvol@imperial.ac.uk

*malariae*, although causing febrile illnesses, rarely lead to severe disease [3] and are only very rarely fatal [4]. Recent evidence of wide scale confusion of a monkey (simian) malaria, *Plasmodium knowlesi*, with *P malariae* in humans in Borneo suggests a larger range of possible infecting *Plasmodium* species [5]. In the United Kingdom, for example, the proportion of *P falciparum* infections has been increasing and now approaches almost 75% of all imported malaria. Of all cases of falciparum malaria, around 10% can be classified as severe [6], between which the mortality is 10% but may rise to as high as 50% [7–9]. The overall mortality of all cases of *P falciparum* malaria in travelers ranges between 1% and 3% [10]. Any form of complicated or severe falciparum malaria must be regarded as a life-threatening medical emergency.

## Pathogenesis of falciparum malaria relevant to clinical practice

Since the 1970s, research into the molecular mechanisms involved in the specific cellular interactions responsible for the pathogenesis of severe malaria has yielded much interesting information about possible pathophysiologic processes. There are, however, many unanswered questions about why some patients become seriously ill and die [11,12].

Infections with plasmodia other than *P falciparum* rarely lead to death except from splenic rupture, severe chronic anemia, or in immunocompromised patients who develop unusually high parasitemia following blood transfusion–acquired malaria. Occasional reports of cerebral and other severe forms of malaria associated with species other than *P falciparum* suggest undiagnosed mixed infection. Polymerase chain reaction is helpful in resolving such enigmas [13]. Tumor necrosis factor seems to play a pivotal role in the pathogenesis of severe disease [14]. Although in *P vivax* infections blood levels of tumor necrosis factor may be equal to or even greater than those with falciparum malaria, two features seem unique to *P falciparum*. First, *P falciparum* can achieve far higher parasitemia than other species: parasitemia can be as high as 80% of all red cells infected, whereas for the other malarias rarely more than 5% of red cells are infected. This multiplicative ability seems to be related to the fact that *P falciparum*, although retaining a preference for younger red cells under most conditions, is able to invade red cells of all ages. Unlike *P vivax*, *P falciparum* is not restricted to reticulocytes, an important determinant of malaria infection dynamics [15]. Among *P falciparum* genotypes (strains), there is evidence that parasites with higher multiplication rates are associated with severe disease [16]. Moreover, examination of the proportion of multiply infected cells has shown that the distribution of parasites within the whole red cell population in severe disease becomes less restrictive [17]. In severe disease red cells across all the different age groups become susceptible to invasion, whereas in mild disease there is a predilection for younger red cells [18]. The result is that *P falciparum* can achieve high parasitemia in severe disease.

The second distinguishing feature of *P falciparum* is the ability of erythrocytes containing more mature forms to lodge or sequester in the venules of critical organs, such as brain, liver, heart, kidneys, gastrointestinal tract, skin, and so forth. Sequestration is the result of (1) cytoadherence in which the parasitized red cells bind specifically to receptors on the surface of endothelial cells [19]; (2) rosetting, which is binding of the parasitized red cell to several other uninfected cells, perhaps retarding transition through capillary beds [20]; and (3) decreased deformability of red cells containing the maturing parasites leading to its retention in capillaries [21]. As a consequence of sequestration, peripheral parasitemia does not reflect the total parasite burden. By obstructing blood flow and by concentrating cellular effects of the infected erythrocytes in specific organs, sequestration leads to severe disease. Certainly the induction of maximal amounts of tumor necrosis factor at the time of schizont rupture, for example, requires the close apposition of parasitized red cell and responding cell (eg, monocyte-macrophage), and may well explain the localization of pathologic effects to certain organs where parasites have sequestered [22].

## Distinguishing features of malaria in travelers

When formulating recommendations for the management of imported malaria in travelers, it must be acknowledged that most of the data on severe disease have been acquired studying patients in malaria-endemic areas, especially African children and relatively young previously healthy adult men in South East Asia rather than in travelers. Some of these observations may not be applicable to expatriate travelers of diverse ages, ethnicities, background immunity, and underlying medical conditions. Most cases of imported falciparum malaria in industrialized countries occur in settled immigrants who have revisited their countries of origin in Africa and South East Asia, in tourists, in business travelers, and in foreign visitors. Indeed, for many reasons it has been said that "travellers from industrialized countries and children in malarious regions represent two worlds of malaria" [1].

### *Age and sex*

Travelers with malaria are usually adults, both male and female, who may be elderly [23]. Among European patients, the risk of hospitalization, severe disease, or death from falciparum malaria increased significantly with each decade of life and women seem more susceptible to cerebral complications [24]. Cases among children are less frequent [25].

### *Genetic resistance and susceptibility*

Many genetic polymorphisms that confer some degree of resistance to malaria have been described in malaria-endemic populations [26], notably the hemoglobinopathies, such as sickle cell trait and the thalassemias. There are clearly many more as yet undiscovered, however, which may modify the course of disease in different ethnic groups. Most deaths in malaria, among those who have not been exposed before, occur in Europeans [27].

*Prophylaxis*

Although many travelers take chemoprophylaxis, which does not provide absolute protection, some take none, and others take it inconsistently. With increasing drug resistance, breakthrough malaria is not uncommon. Some travelers are given inappropriate prophylaxis (eg, chloroquine alone for travel to Africa). Inadequate prophylaxis often suppresses parasitemia, making diagnosis more difficult, and certain antibiotics (eg, ciprofloxacin, clindamycin, sulfonamides, and tetracyclines) taken for other reasons may also modify clinical presentation [28]. Most cases of severe malaria and those who die occur in travelers who have not taken antimalarials or have been poorly adherent [8,29].

*Pre-existing acquired immunity*

The acquisition of immunity to malarial infection requires repeated infection, although resistance to severe disease may be acquired after relatively few infections [30]. Nonimmunes (those who have never before been exposed to malaria) are susceptible to severe disease, which they may develop at relatively low parasitemia.

*Underlying disorders*

These days, many travelers to malarious areas have underlying disorders, such as ischemic heart disease, diabetes mellitus, hypertension, and chronic liver and renal disease. They might have had their spleen removed or be on immunosuppressive drugs. These disorders may increase the severity of the disease and make the patient more vulnerable to side effects of antimalarial drugs. Although any direct relationship between HIV infection and susceptibility to malaria has been difficult to demonstrate, apart from in pregnancy [31–33], a recent report from South Africa showed that HIV infection was associated with both severe malaria and death from malaria [34].

*Low clinical suspicion*

In endemic areas, malaria is such a common cause of fever that presumptive antimalarial treatment may be prescribed without even confirming the diagnosis. By contrast, medical personnel in industrialized countries are unfamiliar with malaria, and may miss the diagnosis. In febrile patients, a travel history is often omitted. Malaria is commonly mistaken either by the patient or by medical personnel for influenza, other upper respiratory tract infections, travelers' diarrhea, viral hepatitis, or encephalitis. For this reason the diagnosis is often delayed, a major factor leading to rapid progression to severe disease. A single blood film, examined perfunctorily in a busy hematology service, is often insufficient. Up to three daily (or twice daily) thick and thin blood films may be required before a specific diagnosis can be made. Patients need to stop their antimalarial prophylaxis while a diagnosis is being sought because inadequate prophylaxis may suppress patent peripheral parasitemia. If antimalarials are not recommenced once the diagnosis has been excluded, patients should be told to contact medical help should they subsequently develop a fever. The minimal incubation period for *P falciparum* is 7 days, and although most cases present within the first 6 weeks after return (87% of 182 cases in one study), a few occur between 6 weeks and 6 months (11.4%, 21 cases) and a few beyond (1.6%, 3 cases) [35]. In the United States between 1998 and 2002, of 2099 cases of falciparum malaria, 93% presented in the first month, 6% in the second and third months, and 1% after 6 months [36]. Delayed presentation may result from ineffective prophylaxis (especially with mefloquine [37]) or partial treatment. Many of the manifestations of malaria are nonspecific and include fevers with rigors, headache, backache, myalgias, lethargy, postural hypotension, nausea, vomiting, abdominal pain, and diarrhea. Progression to life-threatening conditions can be frighteningly rapid, with an interval of only 24 hours between the first symptom and death [38,39]. Falciparum malaria, sometimes severe, may quite unexpectedly arise in the context of transmission by blood transfusion [40,41], in a hospital [42,43], or by so-called "airport" malaria [44,45].

## Clinical presentations

Strict definitions of severe disease are essential for research purposes, to allow comparisons between different patient populations (Table 1) [39]. In clinical practice, however, any patient with suspected malaria who demonstrates prostration, any impairment of consciousness, convulsions, or any manifestation of shock, decreased urinary output, respiratory distress, or abnormal bleeding should be treated as an emergency. Some argue that, in the presumed nonimmune traveler, fever with no features of severity but a *P falciparum* peripheral parasitemia of 2% (or greater) should be taken seriously, because deterioration can occur rapidly and sometimes unexpectedly (eg, convulsions and coma). Whereas pulmonary edema and acute renal failure are more common in adults, children may present with vomiting, convulsions, respiratory distress, hypoglycemia, and hyperpyrexia. The author has noted protracted hiccups in a number of patients treated on his unit for severe malaria; it is unclear whether this is caused by diaphragmatic or cerebral irritation.

Table 1
Case definitions of severe falciparum malaria

| | |
|---|---|
| Cerebral malaria | Unrousable coma (GCS <11/15), with peripheral *P falciparum* parasitemia after exclusion of other causes of encephalopathy |
| Severe anemia | Normocytic anemia with hemoglobin <5 g/dL (hematocrit <15%) in presence of parasitemia >10,000/mL |
| Respiratory distress | Pulmonary edema or adult respiratory distress syndrome; also includes rapid labored acidotic breathing sometimes abnormal in rhythm |
| Renal failure | Urine output of less than 400 mL in 24 h (or <12 mL/kg in children) and a serum creatinine >265 mmol/l (>3 mg/dL) |
| Hypoglycemia | Whole blood glucose <2.2 mmol/L (40 mg/dL) |
| Circulatory collapse (shock) | Systolic blood pressure <70 mmHg or core-skin temperature difference >10°C |
| Coagulation failure | Spontaneous bleeding or laboratory evidence of disseminated intravascular coagulation |
| Impaired consciousness of any degree, prostration, jaundice, intractable vomiting, parasitemia ≥2% | In nonimmune individuals should be managed as severe malaria (ie, with parenteral antimalarials) |

*Data from* World Health Organization. Severe falciparum malaria. World Health Organization, Communicable Diseases cluster. Trans R Soc Trop Med Hyg 2000;94(Suppl 1):S1–90.

Cerebral malaria is one of the most dramatic presentations of severe falciparum malaria and should be considered in any patient with malaria, proved or suspected, with any decrease in conscious level. Other neurologic manifestations include increased muscle tone, brisk tendon reflexes, absent abdominal and other superficial reflexes, ankle clonus, extensor plantar responses, and other features of a symmetric upper motor neuron lesion especially in adults. Children may exhibit flaccid muscle tone. Retinal changes (Roth's spots–like hemorrhages and, more rarely, edema, exudates, and papilledema), disconjugate gaze, clenching of the jaws and grinding of the teeth (bruxism), or a brisk jaw jerk reflex are frequently observed. Especially in children, abnormalities of the brainstem (oculocephalic, oculovestibular, pupillary, and corneal) reflexes may occur.

**Differential diagnosis**

Malaria must be distinguished from other potentially imported febrile illnesses including viral illnesses (eg, dengue fever and influenza); typhoid; brucellosis; and respiratory and urinary tract infections. Less common causes of tropical fevers include visceral leishmaniasis, trypanosomiasis, rickettsial infections, and relapsing fevers. The acute coma of cerebral malaria must be distinguished from viral encephalitis (herpes simplex, HIV, enteroviral, mumps, arboviral [eg, West Nile]); bacterial meningoencephalitis (pyogenic and rarely tuberculous); fungal and protozoal meningoencephalitis (African trypanosomiasis); cerebral typhoid; brain abscess; heat stroke; cerebrovascular events; hypertensive encephalopathy; intoxications with drugs and poisons; and other causes of coma. The renal failure of malaria must be distinguished from renal impairment caused by other febrile illnesses, such as leptospirosis; traditional herbal medicines and snakebite; glomerulonephritis; and hypertension. The jaundice and hepatomegaly of malaria should not be confused with that of viral hepatitis (A, B, and E); yellow fever; cytomegalovirus and Epstein-Barr virus infections; leptospirosis; biliary disease; drug-induced diseases; and alcohol. Because cough and diarrhea are common symptoms, malaria must not be mistaken for an upper respiratory tract infection or gastroenteritis. Especially in malaria-endemic areas, malarial parasitemia may be detected in patients with other acute pathology, such as bacterial meningitis and hepatitis.

### Diagnosis and blood film examination

The definitive diagnosis of malaria is made by microscopic examination of both thick and thin blood films. These techniques have been well described elsewhere [46]. More recently, antigen capture tests [47] and polymerase chain reaction [13] have been developed, but they have not yet displaced careful examination of a thin film as the gold standard method of diagnosis, especially in cases of severe disease.

The thin blood film can give valuable information in cases of falciparum malaria:

1. The intensity of infection or parasitemia (usually measured by the percentage of red cells infected): Although parasitemia does not always correlate with disease severity, patients with higher parasitemia deserve consideration for quinine loading dose, exchange transfusion, and other urgent interventions.
2. Parasite maturity: The presence of more mature ring forms, trophozoites with pigment, or schizonts is associated with a worse prognosis than in those patients with only tiny rings in the peripheral blood film [48].
3. Neutrophils containing malarial pigment (hemozoin): The presence of malarial pigment in peripheral blood polymorphs reflects a prolonged infection and a large sequestered parasite burden. Hemozoin is produced by maturing malarial parasites and is the end-product of hemoglobin digestion, consisting of a polymer of heme groups. Hemozoin appears as a clump of golden brown pigment on Giemsa stain (Fig. 1). The finding of greater than or equal to 5% of polymorphs containing hemozoin is associated with a poorer prognosis [49,50].

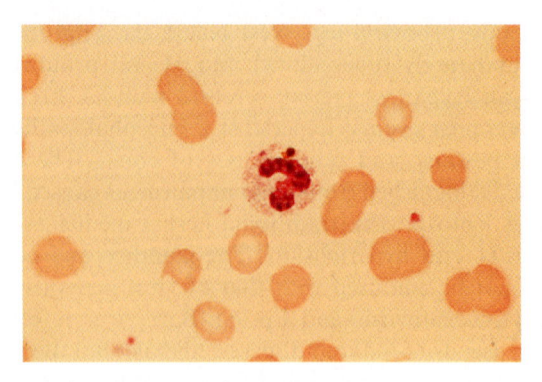

Fig. 1. Giemsa stain showing hemozoin appearing as a clump of golden brown pigment (Original magnification, ×1,000.).

4. Monitoring the effect of treatment: Peripheral blood films should be carefully examined at least twice daily in severe malaria until the parasitemia is undetectable or at least less than 1%, when it may be performed once daily. An initial increase in parasitemia is not uncommon during the first 18 to 24 hours of treatment and paradoxically may be of favorable prognostic significance [51]. Such a rise should not necessarily be interpreted as treatment failure leading to a change of antimalarial therapy, nor should it on its own serve as an indication for exchange transfusion [52].

## Management

Any patient with severe (complicated) falciparum malaria must be considered as a medical emergency and managed at the highest possible level of clinical care, which in industrialized countries is an ICU [53,54]. A venous cannula should be inserted and bloods taken for the investigations as shown in Table 2. Commonly omitted investigations are calcium, magnesium, phosphate, glucose, creatine kinase [55] and lactate, arterial blood gases, and blood cultures. In patients with impaired consciousness, other causes of encephalopathy, especially meningoencephalitis and viral encephalitis, must be excluded. HIV infection, which initiates a differing management algorithm, early on must be excluded. Hypoglycemia must be excluded by bedside measurement of blood glucose and corrected promptly. The level of consciousness should be recorded frequently using the Glasgow Coma Score in adults and Blantyre Coma Score in children [39,56,57].

The state of hydration must be carefully assessed. Patients with severe malaria, especially children, are likely to be dehydrated and hypovolemic to some degree as a result of fever, sweating, vomiting, diarrhea, and lack of fluid intake [58]. Hypovolemia exaggerates shock, renal impairment, and lactic acidosis. Rehydration needs to be performed carefully, however,

Table 2
Investigations relevant in the management of malaria

| Investigation | Relevance | Management |
| --- | --- | --- |
| Blood film for malaria parasites | Essential for diagnosis; assists in assessment of severity and prognosis [46] | See text |
| Full blood count | | |
| Hemoglobin | Often not anemic on presentation; an indicator of duration of infection | Generally threshold for transfusion is high (eg, <7 g/dL in adults [109]; self-recovery generally rapid once parasites cleared |
| White blood cells | Normal in uncomplicated cases; often lymphopenic; in severe malaria often neutrophil leukocytosis | Generally none; when neutrophil leukocytosis present raises possibility of secondary bacterial infection [94] |
| Platelets | Usually low; bleeding in absence of DIC uncommon except for petechiae or purpura | In absence of overt bleeding and platelets >10x10$^9$/μL no need for platelet replacement |
| Blood film and parasite count | Essential for diagnosis and continuing management if high; more mature forms [48] pigment in ≥5% neutrophils or peripheral schizontemia indicates poor prognosis [49] | Depending on facilities and severity might require exchange transfusion [114] |
| Electrolytes | | |
| Sodium | Often low; usually salt-depleted or dilutional; some cases caused by syndrome of inappropriate antidiuretic hormone secretion, cerebral salt-wasting, or the inability to secrete free water | Usually self correcting with treatment |
| Potassium | Normal unless high in presence of acute renal failure | Dialysis may be necessary especially in oliguric or anuric renal failure |
| Creatinine | Normal or high | Dialysis may be necessary |
| Calcium | Often low in severe cases | May need replacement especially if prolongation of QTc on ECG |
| Magnesium | Can be low | May need replacement especially if prolongation of QTc on ECG |
| Glucose and lactate | | |
| Glucose | Often low in severe cases in children, also during quinine administration to adults [60]; often absence of classical symptoms and signs of hypoglycemia | Regular monitoring of glucose in severe cases especially during quinine infusion; immediate administration of 50 mL 50% glucose then 10% dextrose |

(*continued on next page*)

Table 2 (*continued*)

| Investigation | Relevance | Management |
|---|---|---|
| Lactate | Raised in severe cases; good prognostic and progress marker from hour to hour; important to measure CSF lactate if LP performed [126,127] | Important to ensure good tissue and perfusion by adequate hydration, blood, and in some cases ventilation |
| Coagulation | | |
| Including prothrombin time, thrombin time, D-dimers (or fibrinogen degradation products) and platelets | Activated in almost all cases of malaria to some degree [106] | Might require fresh frozen plasma or platelets if clinical evidence of bleeding and platelets below 10x109/μL |
| Liver function tests | | |
| Albumin | Often low in acute infection as part of the acute phase response | Does not require correction unless clinically relevant; danger of fluid overload and pulmonary edema |
| Bilirubin | Often raised because of hemolysis but in severe disease can reflect liver damage; can be resolved by measurement of conjugated and unconjugated forms | May require reduction of quinine dosage because drug is about 80% cleared by the liver |
| Transaminases | Can be moderately raised; if very high consider other concomitant infections (eg, hepatitis A,B,C, or E) | May require reduction of quinine dosage because drug is about 80% cleared by the liver |
| Alkaline phosphatase | Not raised in malaria | If raised think of other causes |
| Creatine kinase | Indicates skeletal muscle damage [55] | Should pre-empt monitoring and management strategies aimed at preserving renal function including renal dialysis |
| C-reactive protein | Raised in acute attack | Useful for daily monitoring in severe cases |
| Procalcitonin | Raised [128] | Correlates with parasite density |
| Blood gases | | |
| pH | Acidosis important in prognosis of severe cases [87] | Requires adequate fluid replacement, possible blood transfusion in anemic cases, and avoidance (if possible) of adrenaline if inotropes are required |
| $Po_2$ | Hypoxia uncommon unless pulmonary edema or infection present | Oxygen or ventilation |

Table 2 (*continued*)

| Investigation | Relevance | Management |
|---|---|---|
| $P_{CO_2}$ | Can be low in presence of acidosis | |
| Bicarbonate | Low in acidosis | Replacement unlikely to help in academia; may need dialysis against a bicarbonate-containing buffer [90] |
| Others | | |
| Quinine levels | Free rather than total quinine levels relevant to efficacy and toxicity; α1-acid glycoprotein is the main quinine-binding plasma protein | Not generally helpful in management; maintain between 10 and 15 mg/L according to parasite sensitivity; for quinidine (4–6 mg/L) |
| ECG monitoring | | |
| QTc interval | Can be prolonged in nonimmune patients especially if underlying cardiac disorder | Reduction of quinine dosage may be necessary if QTc increases by over 25% of baseline |
| Blood and urine culture | Patients often acquire a secondary infection (most commonly respiratory, renal tract, or septicemia) because of immunosuppression of malaria | May require systemic broad-spectrum antibiotics |
| Lumbar puncture | Relevant in very young and elderly and where other causes of encephalopathy, especially meningitis, need to be excluded; in malaria apart from an increased opening pressure (children) and raised lactate [126], the CSF examination is normal | Appropriate antimicrobial chemotherapy |
| Chest radiograph | Often normal; helps in the differential diagnosis of respiratory distress | Requires oxygen and consideration of mechanical ventilation [84] |
| CT or MRI brain | Might demonstrate cerebral edema, a space-occupying lesion, and exclude other causes of decreased consciousness | Might support the use of mannitol if cerebral edema revealed [79] |

*Abbreviations:* CSF, cerebrospinal fluid; DIC, disseminated intravascular coagulation; LP, lumbar puncture; QTc, corrected QT interval.

especially in adults, because overhydration can induce sometimes fatal pulmonary edema. All unconscious patients should have a urinary catheter.

**Antimalarials**

All patients with any form of complicated disease should be treated parenterally. Gastrointestinal absorption of drugs is variable and the drugs themselves may induce vomiting. Although there are no specific studies that have been performed to establish a threshold for parenteral treatment in nonimmune patients, any patient with a falciparum parasitemia greater than or equal to 2% should be treated with parenteral antimalarials. The choice of drugs, according to availability and licensing, lies between the cinchona alkaloids (ie, quinine or quinidine [in the United States]) or one of the artemisinin derivatives, usually intramuscular artemether or intravenous artesunate (Table 3).

Ideally, quinine is given by slow intravenous infusion, but in an emergency may be given intramuscularly as has been done in children [59]. In most cases, where patients are young and otherwise healthy, a loading dose of 20 mg/kg of quinine dihydrochloride is recommended [60]. To achieve and maintain therapeutic blood quinine concentrations safely and rapidly, an alternative consecutive-infusion regimen (7 mg of salt per kilogram of body weight over 30 minutes followed by 10 mg of salt per kilogram of body weight over 4 hours) based on pharmacokinetic parameters in cerebral malaria has been suggested for use in an ICU (see Table 3) [61].

Unlike children and individuals living in endemic areas, however, there is some indication that particularly in the elderly and those with underlying cardiovascular disease, quinine may induce life-threatening cardiac arrhythmias [62]. In younger otherwise healthy patients in endemic areas arrhythmias seem not to be a problem [63]. This may be because of the difference in binding kinetics of quinine to $\alpha$1-acid glycoprotein (orosomucoid), the main polymorphic, quinine-binding protein in plasma [64], leading to excessively high levels of free drug, responsible not only for the antiparasitic, but also the toxic effects [65]. There are good theoretical arguments for the loading dose especially when attaining therapeutic parasiticidal drug concentrations as rapidly as possible in the face of a rapidly evolving and potentially fatal infection [66]. In the situation of an ICU where exchange transfusion (ET) is feasible, however, it could be argued that the most rapid means to reduce parasitemia safely is by physical methods of red cell removal (ie, ET or erythrocytapheresis) [67]. In the largest series of case-definition severe malaria (93 cases) in a nonendemic country (Hôpital Bichat-Claude Bernard, Paris, France) only 21.7% of the patients received a loading dose of quinine, presumably because most had received quinine, mefloquine, or halofantrine before admission to the ICU (none received ET) [8].

Table 3
Antimalarial treatment regimens in severe malaria

| Drug | Dose | Comments |
|---|---|---|
| Quinine dihydrochloride | 10 mg (salt)/kg by infusion over 4 h in 500 mL 5% dextrose, every 8 h until parasites less than 1% and the patient can take by mouth, then quinine sulphate, 600 mg three times a day orally, until parasites have cleared, then doxycycline, 200 mg daily orally for 7 d | Can induce hypoglycemia and cardiac arrhythmias. A loading dose 20 mg over 4 h in 500 mL 5% dextrose should be given to young otherwise healthy patients and where hyperparasitemia cannot be treated by exchange transfusion. Special caution should be taken when used in the elderly and those with underlying cardiovascular disease. The loading dose should not be given to patients who have received quinine, quinidine, or mefloquine in the previous 24 h |
| Quinine dihydrochloride (rapid-loading dose) [61] | 7 mg (salt)/kg by infusion pump over 30 min followed immediately by 10 mg/kg over 4 h in 5% dextrose, then 10 mg/kg by infusion over 4 h in 500 mL 5% dextrose every 8 h until the parasitemia is less than 1% and the patient can take by mouth, then quinine sulphate, 600 mg three times a day orally until parasites have cleared, then doxycycline, 200 mg daily orally for 7 d | As above. |
| Quinidine gluconate | 24 mg quinidine salt/kg (equivalent to 15 mg/kg base) infused over 4 h followed by 12 mg/kg salt (7.5 mg base) over 4 h every 8 h until parasites less than 1% and the patient can take by mouth. Then quinine sulphate, 600 mg three times a day orally, until parasites have cleared, then doxycycline, 200 mg daily orally for 7 d | In an emergency and in the United States where quinine may not always be available. The same precautions as outlined above with quinine apply. |

*(continued on next page)*

Table 3 (*continued*)

| Drug | Dose | Comments |
|---|---|---|
| Quinidine gluconate (continuous infusion) | 10 mg salt/kg (equivalent to 6.25 mg base/kg) infused over 2 h followed by a continuous infusion of 0.02 mg salt/kg/min (0.0125 mg base/kg/min quinidine) until parasites less than 1% and the patient can take by mouth. Then quinine sulphate, 600 mg three times a day orally, until parasites have cleared, then doxycycline, 200 mg daily orallyfor 7 d | In an emergency and in the United States where quinine may not always be available. The same precautions as outlined above with quinine apply. |
| Artemether (a qinghaosu [artemisinin] derivative) | 3.2 mg/kg intramuscularly on the first day, followed by 1.6 mg/kg daily (usual adult dose 160 mg followed by 80 mg daily for 6 d) until parasites cleared and the patient can take by mouth. Then doxycycline, 200 mg daily orally for 7 d | Alternative to quinine. Usually intramuscular. Requires doxycycline as recrudescences are common |
| Artesunate | 2.4 mg/kg intravenously followed by 1.2 mg/kg at 12 and 24 h; then 1.2 mg/kg daily (usual adult dose 120 mg followed by doses of 60 mg daily for 6 d) until parasites cleared. Then doxycycline, 200 mg daily by mouth for 7 d | Can be given intravenously because it is water soluble. Also requires doxycycline because recrudescences are common |
| Doxycycline | 200 mg daily orally for 7 d | To be used in conjunction with quinine-quinidine after parasite clearance and the patient can take by mouth |
| Clindamycin | 450 mg three times a day orally for 7 d | To be used in conjunction with quinine-quinidine after parasite clearance and the patient can take by mouth |

Northwick Park Hospital, a referral center from London's Heathrow Airport, has treated 622 cases of malaria since 1991, of which 420 (68%) have been caused by *P falciparum*. Of these, 51 (8%) have been severe cases and 11 of these received a loading dose; 40 did not. Five patients (10%) with severe malaria died, two of who received a loading dose. One of these patients given a loading dose (admitted with a 5% parasitemia and nonsevere disease) died in ventricular asystole. Abnormally high free concentrations of quinine, 9.01 mg/L (despite a normal total therapeutic level at the time of 13.16 mg/L), were documented [62]. The second, a 73-year-old man with a 1% parasitemia, died with bradycardia, hypotension, and acute respiratory distress syndrome (ARDS). A further nine cases with severe disease received the loading dose. The loading dose should certainly not be given to patients who have received quinine, quinidine, or mefloquine in the previous 24 hours. Quinine levels may provide a rough guide but are generally not promptly available and reflect total, not free, quinine levels, the latter of which are responsible for both the therapeutic and toxic side effects [68].

Quinidine gluconate is used in the United States where quinine is unavailable (see Table 3) [69]. The recommended dosage is 10 mg salt/kg (equivalent to 6.25 mg base/kg) infused over 2 hours followed by a continuous infusion of 0.02 mg salt/kg/min (0.0125 mg/kg/min quinidine base). An alternative regimen involves 8 hourly intravenous infusions (see Table 3).

Once the parasitemia is less than 1% and the patient is able to take drugs by mouth, treatment may be completed with oral quinine at a dose of 10 mg salt/kg (usually 600 mg every 8 hours). Quinine can be discontinued once the patient is aparasitemic for two consecutive blood films, taken 24 hours apart; however, it is essential to complete the treatment usually with oral doxycycline, 200 mg daily for 7 days, or in the case of pregnant women and children, with clindamycin, 5 mg/kg base orally three times a day (usual dose in adults, 450 mg three times a day for 7 days) [70]. These drugs prevent recrudescent infection, which is common after monotherapy with quinine. Sulfadoxine-pyrimethamine (Fansidar) is no longer recommended because of increasing resistance and lack of availability. Some clinicians prefer to continue with quinine for a full 7 days, but this is often poorly tolerated leading to symptoms of cinchonism (tinnitus, deafness, nausea, vomiting, ataxia, and blurring of vision). In any event, even after a 7-day course of quinine without a tetracycline, recrudescence may still occur.

Although in young children and healthy males in tropical areas use of the cinchona alkaloids has not been shown to have major cardiac arrhythmogenic effects, such effects (notably QT interval prolongation) have been noted in nonimmune travelers. When using the cinchona alkaloids especially in the elderly and nonimmune, a baseline electrocardiogram should be obtained with careful observation of the rhythm and corrected QT interval. Any prolongation greater than 25% over baseline should require careful observation for both arrhythmias and hypotension and possible tailoring of the dosage of quinine. Because cinchona alkaloids, both quinine and quinidine, are potent stimulants of insulin secretion, glucose should be carefully monitored especially in pregnant women [71].

Theoretical arguments favoring artemisinin derivatives over cinchona alkaloids have not resulted in studies demonstrating significantly reduced mortality in the use of artemisinins. Artemisinin and its derivatives, especially artemether or artesunate, result in more rapid parasite clearance (being active on the immature parasite forms [72]), but this does not translate into a significantly improved outcome in studies performed so far, although the results have favored the artemisinins [73]. In many developed countries artemisinin derivatives are not licensed and can only be used on a named patient basis. The toxicity profile favors the use of artemisinins in severe disease, however, and they can be used as second-line drugs in settings where quinine or quinidine toxicity precludes the use of the cinchona alkaloids (eg, in cinchona alkaloid–induced arrhythmias; hypoglycemia; or blackwater fever, although no published information is available on the frequency of this complication with the artemisinin derivatives). The more readily controlled intravenous route of administration of artesunate favors its use over intramuscular artemether [74].

**Management of other manifestations**

Administration of an antimalarial drug is the only intervention of proved efficacy in severe malaria. Other supportive measures, however, may be required.

*Cerebral malaria*

Unrousable coma may persist for up to 72 hours and longer in adults. A few long-term neurologic sequelae of cerebral malaria have been reported in nonimmune travelers, such as focal epilepsy, memory impairment, and diffuse white matter damage detected by MRI [75]. Patients who are unconscious should be nursed in the appropriate position, their stomach drained with a nasogastric tube with an endotracheal tube inserted. Regular neurologic observations should be recorded. Mechanical ventilation may be necessary.

The use of steroids in the context of cerebral malaria is perhaps one area in which there is little or no controversy. In the past, believing that cerebral malaria might reflect an overexuberant immunologic response to infection, corticosteroids were used in treatment. In two well-conducted studies, however, dexamethasone not only failed to improve case fatality of cerebral malaria but also lengthened the period of unconsciousness and the risk of infection and gastrointestinal bleeding [76,77]. The value of corticosteroids in ARDS or severe Coombs-positive anemia caused by malaria has not been explored.

In children with cerebral malaria and evidence of raised intracranial pressure [78], mannitol (1 g/kg infused over 30 minutes as a 10% or 20% solution) has been shown to control intermediate intracranial hypertension, but not when severe (>40 mm Hg) [79]. Serum osmolality must be monitored if repeated doses are used. Mannitol should not be given if the serum osmolality rises above 330 mOsm/L. The use of mannitol, however, has not been systematically studied in malaria in adults.

*Convulsions*

Convulsions in malaria occur particularly in children and may be partly caused by hyperpyrexia. Tepid sponging, fanning, and paracetamol are effective. Aspirin is contraindicated in children because of its association with Reye's syndrome, acidosis [80], and gastrointestinal bleeding. The use of prophylactic phenobarbitone reduced the frequency of seizures but increased case fatality [81]. In patients with cerebral malaria, seizures must be treated promptly with a benzodiazepine, such as diazepam or lorazepam, but these drugs carry the risk of respiratory depression. Continuous seizure activity may be covert or clinically unapparent in children and evidenced only by subtle signs, such as deviation of the eyes, twitching of a corner of the mouth, or posturing of one arm. Such seizure activity may be confirmed by electroencephalogram or a test dose of anticonvulsant, which may result in a dramatic recovery of full consciousness [82].

*Respiratory distress*

Respiratory distress is an important complication of severe malaria in children [83], but can also accompany disease in adults. Respiratory distress (ie, the observation of deep labored breathing), however, may have a number of causes, most importantly acidosis, but also infection, aspiration pneumonia, fluid overload, anemia, acute lung injury, and ARDS [84]. Because each of these entities require a different modality of treatment, it is important that the clinician considers all these possibilities when embarking on treatment decisions for respiratory distress.

*Acidosis*

Acidosis is emerging as a major complication in severe malaria, with a multifactorial origin and a major impact on outcome [85–87]. Tissue hypoxia, liver dysfunction, and impaired renal handling of bicarbonate all contribute. The management of acidosis involves principles of overall care with the administration of antimalarials, oxygen, fluids, and electrolytes where appropriate. In the author's experience the administration of intravenous bicarbonate to acidotic malarial patients seldom helps and can lead to both hypernatremia and hyperosmolarity [88]. In severely anemic and acidotic children, blood transfusion seems to improve acidosis by correcting the oxygen debt, as does ventilation [89]. If undertaking hemofiltration in the context of acute renal failure and lactic acidosis, it is judicious to dialyze against bicarbonate rather than the more conventional lactate-buffered dialysate [90]. In the study by Hilton et al [90], it was possible (where previously intravenous sodium bicarbonate had failed) to correct the acidosis of 200 patients with lactic acidosis (of varying cause) using bicarbonate buffered dialysate without causing extracellular volume expansion or hypernatremia. Of the cardiac catecholamine inotropes, epinephrine (adrenaline) should be avoided if at all possible because unlike other inotropic agents, such as dopamine, dobutamine, and norepinephrine, it increases lactate and exacerbates acidosis [85].

*Respiratory tract infection*

Pneumonia is not infrequent, either as a result of aspiration in the comatose patient or as a complication of the transient immunosuppression that complicates malaria [91]. It should be considered especially in the face of deteriorating respiratory function with newly evolving localized radiographic changes, a neutrophil leukocytosis, a rising C-reactive protein, and persisting fever despite parasite clearance. There should be a low threshold for adding broad-spectrum antibiotics in such a situation.

*Fluid overload*

Fluid overload is a risk, especially when patients have been transferred between hospitals and fluid resuscitation is repeated without proper examination of the medical case notes. Profound hypoalbuminemia, the result of the catabolic effects of the acute infection, potentiates this process. Fluid replacement should be meticulously monitored by observing central venous pressure; a central venous–right atrial pressure of +10 cm $H_2O$ should not be exceeded. The use of albumin as replacement in severe malaria is unresolved and apart from its expense, runs the risk of fluid overload. Overload pulmonary edema should be treated with oxygen; potent diuretics; upright posture; and, in extreme cases, by controlled venesection.

*Acute lung injury and acute respiratory distress syndrome*

Acute lung injury and ARDS occur suddenly and unpredictably in malaria as in any other severe septic condition [84]. Acute lung injury has been defined according to new international criteria as the acute onset of bilateral pulmonary infiltrates with a $Pao_2$–fraction of inspired oxygen ($Fio_2$) less than or equal to 300 mm Hg (40 kPa) regardless of positive end-expiratory pressure and a pulmonary artery occlusion pressure less than or equal to 18 mm Hg (2.4 kPa). ARDS is defined as a $Pao_2$-$Fio_2$ less than or equal to 200 mm Hg (approximately 27 kPa) [92]. Pathogenesis is related to neutrophil adherence and complement-mediated neutrophil degranulation in the pulmonary capillaries leading to increased permeability and formation of pulmonary edema in the absence of raised right-sided cardiac pressures. As in the case of ARDS in other severe infections, the use of corticosteroids is unsupported by convincing evidence, although mechanical ventilation with positive end-expiratory pressure is effective in some cases.

*Secondary bacterial, viral, or fungal infection*

Secondary bacterial infection is an important complication of severe malaria, which can be profound, occurring early in the disease and leading to shock and multiorgan failure [93,94]. Bacterial infection can lead to septicemia, bacterial pneumonia, urinary tract infections, or meningitis. Common organisms include pneumococci, salmonella, *Escherichia coli*, and other gram-negative organisms. Fever blisters (cold sores) caused by herpes simplex are a common accompaniment of malarial infection, and two cases of fatal invasive aspergillosis in nonimmune European adults without underlying disease have been reported [95].

*Hypoglycemia*

Hypoglycemia is less frequently observed at presentation in nonimmune travelers with severe disease than in African children and pregnant women in malaria-endemic areas, partly reflecting differences in nutritional status [96]. Quinine or quinidine-induced hyperinsulinemic hypoglycemia may occur in all groups of patients [71]. Any patient with a blood glucose level below 2.2 mEq/L should be treated immediately with an intravenous bolus of 50% dextrose solution, 1 mL/kg, followed by a continuous infusion of 10% dextrose. Profound hypoglycemia can break through such treatment [97], however, and meticulous surveillance of blood glucose levels using bedside reagent "stix" methods should be used during quinine infusion. Undetected hypoglycemia can cause irreversible neurologic damage. Quinine or quinidine-induced hypoglycemia may develop late in the clinical course, when the patient seems to be recovering and parasitemia has been eliminated. It should be suspected in any patient who is convulsing, unconscious, or whose Glasgow Coma Score is deteriorating. Clinical manifestations of hypoglycemia, such as anxiety, tachypnea, tachycardia, sweating, and other autonomic signs, involuntary movements, and abnormal posturing, can all too easily be misinterpreted as features of malaria itself rather than this common and important complication of the disease and its treatment.

*Hypotension and shock*

Hypotension and shock in severe malaria (algid malaria) is usually indicative of a complicating bacterial infection [94] but more rarely splenic rupture or gastrointestinal bleeding. In the patient with severe malaria in an

ICU, treatment of hypotension demands a balance between adequate circulation and renal perfusion and the risk of inducing fluid overload and pulmonary edema by excessive volume replacement. The threshold to use antibiotics in this setting should be low and the initial addition of a broad-spectrum antibiotic is appropriate.

*Fluid and electrolyte disturbances*

Most patients with severe malaria become hyponatremic. In most cases this is attributable to salt depletion and dilution, exacerbated by the infusion of dextrose-containing solutions without saline. A few cases are caused by the syndrome of inappropriate antidiuretic hormone secretion [98] and cerebral salt-wasting syndrome (in which there is excessive natriuresis in patients with intracranial disease) [99], whereas others are cause by the inability to secrete free water. Sometimes hyponatremia develops suddenly and unexpectedly in the course of treatment of seemingly uncomplicated disease in the absence of hypoglycemia or renal impairment [100]. Adequate fluid rehydration alone usually allows correction of hyponatremia. Hypertonic saline is not indicated. Hypocalcemia is also a common feature of severe disease, often attributable to hypoalbuminemia. In patients without renal failure it seems to be caused by parathyroid gland dysfunction, because parathyroid hormone levels are inappropriately low, whereas in the presence of renal failure it is thought to be caused by skeletal resistance to the action of parathyroid hormone resulting from the combination of phosphate retention and reduced 1,25-dihydroxyvitamin D levels, which occur in renal failure [101]. Careful attention should be paid to plasma potassium, calcium, magnesium, and phosphate concentrations especially when using cinchona alkaloids, which cause hyperinsulinemia, and glucose solutions, which encourage potassium and phosphate to enter cells. Resulting electrolyte abnormalities can exacerbate cardiac arrhythmias.

*Blackwater fever*

Some patients, particularly semi-immunes, develop massive intravascular hemolysis and hemoglobinuria (blackwater fever) as a complication of falciparum malaria especially when given quinine. The mechanism remains unknown. Blackwater fever does not in itself indicate severe renal impairment but more reflects the presence of massive hemolysis. In some cases it may be associated with an underlying hemolytic tendency (eg, glucose-6-phosphate dehydrogenase deficiency) [102]. When associated with renal impairment the prognosis is far worse.

*Acute renal failure*

The acute renal failure of malaria occurs either as a component of severe disease with multiorgan failure and a poor prognosis, or when parasitemia is declining or has even been cleared [103,104]. The renal failure of malaria is often nonoliguric but in some cases may be oliguric (urine output <400 mL per 24 hours) or anuric. Hemofiltration has proved superior to peritoneal dialysis [105]. In the ICU setting, hemofiltration or hemodiafiltration (the combination of hemodialysis and hemofiltration either simultaneously or sequentially) and in a few cases hemodialysis may be required.

*Hemostatic disorders*

In severe malaria, blood coagulation pathways are almost always activated [106], but spontaneous bleeding or disseminated intravascular coagulation is relatively uncommon. This is particularly surprising in view of accompanying thrombocytopenia. Patients with malaria rarely bleed with platelet counts above $10 \times 10^9/\mu L$. Aspirin and corticosteroids should be avoided lest they exaggerate this tendency. In the ICU, patients should be given a histamine-2 antagonist (eg, intravenous cimetidine or ranitidine) to reduce the risk of gastrointestinal bleeding. If there are prolonged clotting times with overt bleeding, fresh frozen plasma and platelets may be given as in any other bleeding disorder. Vitamin K (10 mg) can be given intravenously for 3 days. Conversely, some patients have a hypercoagulable state: cerebral venous and dural thrombosis has been reported as a rare complication of severe malarial disease [107].

*Hyperparasitemia*

The decision at what level of parasitemia to treat falciparum malaria parenterally in travelers remains arbitrary. In travelers, most guidelines at specialist hospitals in the United Kingdom recommend parenteral treatment for parasitemia greater than or equal to 2%. Hyperparasitemia in itself does not necessarily have major prognostic significance in semi-immune individuals (individuals living in an endemic area and exposed on a number of occasions to malaria) but in nonimmune travelers is an indicator of potentially severe disease [8]. It is also an important factor when considering ET (see later).

*Anemia*

Travelers with severe malaria rarely present with profound anemia. Normocytic anemia of some degree (and sometimes severe) almost always occurs during the course of treatment after a delay of a few days, however, and is caused by a combination of hemolysis and dyserythropoiesis [108]. Once parasitemia has cleared there is almost always a vigorous marrow erythroid response with brisk reticulocytosis in patients who are not deficient in hematinics (iron and folate), neither of which are caused by malaria per se. For this reason, patients with malaria rarely need blood transfusion when the hemoglobin is above 7 g/dL, but this raises yet another controversy in management of severe disease. General studies on the reduced use of blood transfusion in the ICU have been reported: in critically ill patients on an ICU (none of whom had malaria), a restrictive strategy of red-cell transfusion (transfusing only when hemoglobin fell below 7 g/dL) was at least as effective as, and possibly superior to, a liberal strategy, with the possible exception of patients with acute myocardial infarction and unstable angina [109]. In the setting of young, relatively fit travelers with the anemia of malaria who are not hematinic deficient, it is appropriate to retain this relatively conservative policy for the use of transfusion and to restrict transfusion in severe malaria to hemoglobin concentrations below 7 g/dL. This considerably reduces all the known and unknown risks especially of infection that accompany blood transfusion. Clearly, such a decision whether to transfuse or not is modified by other factors, such as any underlying condition (eg, respiratory or cardiac disease) or the availability of safe blood.

*Splenic rupture*

Splenic rupture should be considered in any patient with falciparum malaria who develops abdominal pain or shock [110]. Ultrasound or CT scanning together with a surgical opinion is essential for diagnosis and management.

**Further treatment modalities in malaria in travelers: transfusion, ventilation, and dialysis**

Clearly within the sophisticated environment of an ICU in industrialized countries technologies for the management of severe malaria are available and include ET, mechanical ventilation, and dialysis.

*Exchange transfusion*

There are compelling theoretical reasons for the use of ET in malaria, an intraerythrocytic infection [67]. ET not only removes parasitized red cells but also toxic products, debris, harmful metabolites, uninfected red cells with reduced deformability, and cytokines, but also corrects anemia and acidosis. ET with fresh blood also replaces red cells, platelets, and clotting factors and has been used successfully in a limited number of cases [111]. Despite all these advantages, ET has not been shown to improve outcome in all studies [112]. A meta-analysis of the use of ET in severe malaria could not endorse the use of this modality of treatment on a routine basis [113]. There were limitations in this analysis, however, the most important being that patients in the exchanged group were overall much more ill than those in the nonexchanged controls.

The author has developed a practical set of indications, which considers all patients with an arbitrary parasitemia of greater than or equal to 30% as appropriate for ET [114]. This threshold can be lowered for patients who have other manifestations of severe complicated malaria (see Table 1), have underlying medical conditions, or are elderly or pregnant. Below 30%, hyperparasitemia on its own is not sufficient to justify ET. At Northwick Park Hospital 26 of 51 cases of severe malaria had hyperparasitemia ($\geq$10% [ie, $\geq$ approximately 500,000 parasites/$\mu$L]). Five received ET. Three had parasitemia greater than 30%; all three were exchanged, one of who died. The remaining 23 with hyperparasitemia all survived, a further two receiving ET.

Erythrocytapheresis in which the red blood cell fraction is removed by apheresis and the plasma, leukocyte, and platelet fractions are returned to the patient has also been used to good effect in severe disease [115,116]. Erythrocytapheresis has advantages over ET because of speed, efficiency, hemodynamic stability, and retention of plasma components, such as clotting factors, but is only available in specialized centers and lacks the advantage of ET of removing and replacing plasma. Because the apparent volume of distribution of the cinchona alkaloids is so great, neither the dose nor frequency of dosing need be changed during ET or erythrocytapheresis.

*Mechanical ventilation*

The respiratory indications for mechanical ventilation in malaria are not specifically different from other medical conditions and include poor respiratory effort, acute pulmonary edema, aspiration pneumonia, and ARDS. Mechanical ventilation may also be used to reduce acidemia (pH < 7.3) or raised intracranial pressure. Mechanical ventilation and renal replacement have probably been the two most important factors that have reduced mortality in the treatment of severe malaria in industrialized countries [117].

*Renal dialysis and hemofiltration*

In adults renal impairment is an important manifestation of severe disease, and in the absence of dialysis of one sort or another has a very poor outcome. In this regard hemofiltration is preferred over peritoneal dialysis in a study performed in an endemic setting [105].

**Other adjunctive therapies**

*Anti–tumor necrosis factor measures and pentoxifylline*

The basis for anti–tumor necrosis factor agents in severe malaria is compelling, but the reality has been disappointing. Monoclonal anti–tumor necrosis factor antibodies, although reducing fever significantly [118], were not shown to improve outcome; the use of pentoxifylline (a potent anti–tumor necrosis factor drug) has proved equally disappointing [119]. The use of polyclonal anti–tumor necrosis factor antibodies in a small number of patients with severe malaria showed some benefit [120].

*Iron chelators*

In the belief that parasites have an absolute need for iron these drugs have been used in severe disease but been shown not to add any advantage [121].

*Dichloroacetate*

Dichloroacetate has been used for treatment of the lactic acidosis of diabetic ketoacidosis. It stimulates pyruvate dehydrogenase. Hyperlactatemia is an important indicator of poor outcome in malaria. In a limited study the use of dichloroacetate in severe malaria was shown to reduce lactate levels in malaria but not to affect outcome [122,123].

N-*Acetylcysteine*

Oxidative damage to the red cell membrane in malaria is thought to contribute to red cell rigidity and ultimately to pathophysiology [124]. The antioxidant N-acetylcysteine has been used in an initial study, and has been shown to be both safe and of promise as a possible adjunctive therapy for severe malaria [125].

**Summary**

This article emphasizes that for many controversial reasons, severe malaria in travelers differs from that seen in endemic areas. There is no controversy, however, that malaria in individuals living in endemic areas should retain research priority. Some of the questions raised might never be amenable to randomized controlled trials, either because of ethical or logistical restraints. A possibly indulgent wish list of outcome (mortality) studies using currently known treatment modalities, however, includes the loading dose of quinine, vigorous fluid replacement, ET, the artemisinins, mannitol, and N-acetylcysteine in the treatment of severe malaria. There may clearly be many more. The treatment of severe malaria remains a challenge to those with an interest in managing life-threatening disease with complex and fascinating pathophysiology. As challenging as the studies listed previously may seem, however, priority must inevitably be given to research on how one can prevent and treat mild disease in the first place.

## Acknowledgments

I thank Dr. Michael Brown and Dr. Robert Wilkinson and Professor Wallace Peters for their critical comments.

## References

[1] Wellems TE, Miller LH. Two worlds of malaria. N Engl J Med 2003;349:1496–8.
[2] Moore DA, Grant AD, Armstrong M, et al. Risk factors for malaria in UK travellers. Trans R Soc Trop Med Hyg 2004;98:55–63.
[3] Lawn S, Krishna S, Jarvis J, et al. Case reports: pernicious complications of benign tertian malaria. Trans R Soc Trop Med Hyg 2003;97:551–3.
[4] Lobovska A, Rubik I, Holub M, et al. The first death from tertian malaria in the Czech Republic. Cas Lek Cesk 1999;138:52–5.
[5] Singh B, Kim Sung L, Matusop A, et al. A large focus of naturally acquired *Plasmodium knowlesi* infections in human beings. Lancet 2004;363:1017–24.
[6] Kain KC, Harrington MA, Tennyson S, et al. Imported malaria: prospective analysis of problems in diagnosis and management. Clin Infect Dis 1998;27:142–9.
[7] Losert H, Schmid K, Wilfing A, et al. Experiences with severe *P falciparum* malaria in the intensive care unit. Intensive Care Med 2000;26:195–201.
[8] Bruneel F, Hocqueloux L, Alberti C, et al. The clinical spectrum of severe imported falciparum malaria in the intensive care unit: report of 188 cases in adults. Am J Respir Crit Care Med 2003;167:684–9.
[9] Krishnan A, Karnad DR. Severe falciparum malaria: an important cause of multiple organ failure in Indian intensive care unit patients. Crit Care Med 2003;31:2278–84.
[10] Muentener P, Schlagenhauf P, Steffen R. Imported malaria (1985–95): trends and perspectives. Bull World Health Organ 1999;77:560–6.
[11] Pasvol G. Cell-cell interaction in the pathogenesis of severe falciparum malaria. Clin Med 2001;1:495–500.
[12] Miller LH, Baruch DI, Marsh K, et al. The pathogenic basis of malaria. Nature 2002;415:673–9.
[13] Hanscheid T, Grobusch MP. How useful is PCR in the diagnosis of malaria? Trends Parasitol 2002;18:395–8.
[14] Kwiatkowski D, Hill AV, Sambou I, et al. TNF concentration in fatal cerebral, non-fatal cerebral, and uncomplicated *Plasmodium falciparum* malaria. Lancet 1990;336:1201–4.
[15] McQueen PG, McKenzie FE. Age-structured red blood cell susceptibility and the dynamics of malaria infections. Proc Natl Acad Sci USA 2004;101:9161–6.
[16] Chotivanich K, Udomsangpetch R, Simpson JA, et al. Parasite multiplication potential and the severity of falciparum malaria. J Infect Dis 2000;181:1206–9.
[17] Simpson JA, Silamut K, Chotivanich K, et al. Red cell selectivity in malaria: a study of multiple-infected erythrocytes. Trans R Soc Trop Med Hyg 1999;93:165–8.
[18] Pasvol G, Weatherall DJ, Wilson RJ. The increased susceptibility of young red cells to invasion by the malarial parasite *Plasmodium falciparum*. Br J Haematol 1980;45:285–95.
[19] Berendt AR, Ferguson DJ, Gardner J, et al. Molecular mechanisms of sequestration in malaria. Parasitology 1994;108:S19–28.
[20] Carlson J. Erythrocyte rosetting in *Plasmodium falciparum* malaria, with special reference to the pathogenesis of cerebral malaria. Scand J Infect Dis Suppl 1993;86:1–79.
[21] Dondorp AM, Kager PA, Vreeken J, et al. Abnormal blood flow and red blood cell deformability in severe malaria. Parasitol Today 2000;16:228–32.
[22] O'Dea KP, Pasvol G. Optimal tumor necrosis factor induction by *Plasmodium falciparum* requires the highly localized release of parasite products. Infect Immun 2003;71:3155–64.

[23] Schwartz E, Sadetzki S, Murad H, et al. Age as a risk factor for severe *Plasmodium falciparum* malaria in nonimmune patients. Clin Infect Dis 2001;33:1774–7.
[24] Muhlberger N, Jelinek T, Behrens RH, et al. Age as a risk factor for severe manifestations and fatal outcome of falciparum malaria in European patients: observations from TropNetEurop and SIMPID surveillance data. Clin Infect Dis 2003;36:990–5.
[25] Brabin BJ, Ganley Y. Imported malaria in children in the UK. Arch Dis Child 1997;77:76–81.
[26] Hill AV. The immunogenetics of resistance to malaria. Proc Assoc Am Physicians 1999;111:272–7.
[27] Jelinek T, Schulte C, Behrens R, et al. Imported falciparum malaria in Europe: sentinel surveillance data from the European network on surveillance of imported infectious diseases. Clin Infect Dis 2002;34:572–6.
[28] Puri SK, Dutta GP. Antibiotics in the chemotherapy of malaria. Prog Drug Res 1982;26:167–205.
[29] Lewis SJ, Davidson RN, Ross EJ, et al. Severity of imported falciparum malaria: effect of taking antimalarial prophylaxis. BMJ 1992;305:741–3.
[30] Gupta S, Snow RW, Donnelly CA, et al. Immunity to non-cerebral severe malaria is acquired after one or two infections. Nat Med 1999;5:340–3.
[31] Ayisi JG, van Eijk AM, ter Kuile FO, et al. The effect of dual infection with HIV and malaria on pregnancy outcome in western Kenya. AIDS 2003;17:585–94.
[32] Ladner J, Leroy V, Simonon A, et al. HIV infection, malaria, and pregnancy: a prospective cohort study in Kigali, Rwanda. Am J Trop Med Hyg 2002;66:56–60.
[33] Ticconi C, Mapfumo M, Dorrucci M, et al. Effect of maternal HIV and malaria infection on pregnancy and perinatal outcome in Zimbabwe. J Acquir Immune Defic Syndr 2003;34:289–94.
[34] Grimwade K, French N, Mbatha DD, et al. HIV infection as a cofactor for severe falciparum malaria in adults living in a region of unstable malaria transmission in South Africa. AIDS 2004;18:547–54.
[35] Svenson JE, MacLean JD, Gyorkos TW, et al. Imported malaria: clinical presentation and examination of symptomatic travelers. Arch Intern Med 1995;155:861–8.
[36] Shah S, Filler S, Causer LM, et al. Malaria surveillance—United States, 2002. MMWR Surveill Summ 2004;53:21–34.
[37] Reyburn H, Behrens RH, Warhurst D, et al. The effect of chemoprophylaxis on the timing of onset of falciparum malaria. Trop Med Int Health 1998;3:281–5.
[38] Moore DA, Jennings RM, Doherty TF, et al. Assessing the severity of malaria. BMJ 2003;326:808–9.
[39] WHO. Severe falciparum malaria. World Health Organization, Communicable Diseases Cluster. Trans R Soc Trop Med Hyg 2000;94(Suppl 1):S1–90.
[40] Becker JL. Vector-borne illnesses and the safety of the blood supply. Curr Hematol Rep 2003;2:511–7.
[41] Dodd RY. Transmission of parasites and bacteria by blood components. Vox Sang 2000;78(Suppl 2):239–42.
[42] Alweis RL, DiRosario K, Conidi G, et al. Serial nosocomial transmission of *Plasmodium falciparum* malaria from patient to nurse to patient. Infect Control Hosp Epidemiol 2004;25:55–9.
[43] Kirchgatter K, Wunderlich G, Branquinho MS, et al. Molecular typing of *Plasmodium falciparum* from Giemsa-stained blood smears confirms nosocomial malaria transmission. Acta Trop 2002;84:199–203.
[44] Thang HD, Elsas RM, Veenstra J. Airport malaria: report of a case and a brief review of the literature. Neth J Med 2002;60:441–3.
[45] Jafari S, Durand R, Lusina D, et al. Molecular characterisation of airport malaria: four cases in France during summer 1999. Parasite 2002;9:187–91.

[46] Warhurst DC. Laboratory procedures for diagnosis of malaria. In: Abdalla SH, Pasvol G, editors. Malaria: a hematological perspective, vol. 4. London: Imperial College Press; 2004. p. 448.

[47] Craig MH, Bredenkamp BL, Williams CH, et al. Field and laboratory comparative evaluation of ten rapid malaria diagnostic tests. Trans R Soc Trop Med Hyg 2002;96: 258–65.

[48] Silamut K, White NJ. Relation of the stage of parasite development in the peripheral blood to prognosis in severe falciparum malaria. Trans R Soc Trop Med Hyg 1993;87:436–43.

[49] Nguyen PH, Day N, Pram TD, et al. Intraleucocytic malaria pigment and prognosis in severe malaria. Trans R Soc Trop Med Hyg 1995;89:200–4.

[50] Metzger WG, Mordmuller BG, Kremsner PG. Malaria pigment in leucocytes. Trans R Soc Trop Med Hyg 1995;89:637–8.

[51] Gachot B, Houze S, Le Bras J, et al. Possible prognostic significance of a brief rise in parasitaemia following quinine treatment of severe *Plasmodium falciparum* malaria. Trans R Soc Trop Med Hyg 1996;90:388–90.

[52] Mordmuller B, Kremsner PG. Hyperparasitemia and blood exchange transfusion for treatment of children with falciparum malaria. Clin Infect Dis 1998;26:850–2.

[53] Warrell D, Phillips RE, Garrard CS. Intensive care unit management of severe malaria. Clin Intensive Care 1991;2:86–95.

[54] Njuguna P, Newton C. Management of severe falciparum malaria. J Postgrad Med 2004; 50:45–50.

[55] Davis TM, Supanaranond W, Pukrittayakamee S, et al. Progression of skeletal muscle damage during treatment of severe falciparum malaria. Acta Trop 2000;76:271–6.

[56] Molyneux ME, Taylor TE, Wirima JJ, et al. Clinical features and prognostic indicators in paediatric cerebral malaria: a study of 131 comatose Malawian children. QJM 1989;71: 441–59.

[57] Newton CR, Chokwe T, Schellenberg JA, et al. Coma scales for children with severe falciparum malaria. Trans R Soc Trop Med Hyg 1997;91:161–5.

[58] Maitland K, Levin M, English M, et al. Severe *P falciparum* malaria in Kenyan children: evidence for hypovolaemia. QJM 2003;96:427–34.

[59] Pasvol G, Newton CR, Winstanley PA, et al. Quinine treatment of severe falciparum malaria in African children: a randomized comparison of three regimens. Am J Trop Med Hyg 1991;45:702–13.

[60] White NJ, Looareesuwan S, Warrell DA, et al. Quinine loading dose in cerebral malaria. Am J Trop Med Hyg 1983;32:1–5.

[61] Davis TM, Supanaranond W, Pukrittayakamee S, et al. A safe and effective consecutive-infusion regimen for rapid quinine loading in severe falciparum malaria. J Infect Dis 1990; 161:1305–8.

[62] Bonington A, Davidson RN, Winstanley PA, et al. Fatal quinine cardiotoxicity in the treatment of falciparum malaria. Trans R Soc Trop Med Hyg 1996;90:305–7.

[63] Bethell DB, Phuong PT, Phuong CX, et al. Electrocardiographic monitoring in severe falciparum malaria. Trans R Soc Trop Med Hyg 1996;90:266–9.

[64] Wanwimolruk S, Denton JR. Plasma protein binding of quinine: binding to human serum albumin, alpha 1-acid glycoprotein and plasma from patients with malaria. J Pharm Pharmacol 1992;44:806–11.

[65] Winstanley P, Newton C, Watkins W, et al. Towards optimal regimens of parenteral quinine for young African children with cerebral malaria: the importance of unbound quinine concentration. Trans R Soc Trop Med Hyg 1993;87:201–6.

[66] White NJ. Controversies in the management of severe malaria. Baillieres Clin Infect Dis 1995;2:309–30.

[67] Powell VI, Grima K. Exchange transfusion for malaria and Babesia infection. Transfus Med Rev 2002;16:239–50.

[68] Silamut K, Molunto P, Ho M, et al. Alpha 1-acid glycoprotein (orosomucoid) and plasma protein binding of quinine in falciparum malaria. Br J Clin Pharmacol 1991;32:311–5.
[69] Phillips RE, Warrell DA, White NJ, et al. Intravenous quinidine for the treatment of severe falciparum malaria: clinical and pharmacokinetic studies. N Engl J Med 1985;312:1273–8.
[70] Kremsner PG, Radloff P, Metzger W, et al. Quinine plus clindamycin improves chemotherapy of severe malaria in children. Antimicrob Agents Chemother 1995;39:1603–5.
[71] Phillips RE, Looareesuwan S, Molyneux ME, et al. Hypoglycaemia and counterregulatory hormone responses in severe falciparum malaria: treatment with Sandostatin. QJM 1993;86:233–40.
[72] ter Kuile F, White NJ, Holloway P, et al. Plasmodium falciparum: in vitro studies of the pharmacodynamic properties of drugs used for the treatment of severe malaria. Exp Parasitol 1993;76:85–95.
[73] A meta-analysis using individual patient data of trials comparing artemether with quinine in the treatment of severe falciparum malaria. Trans R Soc Trop Med Hyg 2001;95:637–50.
[74] Newton PN, Angus BJ, Chierakul W, et al. Randomized comparison of artesunate and quinine in the treatment of severe falciparum malaria. Clin Infect Dis 2003;37:7–16.
[75] Roze E, Thiebaut MM, Mazevet D, et al. Neurologic sequelae after severe falciparum malaria in adult travelers. Eur Neurol 2001;46:192–7.
[76] Warrell DA, Looareesuwan S, Warrell MJ, et al. Dexamethasone proves deleterious in cerebral malaria: a double-blind trial in 100 comatose patients. N Engl J Med 1982;306:313–9.
[77] Hoffman SL, Rustama D, Punjabi NH, et al. High-dose dexamethasone in quinine-treated patients with cerebral malaria: a double-blind, placebo-controlled trial. J Infect Dis 1988;158:325–31.
[78] Newton CR, Kirkham FJ, Winstanley PA, et al. Intracranial pressure in African children with cerebral malaria. Lancet 1991;337:573–6.
[79] Newton CR, Crawley J, Sowumni A, et al. Intracranial hypertension in Africans with cerebral malaria. Arch Dis Child 1997;76:219–26.
[80] English M, Marsh V, Amukoye E, et al. Chronic salicylate poisoning and severe malaria. Lancet 1996;347:1736–7.
[81] Crawley J, Waruiru C, Mithwani S, et al. Effect of phenobarbital on seizure frequency and mortality in childhood cerebral malaria: a randomised, controlled intervention study. Lancet 2000;355:701–6.
[82] Crawley J, Smith S, Kirkham F, et al. Seizures and status epilepticus in childhood cerebral malaria. QJM 1996;89:591–7.
[83] Marsh K, Forster D, Waruiru C, et al. Indicators of life-threatening malaria in African children. N Engl J Med 1995;332:1399–404.
[84] Gachot B, Wolff M, Nissack G, et al. Acute lung injury complicating imported *Plasmodium falciparum* malaria. Chest 1995;108:746–9.
[85] Day NP, Phu NH, Bethell DP, et al. The effects of dopamine and adrenaline infusions on acid-base balance and systemic haemodynamics in severe infection. Lancet 1996;348:219–23.
[86] Day NP, Phu NH, Mai NT, et al. Effects of dopamine and epinephrine infusions on renal hemodynamics in severe malaria and severe sepsis. Crit Care Med 2000;28:1353–62.
[87] Day NP, Phu NH, Mai NT, et al. The pathophysiologic and prognostic significance of acidosis in severe adult malaria. Crit Care Med 2000;28:1833–40.
[88] Adrogue HJ, Madias NE. Management of life-threatening acid-base disorders. First of two parts. N Engl J Med 1998;338:26–34.
[89] English M, Waruiru C, Marsh K. Transfusion for respiratory distress in life-threatening childhood malaria. Am J Trop Med Hyg 1996;55:525–30.

[90] Hilton PJ, Taylor J, Forni LG, et al. Bicarbonate-based haemofiltration in the management of acute renal failure with lactic acidosis. QJM 1998;91:279–83.
[91] Ho M, Webster HK, Looareesuwan S, et al. Antigen-specific immunosuppression in human malaria due to *Plasmodium falciparum*. J Infect Dis 1986;153:763–71.
[92] Bernard GR, Artigas A, Brigham KL, et al. Report of the American-European consensus conference on ARDS: definitions, mechanisms, relevant outcomes and clinical trial coordination. The Consensus Committee. Intensive Care Med 1994;20:225–32.
[93] Bruneel F, Gachot B, Timsit JF, et al. Shock complicating severe falciparum malaria in European adults. Intensive Care Med 1997;23:698–701.
[94] Berkley J, Mwarumba S, Bramham K, et al. Bacteraemia complicating severe malaria in children. Trans R Soc Trop Med Hyg 1999;93:283–6.
[95] Hocqueloux L, Bruneel F, Pages CL, et al. Fatal invasive aspergillosis complicating severe *Plasmodium falciparum* malaria. Clin Infect Dis 2000;30:940–2.
[96] Manish R, Tripathy R, Das BK. Plasma glucose and tumour necrosis factor-alpha in adult patients with severe falciparum malaria. Trop Med Int Health 2003;8:125–8.
[97] White NJ, Warrell DA, Chanthavanich P, et al. Severe hypoglycemia and hyperinsulinemia in falciparum malaria. N Engl J Med 1983;309:61–6.
[98] Holst FG, Hemmer CJ, Kern P, et al. Inappropriate secretion of antidiuretic hormone and hyponatremia in severe falciparum malaria. Am J Trop Med Hyg 1994;50:602–7.
[99] Betjes MG. Hyponatremia in acute brain disease: the cerebral salt wasting syndrome. Eur J Intern Med 2002;13:9–14.
[100] Ustianowski A, Schwab U, Pasvol G. Case report: severe acute symptomatic hyponatraemia in falciparum malaria. Trans R Soc Trop Med Hyg 2002;96:647–8.
[101] St John A, Davis TM, Binh TQ, et al. Mineral homoeostasis in acute renal failure complicating severe falciparum malaria. J Clin Endocrinol Metab 1995;80:2761–7.
[102] Tran TH, Day NP, Ly VC, et al. Blackwater fever in southern Vietnam: a prospective descriptive study of 50 cases. Clin Infect Dis 1996;23:1274–81.
[103] Trang TT, Phu NH, Vinh H, et al. Acute renal failure in patients with severe falciparum malaria. Clin Infect Dis 1992;15:874–80.
[104] Naqvi R, Ahmad E, Akhtar F, et al. Outcome in severe acute renal failure associated with malaria. Nephrol Dial Transplant 2003;18:1820–3.
[105] Phu NH, Hien TT, Mai NT, et al. Hemofiltration and peritoneal dialysis in infection-associated acute renal failure in Vietnam. N Engl J Med 2002;347:895–902.
[106] Clemens R, Pramoolsinsap C, Lorenz R, et al. Activation of the coagulation cascade in severe falciparum malaria through the intrinsic pathway. Br J Haematol 1994;87:100–5.
[107] Krishnan A, Karnad DR, Limaye U, et al. Cerebral venous and dural sinus thrombosis in severe falciparum malaria. J Infect 2004;48:86–90.
[108] Phillips RE, Pasvol G. Anaemia of *Plasmodium falciparum* malaria. Baillieres Clin Haematol 1992;5:315–30.
[109] Hebert PC, Wells G, Blajchman MA, et al. A multicenter, randomized, controlled clinical trial of transfusion requirements in critical care. Transfusion Requirements in Critical Care Investigators, Canadian Critical Care Trials Group. N Engl J Med 1999;340:409–17.
[110] de Aguirre Z, De Droogh E, Van den Ende J, et al. Splenic rupture as a complication of *P falciparum* malaria after residence in the tropics: report of two cases. Acta Clin Belg 1998;53:374–7.
[111] Miller KD, Greenberg AE, Campbell CC. Treatment of severe malaria in the United States with a continuous infusion of quinidine gluconate and exchange transfusion. N Engl J Med 1989;321:65–70.
[112] Burchard GD, Kroger J, Knobloch J, et al. Exchange blood transfusion in severe falciparum malaria: retrospective evaluation of 61 patients treated with, compared to 63 patients treated without, exchange transfusion. Trop Med Int Health 1997;2:733–40.

[113] Riddle MS, Jackson JL, Sanders JW, et al. Exchange transfusion as an adjunct therapy in severe *Plasmodium falciparum* malaria: a meta-analysis. Clin Infect Dis 2002;34:1192–8.
[114] Wilkinson RJ, Brown JL, Pasvol G, et al. Severe falciparum malaria: predicting the effect of exchange transfusion. QJM 1994;87:553–7.
[115] Macallan DC, Pocock M, Robinson GT, et al. Red cell exchange, erythrocytapheresis, in the treatment of malaria with high parasitaemia in returning travellers. Trans R Soc Trop Med Hyg 2000;94:353–6.
[116] Zhang Y, Telleria L, Vinetz JM, et al. Erythrocytapheresis for *Plasmodium falciparum* infection complicated by cerebral malaria and hyperparasitemia. J Clin Apheresis 2001;16:15–8.
[117] White NJ. The management of severe falciparum malaria. Am J Respir Crit Care Med 2003;167:673–4.
[118] Kwiatkowski D, Molyneux ME, Stephens S, et al. Anti-TNF therapy inhibits fever in cerebral malaria. QJM 1993;86:91–8.
[119] Looareesuwan S, Wilairatana P, Vannaphan S, et al. Pentoxifylline as an ancillary treatment for severe falciparum malaria in Thailand. Am J Trop Med Hyg 1998;58:348–53.
[120] Looareesuwan S, Sjostrom L, Krudsood S, et al. Polyclonal anti-tumor necrosis factor-alpha Fab used as an ancillary treatment for severe malaria. Am J Trop Med Hyg 1999;61:26–33.
[121] Smith HJ, Meremikwu M. Iron chelating agents for treating malaria. Cochrane Database Syst Rev 2003; CD001474.
[122] Krishna S, Supanaranond W, Pukrittayakamee S, et al. Dichloroacetate for lactic acidosis in severe malaria: a pharmacokinetic and pharmacodynamic assessment. Metabolism 1994;43:974–81.
[123] Agbenyega T, Planche T, Bedu-Addo G, et al. Population kinetics, efficacy, and safety of dichloroacetate for lactic acidosis due to severe malaria in children. J Clin Pharmacol 2003;43:386–96.
[124] Dondorp AM, Omodeo-Sale F, Chotivanich K, et al. Oxidative stress and rheology in severe malaria. Redox Rep 2003;8:292–4.
[125] Treeprasertsuk S, Krudsood S, Tosukhowong T, et al. *N*-acetylcysteine in severe falciparum malaria in Thailand. Southeast Asian J Trop Med Public Health 2003;34:37–42.
[126] White NJ, Warrell DA, Looareesuwan S, et al. Pathophysiological and prognostic significance of cerebrospinal-fluid lactate in cerebral malaria. Lancet 1985;1:776–8.
[127] Medana IM, Hien TT, Day NP, et al. The clinical significance of cerebrospinal fluid levels of kynurenine pathway metabolites and lactate in severe malaria. J Infect Dis 2002;185:650–6.
[128] Hollenstein U, Looareesuwan S, Aichelburg A, et al. Serum procalcitonin levels in severe *Plasmodium falciparum* malaria. Am J Trop Med Hyg 1998;59:860–3.

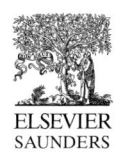

# Cutaneous Leishmaniasis in the Returning Traveler

Alan J. Magill, MD[a,b],*

[a]Walter Reed Army Institute of Research, 503 Robert Grant Avenue,
Silver Spring, MD 20910, USA
[b]Uniformed Services University of the Health Sciences, 4301 Jones Bridge Road,
Bethesda, MD 20814, USA

Infection with protozoan parasites of the genus *Leishmania* leads to a wide variety of clinical disease syndromes called leishmaniasis, or more appropriately the leishmaniases [1]. The three major clinical syndromes are (1) cutaneous leishmaniasis (CL), (2) mucosal leishmaniasis (ML), and (3) visceral leishmaniasis. CL includes typical chronic, ulcerative presentations, and less common nodular, hyperkeratotic, psoriasiform, plaque-like, and verrucous presentations. ML is a destructive or granulomatous reaction seen in the nasal, oral, and hypopharyngeal mucosa that occurs concurrently or more typically, years following CL caused by infection with New World *Leishmania* (subgenus *viannia*) complex parasites. Visceral leishmaniasis is a systemic illness characterized by fever, cachexia, splenomegaly, pancytopenia, and hypergammaglobulinemia. All three of these syndromes have been documented in returning travelers. This article focuses on CL with some comment on ML.

The leishmaniases are a heterogenous collection of clinical diseases caused by many different species of *Leishmania*, each with its own relatively unique geographic distribution, biology, ecology, local mammalian reservoir, and sandfly vector. For example, *Leishmania major*, a common cause of Old World CL, has a wide geographic distribution across North Africa, throughout the Middle East, and Southwest and Central Asia. *L major* exists in a reservoir of various burrow-dwelling rodents and is enzootically transmitted by *Phlebotomus papatasi* sandflies. Humans only become

---

The views of the author do not necessarily reflect the official position of the Department of the Army or the Department of Defense.

* Walter Reed Army Institute of Research, 503 Robert Grant Avenue, Silver Spring, MD 20910.

  *E-mail address:* alan.magill@na.amedd.army.mil

infected when they intrude into the transmission cycle by virtue of their activities. In contrast, *Leishmania tropica*, the other primary etiology of Old World CL that shares a similar geographic distribution, does not have a known animal reservoir. Humans are the reservoir and transmission occurs by way of the bite of *Phlebotomus sergenti* [1–3].

The life cycle of leishmaniasis begins when the promastigote, an elongate, motile form of the parasite found in the sandfly, is transmitted to the unsuspecting human host by the bite of small, delicate female sandflies, which feed from twilight to dawn. Promastigotes invade host macrophages and transform into 3- to 5-μm ovoid amastigotes with a well-defined nucleus and kinetoplast, a rod-shaped specialized mitochondrial structure that contains extranuclear DNA. Visualization of the kinetoplast, which has a characteristic appearance under oil-immersion microscopy (Fig. 1), is required to confirm the diagnosis of leishmaniasis.

The taxonomy of *Leishmania* parasites can be confusing and differences in how parasites are characterized makes comparison of clinical and treatment study outcomes challenging. A simplified, clinically useful taxonomic classification is shown in Fig. 2. Historically, *Leishmania* parasites have been divided into different species based on clinical, biologic, geographic, and epidemiologic criteria. For example, a parasite isolated from a patient with a typical "dry ulcer" in an urban setting in the Middle East was called *L tropica*. Beginning in the early 1970s, intrinsic characteristics, such as biochemical and molecular markers, were identified and used

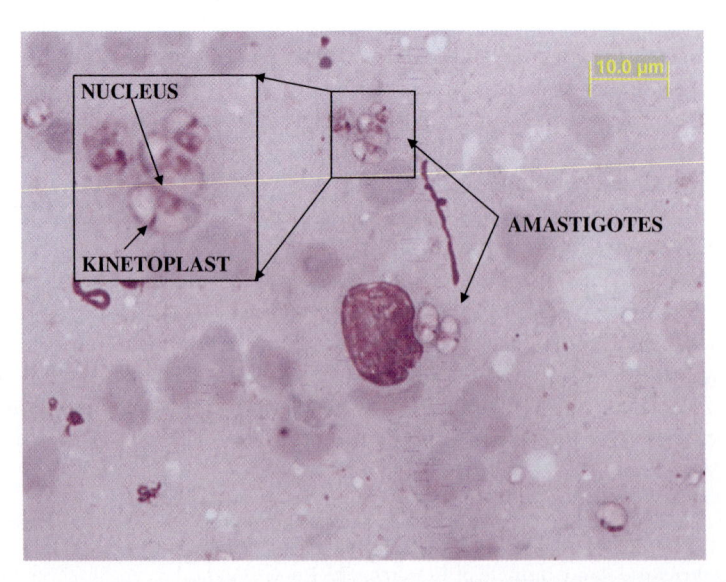

Fig. 1. Tissue smear obtained from a patient with confirmed *Leishmania major* infection. Numerous amastigotes, 3 to 4 μm in width and 4 to 5 μm in length are seen. Note the rod-shaped kinetoplast seen next to the nucleus, enlarged in the inset (Giemsa, original magnification ×1000). (Courtesy of Dr. Pete Weina.)

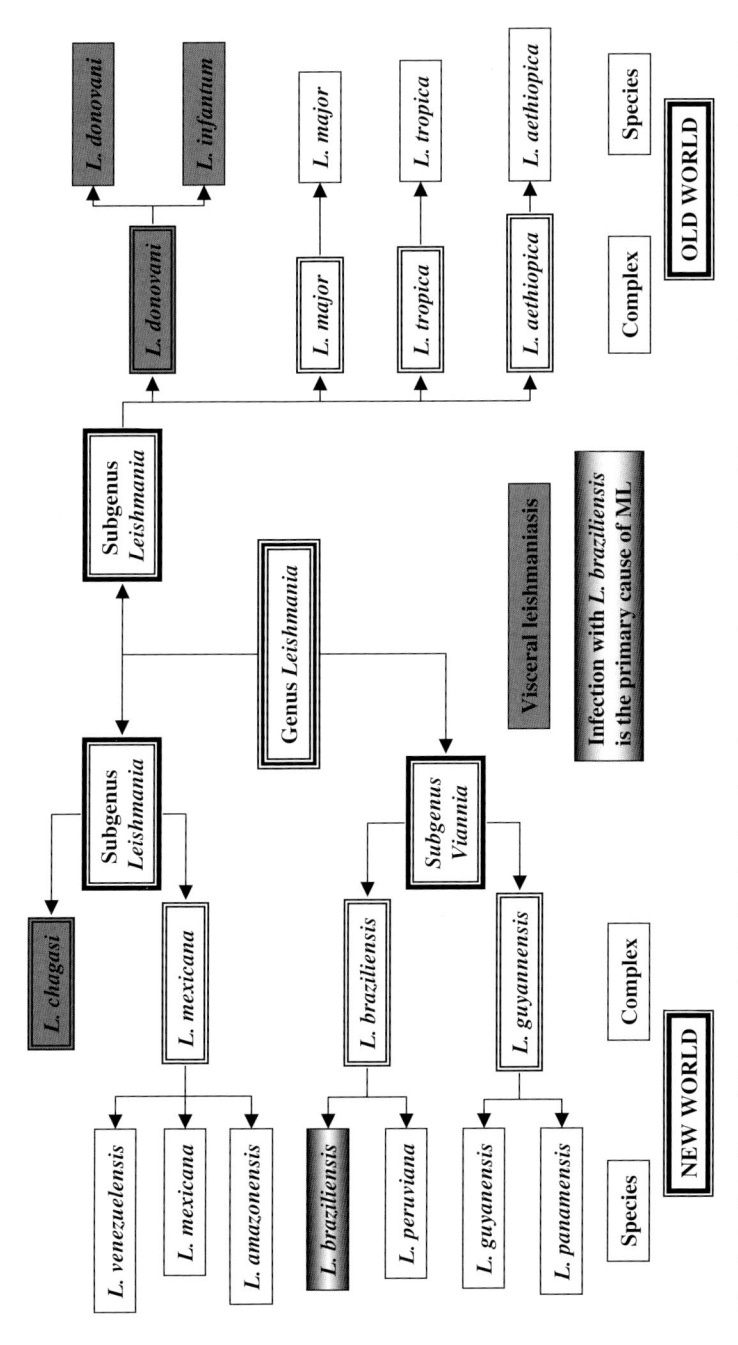

Fig. 2. A clinically useful taxonomic classification based on isoenzyme characterization of the major Leishmania parasites pathogenic for humans. (*Adapted from* Control of the leishmaniases. WHO technical report series No. 793. Geneva: World Health Organization; 1990; with permission.)

to develop classification systems. Isoenzyme analysis by electrophoresis, developed in the 1970s, is widely used as a typing system and still represents a reference technique for *Leishmania* identification. The taxonomic profile determined by isoenzyme electrophoresis is called a zymodeme. Isoenzyme analysis is most often successful with culture amplified parasites. It is time consuming, however, requires specialized laboratory expertise, and usually cannot provide a result to the clinician in a time frame that is meaningful to affect the choice or duration of therapy. Further complicating isoenzyme interpretation is the fact that different research groups have adopted different techniques. The MON (for Montpellier, France) typing system, an authoritative standard from an acknowledged world reference center, uses 15 standardized isoenzyme loci analyzed by starch gel electrophoresis [4]. In contrast, American researchers more commonly use a system of three standardized isoenzyme loci identified by cellulose gel electrophoresis [5]. Intuitively, the use of more isoenzyme loci reveals greater differences between strains. The clinical implications of greater or lesser degrees of characterization are not clearly known, but are likely to be important. For example, *Leishmania panamensis* and *Leishmania guyanensis*, long considered different species, may instead represent clusters within a spectrum of genetic diversity [6].

Other methods of characterizing parasites, such as growth parameters and a host of molecular methods, have led to a unique classification vocabulary to include species, species complex, zymodemes, serodemes, and schizodemes, which makes clinical correlations challenging.

### Epidemiology of cutaneous leishmaniasis in returning travelers

Imported CL has been described in civilian tourists, workers, and expatriates from many nonendemic countries [7–18]. Between 1985 and 1990, the Centers for Disease Control and Prevention (CDC) received 129 requests for sodium stibogluconate ([SSG] Pentostam) to treat civilians with leishmaniasis [11]. A total of 81% (105 of 129) had CL, of which 53% (69 of 129) acquired CL in the Americas, reflecting travel patterns of Americans. Risk estimates varied greatly by destination ranging from a low of 1 per million travelers to Mexico to a high of 1 per 1000 to Suriname. Interestingly, only 19 travelers (32%) were short-term tourists, outside the United States for a median of 20 days (range, 4–182 days). Others risk groups were field researchers, 27 (46%); ornithologists, 11 (19%); tour guides; missionaries; and nature photographers whose activities brought them in contact with sandflies and who remained in high-risk exposure areas for prolonged periods of time. Some specific destinations identified as higher risk were Manu National Park in southern Peru; Tikal National Park in Guatemala; and some destinations in Belize, Suriname, and French Guinea [11]. Between 1991 and 2001, the CDC released SSG over 350 times for the treatment of CL, 75% of the time for New World CL and 17% for Old World CL (Barbara Herwaldt, personal communication, 2004). The continued predominance of New World CL seen in American travelers over the last decade likely reflects the increased numbers visiting tropical areas of the Americas that are participating in ecotourism.

Military operations in endemic countries can also lead to large numbers of nonimmunes being exposed in sort time periods [19]. The recent deployment of tens of thousands of American and other coalition military forces to Iraq in the spring of 2003 has led to the largest epidemic of CL in military forces since World War II [20–22]. Over 600 cases of *L major* acquired in Iraq and a few cases of *L tropica* acquired in Afghanistan have been seen in the United States military.

Reliable predictions of specific high-risk destinations for travelers are difficult to make because infection risk for CL in endemic countries is often focal, seasonal, and subject to year-to-year variation.

## Clinical presentation

Returning travelers present with a nonhealing cutaneous lesion. This is often a chronic, slowly progressive, nonhealing ulcer. Nodules, psoriasiform plaques, verrucous lesions, and sporotrichoid presentations, however, are not uncommon. Examples of CL lesions can be seen in Fig. 3. Almost uniformly patients initially believe it is an "infected insect bite." They become concerned and seek medical attention when the small inflammatory papule enlarges to a nodule that slowly develops a central ulceration. A crust forms that drops off to expose an ulcer base that is painless, usually has a raised or rolled margin, and may have satellite lesions [23–25]. Regional lymphadenopathy proximal to the bite site can be seen, especially with infections caused by *Leishmania viannia braziliensis* acquired in the Americas [17,26,27]. The lymphadenopathy associated with *L braziliensis* infection usually precedes the development of the ulcerative lesion and can be associated with fever, hepatomegaly, and systemic complaints [27,28].

The incubation period is defined as the time of infection until the time of first clinically apparent lesion. For travelers, the time of infection is not known, but often inferred from the exposure window related to travel. Typical incubation periods range from weeks to months after exposure with variability depending on the strain of infecting parasite [1]. Time to first clinical presentation was $9 \pm 5$ weeks in 310 United States military personnel with *L major* infection [20].

The diagnosis of CL is usually not considered at the initial encounter with a health care professional. A short course of antibiotics is often prescribed that has little or no effect. At some point in the course of events, often after a referral to a dermatologist, infectious disease specialist, or a travel medicine specialist, the diagnosis of CL is considered.

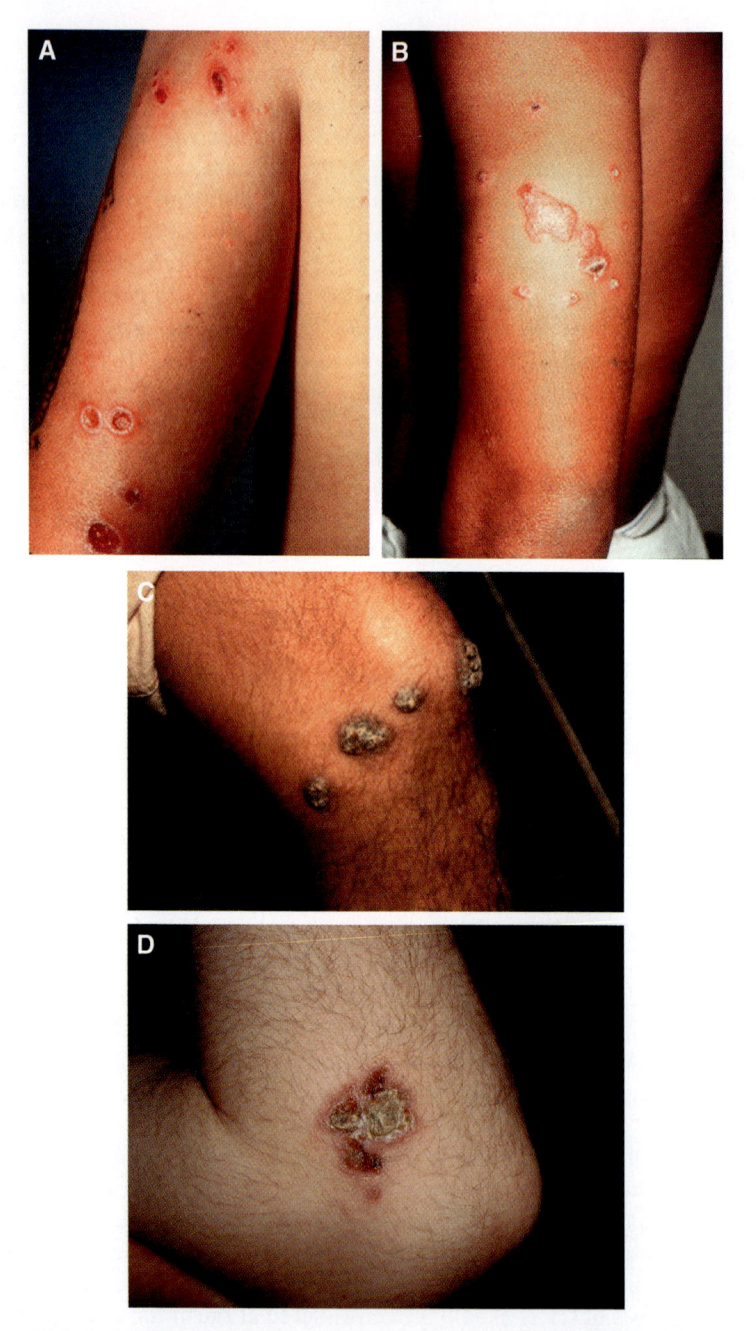

Fig. 3. Clinical presentation of cutaneous leishmaniasis. (*A*) Lymphangitic spread from a distal bite site, *L panamensis*. (*B*) Papular primary with satellite lesions. (*C*) Nodular lesions. (*D*) Crusted exudate over ulcer base, *L major*. (Courtesy of Dr. Pete Weina.)

The ulcers of CL are usually not tender or painful, unless a secondary bacterial infection is also present. Differentiation between a leishmanial ulcer that is superinfected with bacteria and a pyoderma can be difficult and may require microbiologic and histopathologic evaluation. Once amastigotes are visualized, bacterial superinfection is likely if the ulcer is painful or draining pus.

**Diagnosis**

Although a classic clinical presentation along with a history of travel to an endemic area can make the positive predictive value of a clinical diagnosis very high, it is often difficult to distinguish CL from other diagnoses based on clinical criteria alone. A complete differential diagnosis of skin lesions in returning travelers is extensive [29,30], but in practice, the diagnosis in returning travelers is limited to a few of the more common etiologies. Tropical pyoderma is a skin disorder that often presents as a crusted ulcer usually associated with staphylococcal or streptococcal infection. Although it can be very difficult to distinguish from CL [31], a careful history can help distinguish between the two diagnoses. Tropical pyoderma begins as a small pustule, which is moderately painful and pruritic, ruptures with minimal manipulation, and then ulcerates. The entire process from initial pustule to ulceration occurs over days. A leishmanial ulcer begins as a small papule, enlarges into a nodule, and then ulcerates. This process occurs over many days to a few weeks and there is seldom associated pain or pruritus. Tropical pyoderma does not have the typical rolled-up ulcer margin and periulcer induration associated with *Leishmania* infection.

If the history is consistent with tropical pyoderma or if *Leishmania* diagnostic capabilities are not easily available, a 7- to 10-day course of an oral antibiotic, such as amoxicillin-clavulanate or a fluoroquinolone, in conjunction with standard wound care is a reasonable empiric approach. Pyoderma improves with antibiotics over the course of a week, whereas ulcers caused by *Leishmania* do not respond at all, or only modestly improve if bacterial superinfection was present.

Both basal and squamous cell cutaneous carcinomas can be confused with *Leishmania* lesions. Other infectious causes of ulcerative lesions that can appear almost identical to *Leishmania*, such as cutaneous diphtheria, tuberculosis, or tularemia, are exceedingly rare and are only identified in the course of a thorough laboratory evaluation. In those with a sporotrichoid presentation, sporotrichosis [32] and infections caused by *Mycobacterium marinum* need to be considered and require appropriate microbiologic confirmation. CL-sporotrichosis coinfections have been reported in Colombia but not in returning travelers [33].

Once the diagnosis of CL is considered, parasitologic confirmation of *Leishmania* parasites is required before specific treatment can be initiated. Serologic tests are not sensitive for the diagnosis of CL and should not be relied on to confirm or exclude the diagnosis. Detection of delayed-type hypersensitivity to *Leishmania* antigens, usually elicited by use of an intradermal skin test, is used as a diagnostic adjunct in many endemic countries. No *Leishmania* skin test, however, is available or approved for use in the United States or Canada.

Parasitologic confirmation of CL can be made by visualization of the amastigote in thin smears from tissue scrapings or "touch preparations" from biopsies; by identification of amastigotes in standard histopathologic sections; by visualization of promastigotes in in vitro or in vivo culture; and by detection of parasite-specific nucleic acid sequences, usually by polymerase chain reaction–based amplification methodologies. It is important to note that most nonendemic country microbiologic laboratories have little to no experience with this parasite and the accuracy of diagnosis may be limited.

Tissue scrapings can be obtained after the lesions have been cleaned and the eschars and exudate have been removed. Use of 1% lidocaine with epinephrine is recommended (unless contraindicated) to decrease bleeding, allow adequate debridement, and improve the quality of the scraping. A No. 10 scalpel blade is then scraped across the ulcer base with enough pressure to obtain an exudate, but not vigorously enough to elicit bleeding. The dermal tissue is then spread on a glass slide with a circular motion to a 2- to 3-cm diameter area [20]. Standard 2- to 3-mm punch biopsies are useful when the initial tissue scrapings are negative, a diagnosis other than *Leishmania* is likely, background histopathology is needed, or nonulcerative lesions are present. Tissue sections should be cut at 3 to 4 μm and stained with hematoxylin and eosin. The Brown-Hopps modified tissue gram stain highlights the kinetoplast and can be useful in some cases (Dr. Ronald Neafie, personal communication, 2004).

Exclusion of the diagnosis of leishmaniasis based on a single test or specimen is not recommended. More than one test method using multiple specimens improves the diagnostic yield [34,35].

In the United States, there are two sources of diagnostic services available free of charge to requesting physicians. Civilian physicians can request diagnostic assistance from the CDC by calling 770-488-4475 and referring to on-line guidance at http://www.dpd.cdc.gov/dpdx/HTML/DiagnosticProcedures.htm. Military physicians can request diagnostic assistance from the Walter Reed Army Institute of Research by calling 301-319-9956 and referring to on-line guidance at http://www.pdhealth.mil/leish.asp. Expert pathology consultation is also available from the Division of Infectious and Tropical Diseases Pathology, Armed Forces Institute of Pathology (http://www.afip.org/).

## Mucosal leishmaniasis

ML is an uncommon sequelae of infection with New World *L braziliensis* [36–40] or rarely, *L panamensis* [41,42], *L guyanensis* [43,44], or *L amazonensis*

[45]. Ulcerative, granulomatous, or destructive lesions may appear in the nasal, buccal, and orohypopharyngeal mucosa concurrently with the primary cutaneous lesion or more commonly months to years later. Estimates of the risk of developing ML following infection with *L brasiliensis* in endemic countries varies widely, ranging from 2% to 10% in areas of southern Brazil and Bolivia known to be at high risk down to an occasional occurrence in Middle America [39,46].

ML in returning travelers is rare, with only a handful of cases reported worldwide [47–54]. It is not surprising that the diagnosis of ML is delayed in most cases because physicians from nonendemic countries are not aware of the disease. Initial symptoms in travelers may only be nonspecific nasal congestion with minimal involvement of the nasal septum and turbinates [52]. ML should be considered in a patient with chronic nasal congestion and a history of travel to an endemic area of Latin America. The presence of nasal mucosal abnormalities, especially if granulomas are seen on tissue histopathology, should prompt a *Leishmania*-specific evaluation. Once the diagnosis is entertained clinically, parasitologic confirmation is difficult because ML is an oligoparasitic syndrome. Parasites are few in number and amastigotes are not easily visualized in standard smear preparations or histologic sections. Culture may also be unsuccessful. Detection of *Leishmania* DNA by polymerase chain reaction is the most sensitive diagnostic test [17], although validated, reproducible assays remain unavailable to most practicing clinicians. The differential diagnosis for ML includes lymphoma, mid-line granuloma, Wegener's granulomatosis, paracoccidioidomycosis, histoplasmosis, tuberculosis, leprosy, and other uncommon diagnoses [1,51,52]. Expert consultation and otorhinolaryngology evaluation is recommended.

Although ML is rare in travelers, the desire to prevent its occurrence guides all management decisions once CL is confirmed. Infections acquired in the New World are usually treated with parenteral, systemic drugs, unless the infecting parasite is convincingly shown to be *Leishmania mexicana,* which is not associated with ML. Because this information is usually not known when treatment is initiated, a pentavalent antimony (SbV) agent is usually begun. Although there are no convincing data to prove systemic treatment with SbV prevents later development of ML, cases of ML have been associated with incomplete or missing SbV treatment [39,46,47]. Expert opinion clearly favors systemic treatment of all New World acquired *L brasiliensis* infections.

## Treatment

Most CL resolves over time without any specific treatment leaving an atrophic scar. The time course of healing can vary from months to years, however, based on the infecting parasite strain, the host immune status, and the location of the ulcerative lesions. Most individuals are not willing to let nature take its course and seek medical care because the location and number of lesions present major cosmetic concerns, place limitations on activity, or become symptomatic because of secondary bacterial infection.

*The importance of knowing the infecting parasite strain*

CL caused by Old World species, mostly *L major* and *L tropica*, in general leads to a more benign clinical course with self-limiting disease and fewer complications than some New World infecting strains. Chronic persistent *L tropica* infections (leishmaniasis recidivans) occur in endemic countries but rarely in returning travelers. One recent case in an immigrant has been reported [55].

Patients with similar clinical pictures respond differently to treatment based partly on the species of infecting *Leishmania* parasite. For example, the relative efficacy and toxicity of SSG and ketoconazole for the treatment of parasitologically proved CL was compared in a randomized clinical trial conducted in 120 Guatemalan men who were divided into three treatment groups: (1) SSG (20 mg of antimony per kilogram per day intravenously for 20 days); (2) ketoconazole (600 mg per day orally for 28 days); and (3) placebo [56]. Among patients infected with *L braziliensis*, 24 (96%) of 25 in the SSG group but only 7 (30%) of 23 in the ketoconazole group responded. Among *L mexicana* infected patients, only four (57%) of seven in the SSG group but eight (89%) of nine in the ketoconazole group responded.

Even within a species complex thought to be relatively homogenous, such as *L major*, significant enzymatic variation has been described in isolates from different geographic locations [57,58] that has significance in experimental animal models [59] and in clinical presentations in patients [60]. If clinical significance can be linked to small phenotypic differences in a relatively homogenous parasite complex, such as *L major*, the implications for much more heterogenous complexes, such as *L tropica* [61], could be dramatic.

In addition to determining the success of a particular treatment, knowing the infecting species can allow for an optimal drug regimen, limiting unnecessary exposure of patients to poorly tolerated drugs. In a randomized, double-blind, placebo-controlled study of 10 versus 20 days of SSG in United States military personnel who contracted CL while serving overseas, 19 patients received SSG for 10 days (and placebo for 10 days), and 19 patients received SSG for 20 days [62]. Cure rates were 100% (19 of 19 patients) in the 10-day group and 95% (18 of 19 patients) in the 20-day group. As expected, side effects were more common among patients who received 20 days of therapy. In this group of otherwise healthy young adults, SSG at a dosage of 20 mg/kg/d for 10 days seems to have been therapeutically equivalent and less toxic than the standard 20-day course. The range of infecting parasites in this study included 18 *L panamensis*,

6 *L major*, 2 *L braziliensis*, 1 *L viannia naiffi*, 1 *L (Viannia) guyanensis*, and 1 *L tropica*.

## Drug treatment

The treatment of CL in returning travelers has been reviewed recently [63]. Only issues relevant to practicing physicians in North America are dealt with in this article. There are no simple, all-inclusive treatment recommendations for the many different forms of CL. In general, New World CL has been traditionally treated with parenteral SbV, partly out of the belief that systemic treatment prevents the late complication of ML. Old World CL has been viewed by many as a less serious, self-healing disease that usually does not warrant systemic parenteral treatment. Local and physical therapies have been more commonly used in Old World CL.

The goal of targeted drug therapy is a well-tolerated, species-specific treatment that maximizes benefit and minimizes harm in each individual patient. The current reality, however, especially in North America, is a "one size fits all" recommendation based on parenteral SbV. The heterogeneity and diversity of syndromes seen in clinical practice result in patients who present with a complex spectrum of lesions that are associated with cosmetic and functionally important considerations. Evidence-based treatment recommendations that apply to all the leishmaniases do not exist and experts disagree on the optimal individual case management.

## Is any treatment indicated?

When faced with a parasitologically confirmed case of CL, the first management decision concerns whether any specific treatment is indicated. Fig. 4 lists relevant criteria when considering if treatment is indicated. For example, a few small lesions caused by *L major* that are improving by history and are located on easily covered skin surfaces, such as the leg or back, may not require any specific intervention. Patients with multiple lesions, one or more large (>5 cm in diameter) lesions, lesions in cosmetically unacceptable locations, or those that are getting worse by history should usually be offered treatment. Patients with proved or suspected infection caused by a New World parasite associated with ML should always be offered systemic parenteral treatment.

## Local versus systemic treatment?

The decision to offer a local treatment over no treatment can be based on the same criteria as listed in Fig. 4. In practice, these patients have lesions that warrant some intervention, but the toxicity associated with parenteral agents, such as SbV or amphotericin B, outweigh the benefit of using these agents. For example, a single ulcer less than 5 cm in diameter caused by *L major* in a cosmetically troublesome area, such as the dorsum of the hand,

| No Treatment | | Treatment |
|---|---|---|
| Late* | *Stage of lesion(s)* | Early |
| Single (few) | *Number of lesions* | Multiple |
| Uncomplicated | *Complexity* | Complicated** |
| Immunocompetent | *Immune status* | Immunocompromised |
| None | *Mucosal involvement* | Yes |
| Non-exposed | *Skin location* | Exposed |
| Excluded | *L. braziliensis* | Confirmed*** |
| No concern | *How bothersome are the lesions to the patient or his/her family?* | Very bothersome |
| Small (<1 cm) | *Size of lesion(s)* | Very large (> 5 cm) |

* By history, a lesion that is already starting to improve. It is "better" today than it was a few weeks ago
** Location of lesion(s) restricts joint mobility, prevents wearing of clothes or shoes, facial lesions may lead to disfigurement, nose and ear lesions are very slow to heal.
*** confirmed *L. braziliensis* infections should be treated with parenteral SbV or amphotericin B deoxycholate

Fig. 4. Criteria to consider when deciding treatment options for cutaneous leishmaniasis.

which by history is getting worse, is still early in the natural history. Although the ulcer will likely resolve in 6 to 12 months, the patient understandably does not want to wait. Parenteral therapy is efficacious, but the toxicity may not be desirable. These patients are ideal candidates for a local treatment, such as a physical method, topical therapy, or intralesional chemotherapy.

*Physical methods*

CL has been treated with a wide range of physical methods including heat (cauterization, application of local heat by device, or infrared or heat lamps); cold (liquid nitrogen with or without cryoprobe); and surgical excision or curettage in endemic countries. Most reports of physical methods have been uncontrolled studies in Old World CL without parasite characterization, and the choice of the method has generally been based on local preference and customary medical practice. Treatment success of a new drug is hard to quantify without a placebo arm in a controlled study because background cure rates caused by natural healing may confound the interpretation. In general, only cryotherapy is used in North America.

North American dermatologists are quite familiar with cryotherapy and use liquid nitrogen for a number of different indications. In CL it is best suited for small lesions acquired in the Old World that are minimally inflamed. Apply liquid nitrogen with a cotton-tipped applicator using moderate pressure for two freeze-thaw cycles (15- to 20-second freeze followed by a 1-minute thaw) to the whole lesion, reassess at 1- to 2-week intervals, and repeat treatment once or twice as needed. Adequate treatment results when the skin turns white 2 to 3 mm beyond the margins of the lesion. Edema and blistering occur within hours and last for a few days followed by crusting and formation of an eschar. In a large case series (N = 461) reported from an *L tropica*–endemic area of Turkey, one cryotherapy session was sufficient in 90% of cases when applied to lesions less than 1 cm in diameter [64]. There was an 8% relapse rate at 6 months. Hypopigmentation developed after cryotherapy in 68%, but repigmentation usually occurred in 2 to 3 months. In a second series (N = 215) of mixed *L tropica* and *L major* cases reported from Jordan, one to three cryotherapy sessions led to a clinical cure for all but one patient [65]. About 40% of patients resolved with either hypopigmentation or hyperpigmentation and 5% had residual scars.

Local heat treatments have been of interest for years because *Leishmania* species are heat sensitive [66]. A device (ThermoMed; ThermoSurgery Technologies, Inc., Phoenix, AZ) that generates focused and controlled heating of the skin (size and depth), by use of radiofrequency, was cleared by the US Food and Drug Administration (FDA) in May, 2002. Published experience with the device is limited. A placebo-controlled trial in Guatemala with an early prototype device showed healing equivalent with the intramuscular regimen of SbV used in the study, but that regimen is considered suboptimal by today's standards [67]. Recent experience with a current version of ThermoMed in *L tropica* infections in Afghanistan showed 69% efficacy at 3 months following a single treatment (Dr. Richard Reithinger, personal communication, 2004). Use of a topical antibiotic ointment for a few days after heat treatment decreases the number of infectious complications. The usefulness of this device remains to be determined in controlled clinical studies.

*Topical treatments*

Topical preparations of paromomycin phosphate (PP), an aminoglycoside antibiotic, have been used for years for the treatment of Old World CL. Most published experience is with either 15% PP formulated with 12% methylbenzethonium chloride in white soft paraffin, known as "P-ointment" and available commercially in Israel as Leshcutan, or 15% PP formulated with 10% urea in white soft paraffin. Neither preparation is approved or commercially available in the United States. Establishing efficacy is difficult because of the variable dosing regimens tested in both New and Old World CL. P-ointment is modestly effective against *L major*, but not effective against *L tropica* in the Old World [68–72] and somewhat less effective for New World infections in Guatemala and Belize [73,74].

Topical PP is a reasonable option for small, simple ulcerative lesions caused by *L major* and *L mexicana* complex parasites. Nodular or hyperkeratotic lesions, locations on the nose and ears, sporotrichoid presentations, and ulcers caused by *L tropica* and *L braziliensis* are not suitable for topical treatment. Although there are no commercial preparations available in the United States, physicians can request topical PP for an individual patient from a compounding pharmacy. The usual prescription is for 15% PP with 10% urea in white soft paraffin [75]. The efficacy of topical PP preparations has varied widely based on the infecting parasite, geographic location of clinical trials [76], the composition of the formulation [75], dosing regimen [77], and whether an occlusive dressing was used or not. For example, the efficacy of P-ointment, which contains 12% methylbenzethonium chloride, has been attributed at least in part to the methylbenzethonium chloride component [75]. If satisfactory improvement is not seen in a time period of 2 to 4 weeks, an alternative treatment can be considered. A locater for compounding pharmacies in the United States can be accessed at the International Academy of Compounding Pharmacy website (http://www.iacprx.org/referral_service/index.html).

*Intralesional injections*

Intralesional injections with SbV compounds are a primary means of therapy for Old World CL in endemic countries [64,78–84]. Efficacy is reported to be very high but there are few randomized controlled trials. Intralesional injections can be very painful and difficult to administer to children, around digits, and on the face. Lesions on the back or thigh, locations with relatively fewer nerve endings and adequate subcutaneous tissue, are much easier to treat with an intralesional injection than locations on the hand, digits, or face that are rich in nerve endings and have minimal subcutaneous tissue. Current SbV treatment protocols in the United States do not include intralesional as a route of administration and experience is very limited. Recent experience with combined intralesional SbV and cryotherapy shows improved efficacy of the combination over either one alone [85,86].

*Systemic therapy*

*Oral agents*

There are no FDA-approved oral agents with an indication for the treatment of any form of leishmaniasis. The well-known antifungal azole compounds ketoconazole, itraconazole, and fluconazole have antileishmanial activity in vitro and limited efficacy in clinical trials.

In the New World, ketoconazole, 600 mg daily for 28 days, cured eight (89%) of nine patients with *L mexicana* in Guatemala [56], and 16 (76%) of 21 patients with *L panamensis* in Panama [87]. Ketoconazole is not efficacious against *L brasiliensis* in Guatemala [56]. In the Old World, ketoconazole, 600 mg daily for 30 days, cured 57 (89%) of 64 patients in Iran (parasites not characterized, but likely to be *L major*) [88]. In an area of Turkey known to be endemic for *L tropica*, ketoconazole, 400 mg daily for 30 days, failed to cure any of 32 patients [72].

Itraconazole, 4 mg/kg for 6 weeks, cured 10 (67%) of 15 and 7 (70%) of 10 of patients in India (parasites not characterized, but likely to be *L major*) [89,90]. Itraconazole, 7 mg/kg for 3 weeks, cured 59% of patients with *L major* in Iran but the placebo cure rate was 44% [91]. Itraconazole, 200 mg twice daily for 28 days, was no better than placebo in Colombia in treating patients from *L panamensis*–endemic areas [92].

In a randomized, double-blind, placebo-controlled trial in Saudi Arabia, fluconazole, 200 mg daily for 6 weeks, cured 63 (79%) of 80 at 3 months compared with 22 (34%) of 65 in the placebo group [93]. Time to healing was shortened by about 3 weeks in the fluconazole-treated patients in this cohort with *L major* infection. Lesions on the face and ear, which are much more difficult to treat, were excluded from the trial.

Azole drugs have shown modest efficacy against *L major* in the Old World and *L mexicana* complex parasites in the New World, conflicting results in *L panamensis* infections, and are no better than placebo for *L tropica* and *L braziliensis*. They are not recommended for use in patients with *L braziliensis* infections, because there are no data on the efficacy in preventing ML. Many of the trials have been with small numbers, open or uncontrolled in design, lacking standardized outcome measures or definitions of cure, and have little information on optimal dose or schedule. Nevertheless, azoles are used because they are usually well tolerated by patients and are convenient. Patients should be counseled that azoles are not the most efficacious therapy, however, and treatment failures routinely occur.

Many other oral agents including rifampicin [94–96], dapsone [97–99], oral zinc sulfate [100], and allopurinol have been tested in CL both as a single drug and with SSG [101–103]. These agents are not recommended because of limited data and conflicting results. Their use should be considered investigational until further studies are performed.

## Parenteral agents

SSG is the only SbV agent available in the United States but is not an FDA-approved drug. SSG can only be used by physicians in a treatment protocol under an Investigational New Drug application on file with the FDA. Once *Leishmania* infection is parasitologically confirmed, SSG can be obtained at no cost to the requesting physician from the Parasitic Drug Service of the CDC for civilian physicians and from the US Army Medical Material Development Activity for military personnel. Physicians from all branches of the United States military should contact the Infectious Disease Service of the Walter Reed Army Medical Center (202-782-1663) to request assistance with a possible case of leishmaniasis.

SSG can be administered safely to patients with CL on an outpatient basis [104]. It is my recommendation that the drug be given intravenously through a steel butterfly needle that can be inserted into an antecubital vein each day, a strategy that eliminates the possibility of device-related infections. There were four device-related infections, two of which were serious, in 13 patients receiving outpatient SSG by an indwelling catheter in a case series reported from the United Kingdom [104]. The high rate of complications was attributed to lack of asepsis and device manipulation. Intramuscular injections are used in endemic countries, but the large volume required per injection (15–20 mL) is extremely painful and is not likely to be accepted in returning travelers.

SSG has a well-known toxicity profile to include headache; fatigue; musculoskeletal aching; large joint stiffness; and gastrointestinal complaints of anorexia, nausea, vomiting, and mid-epigastric pain associated with pancreatitis [1,105,106]. Nonspecific T wave and ST segment electrocardiographic changes, transient liver enzyme elevations, and bone marrow suppression can also occur [1,105,106]. Systemic complaints and elevations in pancreatic enzymes and aminotransferase levels are seen in the first week of therapy, whereas joint stiffness is dose dependent and tends to worsen as therapy progresses. Detailed monitoring plans are included in treatment protocols associated with the Investigational New Drug application. In general, close clinical, ECG, and laboratory monitoring is required. Drug administration is interrupted frequently when a parameter falls out of range. A few days of a drug holiday are usually all that is required before SSG can be started again. For the SSG inexperienced physician, expert consultation is recommended.

Amphotericin B deoxycholate has long been used for initial treatment of New World CL caused by *L braziliensis* and for second-line treatment of SbV therapeutic failures, although there is surprisingly little published information, no randomized controlled trials, and no consensus on indications, dose, and regimen. Expert opinion favors use of 0.5 to 1 mg/kg/d for 14 to 30 days to a total dose of 1 to 2 g. Although the deoxycholate formulation of amphotericin B is considered highly efficacious for both CL and ML, lipid associated or liposomal formulations of amphotericin B have not been shown to be efficacious in dermatologic manifestations and are not recommended [107].

Clinical cure can be defined as the complete healing and re-epithelialization of the lesion and no evidence of recurrence 6 months after start of treatment. Lesions only partially heal by the end of treatment with SSG. Complete resolution may take an additional several weeks. Evidence of primary failure defined as no improvement or initial improvement followed by recurrence, or relapse after complete healing, is often the appearance of an active margin of the partially healed ulcer. There is no clinical usefulness in trying to demonstrate parasitologic cure of healed lesions because both culture-positive and polymerase chain reaction–positive specimens have been demonstrated in normal-appearing skin, sometimes years after treatment [108].

Patients who fail an initial course of SbV can be retreated with a second course of SbV or treated with amphotericin B. The choice often depends on how well the patient tolerates the drug. Current treatment options and recommendations for CL in returning North American travelers are found in Table 1.

*Clinical pearls*

Leishmanial ulcers or lesions, both primary and reactivation, occurring at sites of previous or recent trauma have been reported on numerous occasions [109,110]. The appearance of lesions along a site of injury is an example of the Koebner phenomenon, also called the isomorphic response, which is well known to dermatologists. Damage to the skin is followed by the development of the disease state in that previously normal skin. A wide variety of seemingly trivial and unrelated trauma, such as abrasions, punctures, blunt trauma, coral cuts, burns, cat scratch, surgical incisions, skin snips, tattoos, shaving cuts, bee stings, and excoriations, have all been associated with the occurrence of leishmanial ulcers from many different species in returning travelers. In these circumstances it is easy to understand why neither the patient nor the physician considers leishmaniasis in the initial differential diagnosis. Patients should be advised against receiving tattoos and cautioned about elective surgery following CL.

Table 1
Treatment recommendations for cutaneous leishmaniasis in returning North American travelers

| Intervention and drugs | Use, dose, regimen | Comment | Level of evidence[a] |
|---|---|---|---|
| Localized heat therapy (ThermoMed) | Single application for 30 seconds at 50°C | Uncomplicated Old World CL<br>Uncomplicated *L mexicana*<br>Use topical antibiotic ointment for several days after treatment | CIII |
| Localized cryotherapy | Topical application of liquid nitrogen for 15–20 second once weekly for 1–3 wk | Uncomplicated Old World CL | BIII [64,65] |
| Topical 15% paromomycin phosphate with 10% urea in white soft paraffin | Apply sufficient amount to cover ulcer twice daily for 3–4 wk | Uncomplicated *L major*<br>Uncomplicated *L mexicana*<br>Ulcerative lesions only<br>Available through compounding pharmacy | CIII[b] |
| Ketoconazole | 600 mg daily for 28 d | *L mexicana* | BI [56] |
|  | 600 mg daily for 28 d | *L panamensis* | BI [87] |
|  | 600 mg daily for 30 d | *L major* | BI [88] |
| Fluconazole | 200 mg daily for 6 wk | Uncomplicated *L major* | BI [93] |
| Pentavalent antimony (SSG) | 20 mg/kg/d for 10–20 d IV | Complicated Old World CL | AI [62] |
|  | 20 mg/kg/d for 20 d IV | *L panamensis*<br>*L braziliensis*<br>Other New World CL | AI [122]<br>AI [56,104,105,123]<br>BIII [63,124,125] |
|  | 20 mg/kg/d for 28 d IV | Mucosal leishmaniasis | BII [126,127] |
|  | 0.1–3 mL IL | *L major*<br>*L tropica* | AII [81,84]<br>BIII |
| Amphotericin B deoxycholate | 0.5–1 mg/kg daily for 14–30 d. Total dose of 1–2 g | Primary treatment for ML SSG failures<br>Patients who do not tolerate SSG | BIII |

*Abbreviations:* CL, cutaneous leishmaniasis; ML, mucosal leishmaniasis; SSG, sodium stibogluconate.

[a] Level of evidence follows the Infectious Disease Society of America Quality Standards for Infectious Diseases [128]. A recommendation is based on both strength and quality of evidence. Strength of evidence for use is given a letter A–C where A is good, B is moderate, and C is poor. Quality of evidence is given a grade of I–III where I is evidence from at least one properly randomized, controlled, trial; II is evidence from a well-designed, nonrandomized trial, from cohort or case-controlled trials, or dramatic results from uncontrolled experiments; and III is expert opinion based on clinical experience, descriptive studies, or reports of expert committees.

[b] Efficacy of individual preparations made by a compounding pharmacy cannot be assessed.

Leishmaniasis is a well-known opportunistic coinfection seen in late stage AIDS patients and other immunocompromised patients. *Leishmania* parasites, especially *L braziliensis* in the New World and *L tropica* in the Old World, are not eradicated with successful drug therapy even in normal hosts [55,108,111]. Because *Leishmania* parasites are not eradicated with drug treatment, there is a risk of developing reactivation disease if the patient becomes immunocompromised with late-stage HIV infection [112,113], use of immunosuppressive drugs associated with transplantation [114], and chronic steroid use [115]. Dermatologic manifestations of *Leishmania* infection in the immunocompromised may be very atypical, and a high degree of clinical suspicion combined with an appropriate laboratory investigation is required to make the correct diagnosis [112].

It has been well documented, but not well known or recognized, that in humans with multiple CL lesions, treatment of one lesion may promote the healing of the other lesions [70,116]. Clinical trials to establish the extent and use of this phenomenon have not been performed. A decision intentionally not to treat all CL lesions with a local therapy, such as a topical drug or a physical method, may be justified on an occasional basis. For example, in a patient with multiple lesions on legs, torso, and face, a physical treatment, such as cryotherapy or intralesional injections, may pose little difficulty on the legs and torso, but facial lesions present a relative contraindication. Treating only the nonfacial lesions initially, with the option to extend or change treatment for the untreated facial lesions if no improvement is observed, may be a clinically appropriate decision in some cases.

SSG therapy leads to a decrease in both total and $CD4^+$ lymphocytes. A typical herpes zoster dermatomal vesicular rash has been documented in several patients during or shortly after completing a course of SSG therapy [104,117]. Incidence ranges from 3% to 7%. Both treating physicians and patients should be made aware of the possibility. There may be diagnostic confusion in the first day or two of prodromal symptoms before the typical zoster vesicular rash occurs.

### A personal perspective

Prevention of infection is the obvious way to decrease the morbidity associated with the leishmaniases. Most of the parasites causing cutaneous syndromes exist as part of enzootic cycles with local mammalian reservoirs throughout endemic subtropical and tropical ecologic zones. Elimination is not feasible and control programs are difficult to sustain. Individual travelers must use standard vector personal protection measures including applying DEET-based repellants; using effective barriers, such as permethrin-based insecticides on clothing and bed-nets; and sleeping in minimal risk locations. Most infections in travelers probably occur as a result of specific behaviors, such as early morning or late evening excursions into the tropical habitat for bird watching or naturalist fieldwork. The most recent epidemic in American soldiers in Iraq was the result of an unprecedented incursion of thousands of nonimmunes into a geographic area with an enzootic cycle of *L major*, small desert rodents, and *P papatasi*.

In most cases, parasitologic confirmation of *Leishmania* with a tissue scraping is successful once the diagnosis of CL is considered. Difficult to confirm cases can be addressed by using additional parasitologic methods available from reference laboratories, expert histopathologic evaluation, or response to empiric treatment. Phenotypic or genotypic characterization of the infecting isolate using isoenzymes or polymerase chain reaction is recommended to assist in making the best management decisions, although many clinical decisions can be made based on knowledge of the geographic origin of infection.

Treatment options for CL, especially in North America, are limited and not satisfactory for optimal management of the individual patient. The diversity of clinical presentations can only be addressed satisfactorily at the extremes of the spectrum with cryotherapy or SSG. Many patients present with lesions not suitable for local or physical methods, but not severe enough for toxic or poorly tolerated systemic treatment. An efficacious, well-tolerated, nonparenteral, systemic treatment is missing. Currently available azoles, such as fluconazole, ketoconazole, and itraconazole, are not very efficacious and do not work against the *Leishmania* parasites responsible for ML.

## Future developments

Miltefosine, originally developed as an anticancer drug, has demonstrated efficacy against Indian visceral leishmaniasis, providing a much-needed oral systemic treatment option for this disease [118,119]. Preliminary efficacy with miltefosine in New Word CL was demonstrated in an open-label, dose escalation, phase I-II trial against *L panamensis* in 72 male Colombian soldiers. A per-protocol cure rate for 50 to 100 mg per day of miltefosine was 66%. The per-protocol cure rate for 133 to 150 mg per day was 94%, similar to the historic per-protocol cure rate for standard injections of antimony of 93% [120].

In a placebo-controlled study of miltefosine against CL in regions of Colombia where *L panamensis* is common, the per-protocol cure rates for miltefosine and placebo were 91% (40 of 44 patients) and 38% (9 of 24) [121]. In regions in Guatemala where *L braziliensis* and *L mexicana* are common, the per-protocol cure rates were 53% (20 of 38) for miltefosine and 21% (4 of 19) for placebo [121]. These results confirm miltefosine as a useful oral agent against CL caused by *L panamensis* in Colombia, but unfortunately not against CL caused by *L braziliensis* in Guatemala, the parasite associated with ML [121]. The results are similar to historic values for the SbV standard of care and placebo in both locations. Miltefosine may yet find a place in the treatment of both severe Old World disease and non–*L braziliensis* disease in the New World; however, the greatest need is for an oral drug in New World *L braziliensis* infections.

## References

[1] Magill A. Leishmaniasis. In: Thomas SG, editor. Hunter's tropical medicine and emerging infectious diseases. 8th edition. Philadelphia: WB Saunders; 2000. p. 665–87.
[2] Reithinger R, Mohsen M, Aadil K, et al. Anthroponotic cutaneous leishmaniasis, Kabul, Afghanistan. Emerg Infect Dis 2003;9:727–9.
[3] Jacobson RL. *Leishmania tropica* (kinetoplastida: trypanosomatidae): a perplexing parasite. Folia Parasitol (Praha) 2003;50:241–50.
[4] Tibayrenc M, Ayala FJ. Evolutionary genetics of *Trypanosoma* and *Leishmania*. Microbes Infect 1999;1:465–72.
[5] Kreutzer RD, Souraty N, Semko ME. Biochemical identities and differences among *Leishmania* species and subspecies. Am J Trop Med Hyg 1987;36:22–32.
[6] Banuls AL, Jonquieres R, Guerrini F, et al. Genetic analysis of leishmania parasites in Ecuador: are *Leishmania (V.) panamensis* and *Leishmania (V.) guyanensis* distinct taxa? Am J Trop Med Hyg 1999;61:838–45.
[7] Nakayama J, Matsumoto T, Asahi M, et al. Imported cutaneous leishmaniasis in Japan. Int J Dermatol 1990;29:670–2.
[8] Naotunne TD, Rajakulendran S, Abeywickreme W, et al. Cutaneous leishmaniasis in Sri Lanka: an imported disease linked to the Middle East and African employment boom. Trop Geogr Med 1990;42:72–4.
[9] Faber WR, Becht M, van Ginkel CJ, et al. Cutaneous leishmaniasis in 49 patients in The Netherlands. Ned Tijdschr Geneeskd 1991;135:229–33.
[10] Melby PC, Kreutzer RD, McMahon-Pratt D, et al. Cutaneous leishmaniasis: review of 59 cases seen at the National Institutes of Health. Clin Infect Dis 1992;15:924–37.
[11] Herwaldt BL, Stokes SL, Juranek DD. American cutaneous leishmaniasis in US travelers. Ann Intern Med 1993;118:779–84.
[12] Viriyavejakul P, Viravan C, Riganti M, et al. Imported cutaneous leishmaniasis in Thailand. Southeast Asian J Trop Med Public Health 1997;28:558–62.
[13] Maguire GP, Bastian I, Arianayagam S, et al. New World cutaneous leishmaniasis imported into Australia. Pathology 1998;30:73–6.
[14] Zlotogorski A, Gilead L, Jonas F, et al. South American cutaneous leishmaniasis: report of ten cases in Israeli travelers. J Eur Acad Dermatol Venereol 1998;11:32–6.
[15] Tan HH, Wong SS, Ong BH. Cutaneous leishmaniasis: a report of two cases seen at a tertiary dermatological centre in Singapore. Singapore Med J 2000;41:179–81.
[16] Harms G, Schonian G, Feldmeier H. Leishmaniasis in Germany. Emerg Infect Dis 2003;9:872–5.
[17] Scope A, Trau H, Anders G, et al. Experience with New World cutaneous leishmaniasis in travelers. J Am Acad Dermatol 2003;49:672–8.
[18] El Hajj L, Thellier M, Carriere J, et al. Localized cutaneous leishmaniasis imported into Paris: a review of 39 cases. Int J Dermatol 2004;43:120–5.
[19] Martin S, Gambel J, Jackson J, et al. Leishmaniasis in the United States military. Mil Med 1998;163:801–7.
[20] Wiena PJ, Neafie RC, Wortmann G, et al. Old World leishmaniasis: an emerging infection among deployed US military and civilian workers. Clin Infect Dis 2004;39:1674–80.
[21] Update: cutaneous leishmaniasis in US military personnel—Southwest/Central Asia, 2002–2004. MMWR Morb Mortal Wkly Rep 2004;53:264–5.
[22] Two cases of visceral leishmaniasis in US military personnel—Afghanistan, 2002–2004. MMWR Morb Mortal Wkly Rep 2004;53:265–8.

[23] Herwaldt BL, Arana BA, Navin TR. The natural history of cutaneous leishmaniasis in Guatemala. J Infect Dis 1992;165:518–27.
[24] Kubba R, Al-Gindan Y, el-Hassan AM, et al. Clinical diagnosis of cutaneous leishmaniasis (oriental sore). J Am Acad Dermatol 1987;16:1183–9.
[25] Dowlati Y. Cutaneous leishmaniasis: clinical aspect. Clin Dermatol 1996;14:425–31.
[26] al-Gindan Y, Kubba R, el-Hassan AM, et al. Dissemination in cutaneous leishmaniasis. 3. Lymph node involvement. Int J Dermatol 1989;28:248–54.
[27] Sousa Ade Q, Parise ME, Pompeu MM, et al. Bubonic leishmaniasis: a common manifestation of *Leishmania* (*Viannia*) *braziliensis* infection in Ceara, Brazil. Am J Trop Med Hyg 1995;53:380–5.
[28] Barral A, Guerreiro J, Bomfim G, et al. Lymphadenopathy as the first sign of human cutaneous infection by *Leishmania braziliensis*. Am J Trop Med Hyg 1995;53:256–9.
[29] Lucchina LC, Wilson ME, Drake LA. Dermatology and the recently returned traveler: infectious diseases with dermatologic manifestations. Int J Dermatol 1997;36:167–81.
[30] Wilson ME. Skin problems in the traveler. Infect Dis Clin North Am 1998;12:471–88.
[31] Mahe A. Bacterial skin infections in a tropical environment. Curr Opin Infect Dis 2001;14:123–6.
[32] Willems JP, Schmidt SM, Greer KE, et al. Sporotrichoid cutaneous leishmaniasis in a traveler. South Med J 1997;90:325–7.
[33] Agudelo SP, Restrepo S, Velez ID. Cutaneous New World leishmaniasis-sporotrichosis coinfection: report of 3 cases. J Am Acad Dermatol 1999;40(6 Pt 1):1002–4.
[34] Navin TR, Arana FE, de Merida AM, et al. Cutaneous leishmaniasis in Guatemala: comparison of diagnostic methods. Am J Trop Med Hyg 1990;42:36–42.
[35] Weigle KA, de Davalos M, Heredia P, et al. Diagnosis of cutaneous and mucocutaneous leishmaniasis in Colombia: a comparison of seven methods. Am J Trop Med Hyg 1987;36:489–96.
[36] Marsden PD. Clinical presentations of *Leishmania braziliensis braziliensis*. Parasitol Today 1985;1:129–33.
[37] Marsden PD. Mucosal leishmaniasis due to *Leishmania* (*Viannia*) *braziliensis* L(V)b in Tres Bracos, Bahia-Brazil. Rev Soc Bras Med Trop 1994;27:93–101.
[38] Zajtchuk JT, Casler JD, Netto EM, et al. Mucosal leishmaniasis in Brazil. Laryngoscope 1989;99:925–39.
[39] Marsden PD. Mucosal leishmaniasis ("espundia" Escomel, 1911). Trans R Soc Trop Med Hyg 1986;80:859–76.
[40] Llanos Cuentas EA, Cuba CC, Barreto AC, et al. Clinical characteristics of human *Leishmania braziliensis braziliensis* infections. Trans R Soc Trop Med Hyg 1984;78:845–6.
[41] Osorio LE, Castillo CM, Ochoa MT. Mucosal leishmaniasis due to *Leishmania (Viannia) panamensis* in Colombia: clinical characteristics. Am J Trop Med Hyg 1998;59:49–52.
[42] Saenz RE, Paz HM, de Rodriguez GC, et al. Mucocutaneous leishmaniasis in Panama: etiologic agent, epidemiologic and clinical aspects. Rev Med Panama 1989;14:6–15.
[43] Naiff RD, Talhari S, Barrett TV. Isolation of *Leishmania guyanensis* from lesions of the nasal mucosa. Mem Inst Oswaldo Cruz 1988;83:529–30.
[44] Santrich C, Segura I, Arias AL, et al. Mucosal disease caused by *Leishmania braziliensis guyanensis*. Am J Trop Med Hyg 1990;42:51–5.
[45] Lucas CM, Franke ED, Cachay MI, et al. Geographic distribution and clinical description of leishmaniasis cases in Peru. Am J Trop Med Hyg 1998;59:312–7.
[46] Jones TC, Johnson WD Jr, Barretto AC, et al. Epidemiology of American cutaneous leishmaniasis due to *Leishmania braziliensis braziliensis*. J Infect Dis 1987;156:73–83.
[47] Blum J, Junghanss T, Hatz C. Erroneous tracks in the diagnosis of cutaneous and mucocutaneous leishmaniasis. Schweiz Rundsch Med Prax 1994;83:1025–9.
[48] Rosbotham JL, Corbett EL, Grant HR, et al. Imported mucocutaneous leishmaniasis. Clin Exp Dermatol 1996;21:288–90.

[49] Lohuis PJ, Lipovsky MM, Hoepelman AI, et al. *Leishmania braziliensis* presenting as a granulomatous lesion of the nasal septum mucosa. J Laryngol Otol 1997;111: 973–5.
[50] Scope A, Trau H, Bakon M, et al. Imported mucosal leishmaniasis in a traveler. Clin Infect Dis 2003;37:e83–7.
[51] Costa JW Jr, Milner DA Jr, Maguire JH. Mucocutaneous leishmaniasis in a US citizen. Oral Surg Oral Med Oral Pathol Oral Radiol Endod 2003;96:573–7.
[52] Ahluwalia S, Lawn SD, Kanagalingam J, et al. Mucocutaneous leishmaniasis: an imported infection among travellers to central and South America. BMJ 2004;329: 842–4.
[53] Singer C, Armstrong D, Jones TC, et al. Imported mucocutaneous leishmaniasis in New York City: report of a patient treated with amphotericin B. Am J Med 1975;59: 444–7.
[54] Galioto P, Fornaro V. A case of mucocutaneous leishmaniasis. Ear Nose Throat J 2002;81: 46–8.
[55] Marovich MA, Lira R, Shepard M, et al. Leishmaniasis recidivans recurrence after 43 years: a clinical and immunologic report after successful treatment. Clin Infect Dis 2001;33: 1076–9.
[56] Navin TR, Arana BA, Arana FE, et al. Placebo-controlled clinical trial of sodium stibogluconate (Pentostam) versus ketoconazole for treating cutaneous leishmaniasis in Guatemala. J Infect Dis 1992;165:528–34.
[57] Ibrahim ME, Evans DA, Theander TG, et al. Diversity among *Leishmania* isolates from the Sudan: isoenzyme homogeneity of *L. donovani* versus heterogeneity of *L. major*. Trans R Soc Trop Med Hyg 1995;89:366–9.
[58] Le Blancq SM, Schnur LF, Peters W. Leishmania in the Old World: 1. The geographical and hostal distribution of *L. major* zymodemes. Trans R Soc Trop Med Hyg 1986;80: 99–112.
[59] Kebaier C, Louzir H, Chenik M, et al. Heterogeneity of wild *Leishmania major* isolates in experimental murine pathogenicity and specific immune response. Infect Immun 2001;69: 4906–15.
[60] Gaafar A, Fadl A, el Kadaro AY, et al. Sporotrichoid cutaneous leishmaniasis due to *Leishmania major* of different zymodemes in the Sudan and Saudi Arabia: a comparative study. Trans R Soc Trop Med Hyg 1994;88:552–4.
[61] Le Blancq SM, Peters W. Leishmania in the Old World: 2. Heterogeneity among *L. tropica* zymodemes. Trans R Soc Trop Med Hyg 1986;80:113–9.
[62] Wortmann G, Miller RS, Oster C, et al. A randomized, double-blind study of the efficacy of a 10- or 20-day course of sodium stibogluconate for treatment of cutaneous leishmaniasis in United States military personnel. Clin Infect Dis 2002;35:261–7.
[63] Blum J, Desjeux P, Schwartz E, et al. Treatment of cutaneous leishmaniasis among travellers. J Antimicrob Chemother 2004;53:158–66.
[64] Uzun S, Uslular C, Yucel A, et al. Cutaneous leishmaniasis: evaluation of 3,074 cases in the Cukurova region of Turkey. Br J Dermatol 1999;140:347–50.
[65] al-Majali O, Routh HB, Abuloham O, et al. A 2-year study of liquid nitrogen therapy in cutaneous leishmaniasis. Int J Dermatol 1997;36:460–2.
[66] Berman JD, Neva FA. Effect of temperature on multiplication of *Leishmania* amastigotes within human monocyte-derived macrophages in vitro. Am J Trop Med Hyg 1981;30: 318–21.
[67] Navin TR, Arana BA, Arana FE, et al. Placebo-controlled clinical trial of meglumine antimonate (glucantime) vs. localized controlled heat in the treatment of cutaneous leishmaniasis in Guatemala. Am J Trop Med Hyg 1990;42:43–50.
[68] El-On J, Weinrauch L, Livshin R, et al. Topical treatment of recurrent cutaneous leishmaniasis with ointment containing paromomycin and methylbenzethonium chloride. BMJ 1985;291:704–5.

[69] Weinrauch L, Katz M, El-On J. Leishmania aethiopica: topical treatment with paromomycin and methylbenzethonium chloride ointment. J Am Acad Dermatol 1987; 16:1268–70.
[70] El-On J, Livshin R, Even-Paz Z, et al. Topical treatment of cutaneous leishmaniasis. J Invest Dermatol 1986;87:284–8.
[71] El-On J, Livshin R, Paz ZE, et al. Topical treatment of cutaneous leishmaniasis. BMJ 1985; 291:1280–1.
[72] Ozgoztasi O, Baydar I. A randomized clinical trial of topical paromomycin versus oral ketoconazole for treating cutaneous leishmaniasis in Turkey. Int J Dermatol 1997;36: 61–3.
[73] Weinrauch L, Cawich F, Craig P, et al. Topical treatment of New World cutaneous leishmaniasis in Belize: a clinical study. J Am Acad Dermatol 1993;29:443–6.
[74] Arana BA, Mendoza CE, Rizzo NR, et al. Randomized, controlled, double-blind trial of topical treatment of cutaneous leishmaniasis with paromomycin plus methylbenzethonium chloride ointment in Guatemala. Am J Trop Med Hyg 2001;65:466–70.
[75] Bryceson AD, Murphy A, Moody AH. Treatment of Old World cutaneous leishmaniasis with aminosidine ointment: results of an open study in London. Trans R Soc Trop Med Hyg 1994;88:226–8.
[76] Armijos RX, Weigel MM, Calvopina M, et al. Comparison of the effectiveness of two topical paromomycin treatments versus meglumine antimoniate for New World cutaneous leishmaniasis. Acta Trop 2004;91:153–60.
[77] Asilian A, Jalayer T, Nilforooshzadeh M, et al. Treatment of cutaneous leishmaniasis with aminosidine (paromomycin) ointment: double-blind, randomized trial in the Islamic Republic of Iran. Bull World Health Organ 2003;81:353–9.
[78] Bogenrieder T, Lehn N, Landthaler M, et al. Treatment of Old World cutaneous leishmaniasis with intralesionally injected meglumine antimoniate using a Dermojet device. Dermatology 2003;206:269–72.
[79] Uzun S, Durdu M, Culha G, et al. Clinical features, epidemiology, and efficacy and safety of intralesional antimony treatment of cutaneous leishmaniasis: recent experience in Turkey. J Parasitol 2004;90:853–9.
[80] Kellum RE. Treatment of cutaneous leishmaniasis with an intralesional antimonial drug (Pentostam). J Am Acad Dermatol 1986;15(4 Pt 1):620–2.
[81] Faris RM, Jarallah JS, Khoja TA, et al. Intralesional treatment of cutaneous leishmaniasis with sodium stibogluconate antimony. Int J Dermatol 1993;32:610–2.
[82] Sharquie KE, Najim RA, Farjou IB. A comparative controlled trial of intralesionally-administered zinc sulphate, hypertonic sodium chloride and pentavalent antimony compound against acute cutaneous leishmaniasis. Clin Exp Dermatol 1997;22:169–73.
[83] Sharquie KE, Al-Talib KK, Chu AC. Intralesional therapy of cutaneous leishmaniasis with sodium stibogluconate antimony. Br J Dermatol 1988;119:53–7.
[84] Tallab TM, Bahamdam KA, Mirdad S, et al. Cutaneous leishmaniasis: schedules for intralesional treatment with sodium stibogluconate. Int J Dermatol 1996;35:594–7.
[85] el Darouti MA, al Rubaie SM. Cutaneous leishmaniasis: treatment with combined cryotherapy and intralesional stibogluconate injection. Int J Dermatol 1990;29:56–9.
[86] Asilian A, Sadeghinia A, Faghihi G, et al. Comparative study of the efficacy of combined cryotherapy and intralesional meglumine antimoniate (Glucantime) vs. cryotherapy and intralesional meglumine antimoniate (Glucantime) alone for the treatment of cutaneous leishmaniasis. Int J Dermatol 2004;43:281–3.
[87] Saenz RE, Paz H, Berman JD. Efficacy of ketoconazole against *Leishmania braziliensis panamensis* cutaneous leishmaniasis. Am J Med 1990;89:147–55.
[88] Salmanpour R, Handjani F, Nouhpisheh MK. Comparative study of the efficacy of oral ketoconazole with intra-lesional meglumine antimoniate (Glucantime) for the treatment of cutaneous leishmaniasis. J Dermatolog Treat 2001;12:159–62.

[89] Dogra J, Aneja N, Lal BB, et al. Cutaneous leishmaniasis in India: clinical experience with itraconazole (R51 211 Janssen). Int J Dermatol 1990;29:661–2.
[90] Dogra J, Saxena VN. Itraconazole and leishmaniasis: a randomised double-blind trial in cutaneous disease. Int J Parasitol 1996;26:1413–5.
[91] Momeni AZ, Jalayer T, Emamjomeh M, et al. Treatment of cutaneous leishmaniasis with itraconazole: randomized double-blind study. Arch Dermatol 1996;132:784–6.
[92] Soto-Mancipe J, Grogl M, Berman JD. Evaluation of pentamidine for the treatment of cutaneous leishmaniasis in Colombia. Clin Infect Dis 1993;16:417–25.
[93] Alrajhi AA, Ibrahim EA, De Vol EB, et al. Fluconazole for the treatment of cutaneous leishmaniasis caused by *Leishmania major*. N Engl J Med 2002;346:891–5.
[94] Kochar DK, Aseri S, Sharma BV, et al. The role of rifampicin in the management of cutaneous leishmaniasis. QJM 2000;93:733–7.
[95] Livshin R, Weinrauch L, Even-Paz Z, et al. Efficacy of rifampicin and isoniazid in cutaneous leishmaniasis. Int J Dermatol 1987;26:55–9.
[96] Do Valle TZ, Oliveira Neto MP, Schubach A, et al. New World tegumentar leishmaniasis: chemotherapeutic activity of rifampicin in humans and experimental murine model. Pathol Biol (Paris) 1995;43:618–21.
[97] Dogra J. A double-blind study on the efficacy of oral dapsone in cutaneous leishmaniasis. Trans R Soc Trop Med Hyg 1991;85:212–3.
[98] Dogra J, Lal BB, Misra SN. Dapsone in the treatment of cutaneous leishmaniasis. Int J Dermatol 1986;25:398–400.
[99] Osorio LE, Palacios R, Chica ME, et al. Treatment of cutaneous leishmaniasis in Colombia with dapsone. Lancet 1998;351:498–9.
[100] Sharquie KE, Najim RA, Farjou IB, et al. Oral zinc sulphate in the treatment of acute cutaneous leishmaniasis. Clin Exp Dermatol 2001;26:21–6.
[101] Martinez S, Gonzalez M, Vernaza ME. Treatment of cutaneous leishmaniasis with allopurinol and stibogluconate. Clin Infect Dis 1997;24:165–9.
[102] Martinez S, Marr JJ. Allopurinol in the treatment of American cutaneous leishmaniasis. N Engl J Med 1992;326:741–4.
[103] Guderian RH, Chico ME, Rogers MD, et al. Placebo controlled treatment of Ecuadorian cutaneous leishmaniasis. Am J Trop Med Hyg 1991;45:92–7.
[104] Seaton RA, Morrison J, Man I, et al. Out-patient parenteral antimicrobial therapy: a viable option for the management of cutaneous leishmaniasis. QJM 1999;92:659–67.
[105] Aronson NE, Wortmann GW, Johnson SC, et al. Safety and efficacy of intravenous sodium stibogluconate in the treatment of leishmaniasis: recent US military experience. Clin Infect Dis 1998;27:1457–64.
[106] Gasser RA Jr, Magill AJ, Oster CN, et al. Pancreatitis induced by pentavalent antimonial agents during treatment of leishmaniasis. Clin Infect Dis 1994;18:83–90.
[107] Wortmann GW, Fraser SL, Aronson NE, et al. Failure of amphotericin B lipid complex in the treatment of cutaneous leishmaniasis. Clin Infect Dis 1998;26:1006–7.
[108] Mendonca MG, de Brito ME, Rodrigues EH, et al. Persistence of leishmania parasites in scars after clinical cure of American cutaneous leishmaniasis: is there a sterile cure? J Infect Dis 2004;189:1018–23.
[109] Wortmann GW, Aronson NE, Miller RS, et al. Cutaneous leishmaniasis following local trauma: a clinical pearl. Clin Infect Dis 2000;31:199–201.
[110] Walton BC. American cutaneous and mucocutaneous leishmaniasis. In: Peters W, Killick-Kendrick K, editors. The leishmaniases in biology and medicine, vol 2. London: Academic Press; 1987. p. 642–4.
[111] Aebischer T. Recurrent cutaneous leishmaniasis: a role for persistent parasites? Parasitol Today 1994;10:25–8.
[112] Puig L, Pradinaud R. Leishmania and HIV co-infection: dermatological manifestations. Ann Trop Med Parasitol 2003;97(Suppl 1):107–14.

[113] Sampaio RN, Salaro CP, Resende P, et al. American cutaneous leishmaniasis associated with HIV/AIDS: report of four clinical cases. Rev Soc Bras Med Trop 2002;35:651–4.
[114] Golino A, Duncan JM, Zeluff B, et al. Leishmaniasis in a heart transplant patient. J Heart Lung Transplant 1992;11(4 Pt 1):820–3.
[115] Motta AC, Arruda D, Souza CS, et al. Disseminated mucocutaneous leishmaniasis resulting from chronic use of corticosteroid. Int J Dermatol 2003;42:703–6.
[116] Bassiouny A, El Meshad M, Talaat M, et al. Cryosurgery in cutaneous leishmaniasis. Br J Dermatol 1982;107:467–74.
[117] Wortmann GW, Aronson NE, Byrd JC, et al. Herpes zoster and lymphopenia associated with sodium stibogluconate therapy for cutaneous leishmaniasis. Clin Infect Dis 1998;27:509–12.
[118] Olliaro PL, Ridley RG, Engel J, et al. Miltefosine in visceral leishmaniasis. Lancet Infect Dis 2003;3:70.
[119] Sundar S, Jha TK, Thakur CP, et al. Oral miltefosine for Indian visceral leishmaniasis. N Engl J Med 2002;347:1739–46.
[120] Soto J, Toledo J, Gutierrez P, et al. Treatment of American cutaneous leishmaniasis with miltefosine, an oral agent. Clin Infect Dis 2001;33:E57–61.
[121] Soto J, Arana BA, Toledo J, et al. Miltefosine for new world cutaneous leishmaniasis. Clin Infect Dis 2004;38:1266–72.
[122] Ballou WR, McClain JB, Gordon DM, et al. Safety and efficacy of high-dose sodium stibogluconate therapy of American cutaneous leishmaniasis. Lancet 1987;2:13–6.
[123] Herwaldt BL, Berman JD. Recommendations for treating leishmaniasis with sodium stibogluconate (Pentostam) and review of pertinent clinical studies. Am J Trop Med Hyg 1992;46:296–306.
[124] Herwaldt BL, Kaye ET, Lepore TJ, et al. Sodium stibogluconate (Pentostam) overdose during treatment of American cutaneous leishmaniasis. J Infect Dis 1992;165:968–71.
[125] Herwaldt BL. Leishmaniasis. Lancet 1999;354:1191–9.
[126] Franke ED, Wignall FS, Cruz ME, et al. Efficacy and toxicity of sodium stibogluconate for mucosal leishmaniasis. Ann Intern Med 1990;113:934–40.
[127] Franke ED, Llanos-Cuentas A, Echevarria J, et al. Efficacy of 28-day and 40-day regimens of sodium stibogluconate (Pentostam) in the treatment of mucosal leishmaniasis. Am J Trop Med Hyg 1994;51:77–82.
[128] Gross PA, Barrett TL, Dellinger EP, et al. Purpose of quality standards for infectious diseases. Infectious Diseases Society of America. Clin Infect Dis 1994;18:421.

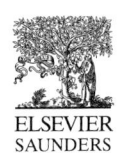

# New Diagnostics in Parasitology
## Peter L. Chiodini, PhD, FRCP, FRCPath[a,b,]*

[a]*Department of Clinical Parasitology, The Hospital for Tropical Diseases, Mortimer Market, London WC1E 6AU, UK*
[b]*London School of Hygiene and Tropical Medicine, Keppel Street, London WC1E 7HT, UK*

Diagnostic parasitology has long relied on classic morphology and light microscopy to demonstrate ova, cysts, or the parasites themselves in a variety of biologic samples. In some cases techniques are used that have changed little in over a century. Performed properly by a well-trained technologist, microscopy still has many advantages:

- Speed: A good microscopist using a rapid stain can make an initial diagnosis of malaria within 20 minutes of specimen receipt.
- Specificity: With experience, demonstration of the characteristic features of an ovum or a cyst is diagnostic.
- Only simple equipment is required: A well-maintained microscope and some simple stains permit accurate diagnosis of a wide range of parasitic infections.

It is against these attributes possessed by microscopy that new methods must be judged, because the laboratory director has a duty not only to provide a high-quality service, but also one that is cost-effective. Advances in biotechnology and long-overdue investment have brought into play new nonmicroscopic methods, some of which are significantly more sensitive and specific than traditional techniques. These must now earn their place in laboratory practice.

This article considers new diagnostics in the context of a diagnostic clinical parasitology laboratory receiving samples from an infectious and tropical disease service. The full content of this article can be found in the online version at: www.theclinics.com, doi:10.1016/j.idc.2004.11.002.

---

Full text of this article can be found at: www.id.theclinics.com; doi:10.1016/j.idc.2004.11.002.

* Department of Clinical Parasitology, The Hospital for Tropical Diseases, Mortimer Market, London WC1E 6AU, UK.
 *E-mail address:* peter.chiodini@uclh.org

## Rapid diagnostics

### Rapid diagnostic tests

Rapid diagnostic tests (RDTs) are based on the use of immunochromatography. An antigen or antibody is immobilized as a line on a nitrocellulose membrane that forms the test strip. The patient sample is then run along the strip by "wicking." As it passes over the test line, any target antigen or antibody present in the specimen (depending on the test configuration) is able to interact with the antibody or antigen immobilized on the membrane. A detecting antibody conjugated to colloidal gold, for example, permits visualization of a positive test reaction.

### Malaria rapid diagnostic tests

RDTs presented in kit form detect malaria antigen. Of the four species infecting humans, RDTs are best at detecting *Plasmodium falciparum* and some kits are designed to identify only this parasite. RDTs are slightly less sensitive for malaria diagnosis than an expert microscopist, but may outperform an inexperienced technologist. They are now well established as adjuncts to malaria diagnosis in many regions of the world, but at the time of writing (2004) are not approved by the US Food and Drug Administration for malaria diagnosis. They do not replace blood films for this purpose.

### Leishmania rapid diagnostic tests

Detection of anti-*Leishmania* antibody is a sensitive indicator of visceral leishmaniasis (kala-azar). The RDT format permits rapid testing in a nonspecialist laboratory. The test is qualitative only, so referral of positives to a reference laboratory for confirmation with a quantitative antibody assay, such as the direct agglutination test, should be undertaken. Negatives should also be referred when the diagnosis is believed to be likely despite a negative *Leishmania* RDT.

### Fecal antigen detection rapid diagnostic tests

Both *Giardia* and *Cryptosporidium* infections can be diagnosed in this way, but it must be remembered that these tests look only for the organism specified, so do not replace fecal microscopy if other parasites are being considered in the differential diagnosis.

### Wuchereria bancrofti *infection*

An RDT for *Wuchereria bancrofti* provides a more convenient method for detecting this organism than filtration of citrated blood because the antigen can be detected by day and by night, obviating the need to disturb patients by taking midnight blood samples.

## Antigen detection ELISA

### Malaria antigens

Histidine rich protein-2 from *P falciparum* or lactate dehydrogenase from all human malarias can be assayed in an ELISA format. They do not replace microscopy for the diagnosis of individual cases, but can be of value in screening large numbers of study samples. Lactate dehydrogenase assays can be adapted for antimalarial drug sensitivity testing.

### Fecal antigens

The fecal cysts of *Entamoeba histolytica* (pathogenic) and *Entamoeba dispar* (nonpathogenic) are morphologically identical. An ELISA for the detection of an *E histolytica*–specific lectin in fecal specimens can be used to differentiate between them and determine which amoebic cyst passers require treatment.

## Immunofluorescence-based fecal microscopy

Fluorescein-conjugated monoclonal antibodies to *Giardia* and *Cryptosporidium* can be used to increase the specificity of fecal microscopy for these organisms and are available commercially in kit form.

## Polymerase chain reaction

### Malaria

For the qualitative detection of malaria parasites, microscopy can no longer be regarded as the gold standard. Polymerase chain reaction (PCR) is at least 10-fold more sensitive than microscopy, and more accurate in speciation and in detection of mixed plasmodial infections. It is not yet able to estimate parasitemia in a way suitable for clinical use, but that will change as methodology improves. The use of PCR to detect antimalarial drug-resistance markers is rapidly expanding and raises the hope of real-time profiling of clinical samples in the future to provide an adjunct to the choice of drug therapy.

### Leishmania

PCR is now the method of choice to confirm a diagnosis of cutaneous leishmaniasis, offering higher sensitivity than both microscopy for amastigotes and culture for promastigotes. It is able to speciate the organism present (impossible by microscopy and very laborious by culture and isoenzyme analysis), itself a major advantage, because the infecting species determines the selection of specific drug therapy.

*Fecal parasites*

PCR is well-established for the speciation of amoebic cysts, to separate *E histolytica* from *E dispar*. Microsporidia can also be detected by PCR, a useful adjunct to diagnosis because microscopy for these organisms is particularly labor-intensive. Microsporidial PCR, however, is currently restricted to specialist centers. PCR-based strain typing of cryptosporidia provides an epidemiologic tool for outbreak investigation, but is not widely deployed for routine clinical diagnosis.

**Summary**

The long-overdue introduction of new technology into parasite diagnostics has produced important tests that are now finding a place in clinical laboratories. It is too early to consider abandoning microscopy; the novel technology will run alongside the more traditional techniques for some years to come. Well-trained microscopists, supported by regular continuing professional development and external quality assessment schemes, are still central to the provision of a reliable diagnostic parasitology service.

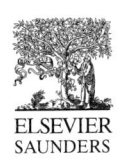

# Index

*Note:* Page numbers of article titles are in **boldface** type.

## A

N-Acetylcysteine
   for malaria, 234
Acidosis
   in malaria
      management of, 227–228
Acquired immunodeficiency syndrome (AIDS)
   travelers with, 36–39
Acute lung injury
   in malaria
      management of, 228–229
Acute myocardial infarction
   in expatriates in Ghana, 86–89
Acute renal failure
   in malaria
      management of, 230–231
Acute respiratory distress syndrome (ARDS)
   in malaria
      management of, 228–229
African trypanosomiasis
   from Tanzania
      detection of, 10–11
   HIV infection and, 126–128
Age
   as factor in adverse effects of yellow fever vaccine, 156
   as factor in malaria in travelers, 213
AIDS. See *Acquired immunodeficiency syndrome (AIDS)*.
Air travel. See also *Air travelers*.
   crib death due to, 78
   during pregnancy, 79–80
   sickness due to, 79
Air travelers. See also *Air travel*.
   aspirin use by, 74–75
   cardiovascular problems in
      automated external defibrillators for, 73–75
   child safety seats for, 77

   face masks for, 67–69
   health risks to, **67–84**
      peanuts, 75–77
      travel delay recommended for, 72–73
   in-flight oxygen for, 69–72
   SARS in, 68
   tuberculosis in, 69
Amphotericin B
   for cutaneous leishmaniasis in returning travelers, 257
Anemia
   in malaria
      management of, 231–232
Antigen(s)
   fecal
      in diagnostic parasitology, 269
   malaria
      in diagnostic parasitology, 269
Antigen detection ELISA
   in diagnostic parasitology, 269
Antimalarial(s)
   for severe malaria in travelers, 222–226
Anti–tumor necrosis factor
   for malaria, 233–234
ARDS. See *Acute respiratory distress syndrome (ARDS)*.
Arthropod(s)
   as vectors, 170
   direct injury due to, 170
   of medical importance
      nonparasitic, 179
      parasites
         of humans, 174–176
            larvae, 176–177
            nest parasites, 177–178
            ticks, 176
      of momentary duration, 178–179
   pre- and post-trip considerations related to, 179–182
   travel medicine guide to, **169–183**

Arthropod(s) (*continued*)
   transmission of, 170–171
      modes of, 171–174

Aspirin
   for air travelers, 74–75

Asplenia
   travelers with, 39–43

Atovaquone-proguanil
   in malaria prevention in travelers, 188–192

Automated external defibrillators
   for air travelers, 73–74

Azithromycin
   in malaria prevention in travelers, 199–201

**B**

Blackwater fever
   in malaria
      management of, 230

Blindness
   intermittent
      with 24-hour history of acute psychosis
         in climber
            case example, 96–99

Blood film examination
   in malaria in travelers, 217–218

Breast-feeding
   by pregnant travelers, 35–36

**C**

Cancer chemotherapy survivors
   traveling by, 39–43

Cardiovascular problems
   in air travelers
      automated external defibrillators for, 73–74

Cerebral malaria
   management of, 226–227

Chagas' disease
   HIV infection and, 128

Chemoprophylaxis
   in malaria prevention in travelers, 187–188, 214

Child safety seats
   for air travel, 77

Children
   young
      traveler's diarrhea in, 25
      traveling with, 16–26. See also *Traveling, with young children.*

Chinese immigrants
   illegal
      falciparum malaria
         detection of, 11

Chloroquine
   in malaria prevention in travelers, 187, 188

Climber(s)
   intermittent blindness with 24-hour history of acute psychosis in
      case example, 96–99

Condom(s)
   in STD reduction in travelers, 111–112

Convulsion(s)
   in malaria
      management of, 227

Counseling
   for travelers visiting friends and relatives in developing countries, 51–52

Crib death
   air travel and, 78

Cutaneous leishmaniasis
   in returning travelers, **241–266**
      clinical presentation of, 245–247
      diagnosis of, 247–248
      epidemiology of, 244–245
      future developments in, 260–261
      mucosal leishmaniasis, 248–249
      personal perspective on, 259–260
      treatment of, 249–259
         amphotericin B in, 257
         drugs in, 251
         fluconazole in, 255
         intralesional injections, 254–255
         itraconazole in, 255
         ketoconazole in, 255
         local *vs.* systemic, 251–253
         oral agents in, 255–256
         parasite strain in, 250–251
         parental agents in, 256–257
         physical methods, 253–254
         SSG in, 256–257
         topical, 254

**D**

Defibrillator(s)
   automated external
      for air travelers, 73–74

Dengue fever
    travel health risks associated with
        surveillance of, 5–6
Developing countries
    travelers visiting friends and relatives
        in
            disease prevention in, **49–65.**
                See also *Traveler(s), visiting
                friends and relatives in
                developing countries.*
            risk assessment for, **49–65.**
                See also *Traveler(s),
                visiting friends and
                relatives in developing
                countries.*
Diabetes mellitus
    in travelers, 30–32
Dialysis
    renal
        for malaria, 233
Diarrhea
    traveler's, **137–149.** See also *Traveler's
        diarrhea.*
Dichloroacetate
    for malaria, 234
Dipstick tests
    for malaria in travelers, 204
Disease(s)
    imported
        travel health risks related to
            surveillance of, **1–13.** See
                also *Travel health
                risks, imported diseases
                and.*
Dominican Republic
    falciparum malaria in
        detection of, 8–10
Drug resistance
    in malaria prevention in travelers,
        187–188

# E
Economy class syndrome, 74
Elderly
    traveling with, 26–30. See also
        *Traveling, with the elderly.*
ELISA
    antigen detection
        in diagnostic parasitology, 269
Encephalitis
    Japanese. See *Japanese encephalitis.*

Exchange transfusion
    for malaria, 232–233
Expatriate(s)
    in Ghana
        acute myocardial infarction in,
            86–89
        international emergency and medical
            evacuation for
                case examples of, **85–101**
        pretravel screening tests in, 88

# F
Face masks
    for air travelers, 67–69
Falciparum malaria
    in Dominican Republic
        detection of, 8–10
    in illegal Chinese immigrants
        detection of, 11
    pathogenesis of, 212–213
Fecal antigen detection RDTs
    in diagnostic parasitology, 268
Fecal antigens
    in diagnostic parasitology, 269
Fever
    typhoid
        in travelers visiting friends
            and relatives in
            developing countries,
            55–56
    yellow. See *Yellow fever.*
Filariasis
    lymphatic
        HIV infection and, 130–131
Fluconazole
    for cutaneous leishmaniasis in
        returning travelers, 255
Fluid and electrolyte disturbances
    in malaria
        management of, 230
Fluid overload
    in malaria
        management of, 228

# G
Gender
    as factor in malaria in travelers,
        213
Genetic resistance and susceptibility
    as factor in malaria in travelers,
        213–214

Geologic engineers
    fever, malaise, and rapidly spreading lesion in
        case example, 92–96
Ghana
    expatriates in
        acute myocardial infarction in, 86–89

# H
Helminth(s)
    intestinal
        HIV infection and, 131–132
Hemofiltration
    for malaria, 233
Hemostatis disorders
    in malaria
        management of, 231
Hepatitis
    A
        in travelers visiting friends and relatives in developing countries, 55
    B
        in travelers visiting friends and relatives in developing countries, 53–54
HIV. See *Human immunodeficiency virus (HIV)*.
HIV infection. See *Human immunodeficiency virus (HIV) infection*.
Human(s)
    parasites of, 174–176
Human African trypanosomiasis
    HIV infection and, 126–128
Human immunodeficiency virus (HIV) infection
    in travelers, 36–39
        medication adherence in, 112–113
        tropical diseases effects of, **121–135**
            Chagas' disease, 128
            human African trypanosomiasis, 126–128
            intestinal helminths, 131–132
            leishmaniasis, 123–126
            liaisis, 130–131
            lymphatic filariasis, 130–131
            malaria, 122–123
            onchocerciasis, 130
            schistosomiasis, 128–130
Hyperparasitemia
    in malaria
        management of, 231

Hypoglycemia
    in malaria
        management of, 229
Hypotension
    in malaria
        management of, 229–230

# I
Illegal immigrants
    Chinese
        falciparum malaria in
            detection of, 11
Immunity
    acquired
        pre-existing
            as factor in malaria in travelers, 214
Immunization(s)
    for travelers
        chlidren, 17–21
        elderly, 27–29
        pregnant, 34
Immunofluorescence-based fecal microscopy
    in diagnostic parasitology, 269
Imported diseases
    travel health risks related to surveillance of, **1–13**. See also *Travel health risks, imported diseases and.*
Infection(s). See also specific types.
    secondary
        in malaria
            management of, 229
In-flight oxygen
    for air travelers, 69–72
International Airlines Transport Association, 73
International emergency and medical evacuation procedures
    for expatriates, refugees, disaster relief workers, and Peace Corps volunteers, **85–101**. See also specific group, e.g., *Expatriate(s)*.
Intestinal helminths
    HIV infection and, 131–132
Iron chelators
    for malaria, 234
Itraconazole
    for cutaneous leishmaniasis in returning travelers, 255

## J

Japanese encephalitis, **157–166**
  described, 157–159
  travelers' risk for, 163–164
  vaccine for
    adverse effects of, 161–163
    described, 159–160
    for travelers, 165–166
    neurologic disease associated with, 162–163

## K

Ketoconazole
  for cutaneous leishmaniasis in returning travelers, 255

## L

Larva(ae)
  duration of stay of, 176–177

Leishmania RDTs
  in diagnostic parasitology, 268

Leishmaniasis(es)
  cutaneous
    in returning travelers, **241–266**. See also *Cutaneous leishmaniasis, in returning travelers.*
    described, 241–244
    geographic distribution of, 241–242
    HIV infection and, 123–126
    life cycle of, 242
  mucosal
    in returning travelers, 248–249
  taxonomy of, 242–244

Liaisis
  HIV infection and, 130–131

Lung injuries
  acute
    in malaria
      management of, 228–229

Lymphatic filariasis
  HIV infection and, 130–131

## M

Malaria
  cerebral
    management of, 226–227
  falciparum. See *Falciparum malaria.*
  HIV infection and, 122–123
  in travelers
    age and, 213
    chemoprophylaxis and, 214
    elderly, 29
    epidemiology of, 185–186, 211–212
    features of, 213–215
    gender and, 213
    genetic resistance and susceptibility and, 213–214
    in developing countries, 57–59
    pre-existing acquired immunity and, 214
    pregnant, 34–35
    prevention of, **185–210**
      atovaquone-proguanil in, 188–192
      azithromycin in, 199–201
      chemoprophylaxis in, 187–188
      drug resistance in, 187–188
      personal protective measures in, 204–205
      primaquine in, 192–195
      standby treatment in, 201–204
      surveillance strategies in, 186–187
      tafenoquine in, 195–199
  rapid diagnostics for, 204
  relief workers with, 89–92
  severe
    acidosis in
      management of, 227–228
    acute lung injury in
      management of, 228–229
    acute renal failure in
      management of, 230–231
    anemia in
      management of, 231–232
    ARDS in
      management of, 228–229
    blackwater fever
      management of, 230
    convulsions in
      management of, 227
    fluid and electrolyte disturbances in
      management of, 230
    fluid overload in
      management of, 228
    hemostatis disorders in
      management of, 231
    hyperparasitemia in
      management of, 231
    hypoglycemia in
      management of, 229

Malaria (continued)
    hypotension in
        management of, 229–230
    in travelers
        antimalarials for, 222–226
        blood film examination in, 217–218
        clinical presentations of, 215–216
        diagnosis of, 217–218
        differential diagnosis of, 216–217
        low clinical suspicion and, 214–215
        management of, 218–222
        underlying disorders and, 214
    respiratory distress in management of, 227
    respiratory tract infection in management of, 228
    secondary infections in management of, 229
    shock in
        management of, 229–230
    splenic rupture in
        management of, 232
    treatment of, **211–240**
        *N*-acetylcysteine in, 234
        anti–tumor necrosis factor measures in, 233–234
        dichloroacetate in, 234
        exchange transfusion in, 232–233
        hemofiltration in, 233
        iron chelators in, 234
        mechanical ventilation in, 233
        pentoxifylline in, 233–234
        renal dialysis in, 233
    travel health risks associated with surveillance of, 3–5
    traveling with young children and, 21–25
    treatment of, **211–240**

Malaria antigens
    in diagnostic parasitology, 269

Malaria RDTs
    in diagnostic parasitology, 268

Mechanical ventilation
    for malaria, 233

Mefloquine
    in malaria prevention in travelers, 187

Microscopy
    fecal
        immunofluorescence-based in diagnostic parasitology, 269

Mucosal leishmaniasis
    in returning travelers, 248–249

Myocardial infarction
    acute
        in expatriates in Ghana, 86–89

## N

Nest parasites, 177–178

Neurologic disease
    Japanese encephalitis vaccine–related, 162–163
    yellow fever vaccine–related, 154

Nonxynol-9
    in STD reduction in travelers contraindications to, 112

## O

Onchocerciasis
    HIV infection and, 130

Oxygen
    in-flight
        for air travelers, 69–72

## P

Parasite(s)
    duration of stay of, 176–177
    human, 174–176
    nest, 177–178
    of momentary duration, 178–179

Parasitology
    new diagnostics in, **1–4**
        antigen detection ELISA, 269
        fecal antigen detection RDTs, 268
        for *Wucheria bancrofti* infection, 268
        immunofluorescence-based fecal microscopy, 269
        leishmania RDTs, 268
        malaria RDTs, 268
        PCR, 269–270
        rapid diagnostics, 268
        RDTs, 268

PCR. See *Polymerase chain reaction (PCR)*.

Peanut(s)
   allergy to
      in air travelers, 75–77

Pentoxifylline
   for malaria, 233–234

Polymerase chain reaction (PCR)
   in diagnostic parasitology, 269–270

Pre-existing acquired immunity
   as factor in malaria in travelers, 214

Pregnancy
   air travel during, 79–80
   traveling during, 32–36
      breast-feeding and, 35–36
      immunizations for, 34
      malaria and, 34–35
      precautions for, 33–34
      traveler's diarrhea and, 35

Primaquine
   in malaria prevention in travelers, 187, 192–195

Proguanil
   in malaria prevention in travelers, 187

Psychosis(es)
   acute
      climber with intermittent blindness and 24-hour history of
         case example, 96–99

# R

Rapid diagnostic tests (RDTs)
   in diagnostic parasitology, 268

RDTs. See *Rapid diagnostic tests (RDTs)*.

Relief workers
   malaria in, 89–92
   schistosomiasis in, 89–92

Renal dialysis
   for malaria, 233

Renal failure
   acute
      in malaria
         management of, 230–231

Respiratory distress
   in malaria
      management of, 227

Respiratory tract infection
   in malaria
      management of, 228

Rupture
   splenic
      in malaria
         management of, 232

# S

Safety
   of elderly traveling, 27

SARS. See *Severe acute respiratory syndrome (SARS)*.

Schistosomiasis
   HIV infection and, 128–130
   relief workers with, 89–92

Secondary infections
   in malaria
      management of, 229

Seizure disorders
   travelers with, 43–44

Severe acute respiratory syndrome (SARS)
   air travel and, 68

Sex
   as factor in malaria in travelers, 213

Sexual tourism, **103–120**

Sexually transmitted diseases (STDs)
   in travelers
      experiences of, 113–116
      risk assessment for
         before travel, 107–113
      risk-reduction behavior related to
         condoms, 111–112
         counseling, 110
         educational messages related to, 110–111
         nonxynol-9
            contraindications to, 112
      screening tests for
         before travel, 107–113
      travel and
         connections between, 104–107, 116–117

Shock
   in malaria
      management of, 229–230

Splenic rupture
   in malaria
      management of, 232

STDs. See *Sexually transmitted diseases (STDs)*.

# INDEX

## T

Tafenoquine
  in malaria prevention in travelers, 195–199
Tanzania
  African trypanosomiasis from detection of, 10–11
$T_H1$-$T_H2$ balance
  review of, 124–125
Thymus disease
  yellow fever vaccine and, 157
Tick(s)
  duration of stay of, 176
Tourism
  sexual, **103–120**
Transformation(s)
  exchange
    for malaria, 232–233
Transplantation(s)
  travelers with, 39–43
Travel
  STDs and, 104–107, 116–117
Travel clinic
  challenging scenarios in, **15–47**
    cancer chemotherapy survivors, 39–43
    diabetic travelers, 30–32
    pregnant travelers, 32–36
    transplant-recipient travelers, 39–43
    travelers with asplenia, 39–43
    travelers with HIV and AIDS, 36–39
    travelers with seizure disorders, 43–44
    traveling with the elderly, 26–30
    traveling with young children, 16–26
Travel delay recommendations
  health risks and, 72–73
Travel health risks
  imported diseases and
    African trypanosomiasis from Tanzania, 10–11
    dengue fever, 5–6
    falciparum malaria
      in Dominican Republic, 8–10
      in illegal Chinese immigrants, 11
    malaria, 3–5
    risk estimates, 6–8
  sentinel events detection in, 8–11
  surveillance of, **1–13**
  systematic observations of, 3–6
Travel medicine guide
  to arthropods of medical importance, **169–183**. See also *Arthropod(s), of medical importance.*
Traveler(s)
  air
    health risks to, **67–84**. See also *Air travelers, health risks to.*
  complex
    advice for, **15–47**. See also *Travel clinic, challenging scenarios in.*
  diabetic, 30–32
  HIV infection in, 112. See also *Sexually transmitted diseases (SDTs).*
  Japanese encephalitis in
    risk factors for, 163–164
    vaccine for, 165–166
  malaria in. See *Malaria, in travelers.*
  pregnant, 32–36
  returning
    cutaneous leishmaniasis in, 241–266. See also *Cutaneous leishmaniasis, in returning travelers.*
  visiting friends and relatives in developing countries
    disease prevention in, **49–65**
      new approach to counseling in, 51–52
    hepatitis A in, 55
    hepatitis B in, 53–54
    high-risk diseases in, 53–61
    malaria in, 57–59
    morbidity associated with, 50–51
    risk assessment for, **49–65**
      general recommendations, 52–53
    routine childhood vaccine–preventable diseases in, 53
    tuberculosis in, 59–61
    typhoid fever in, 55–56
    varicella in, 56–57
Traveler's diarrhea, **137–149**
  causes of, 142–143
  diagnosis of, 143–144
  in pregnant travelers, 35
  in the elderly, 29
  in young children, 25
  prevention of
    nonantibiotic methods in, 142

personal hygiene precautions in, 139–141
vaccines in, 146
treatment of, 144–145

Traveling
with the elderly, 26–30
immunizations for, 27–29
malaria, 29
safety of, 27
traveler's diarrhea in, 29
with young children, 16–26
immunizations, 17–21
malaria, 21–25
preparation for, 17
traveler's diarrhea, 25

Tropical diseases
HIV infection effects on, **121–135**. See also *Human immunodeficiency virus (HIV) infection, tropical diseases effects of.*

Trypanosomiasis
African
from Tanzania
detection of, 10–11
HIV infection and, 126–128

Tuberculosis
in air travelers, 69
in travelers visiting friends and relatives in developing countries, 59–61

Typhoid fever
in travelers visiting friends and relatives in developing countries, 55–56

## V

Vaccine(s)
for traveler's diarrhea, 146
for yellow fever, **151–157**. See also *Yellow fever, vaccine for.*

Varicella
in travelers visiting friends and relatives in developing countries, 56–57

Ventilation
mechanical
for malaria, 233

Viscerotropic disease
yellow fever vaccine–related, 154–155

## W

*Wucheria bancrofti* infection
RDTs for, 268

## Y

Yellow fever
described, 151–153
vaccine for, **151–157**
adverse effects of, 153–155
age-related, 156
risks factors for, 156–157
described, 153
neurologic disease associated with, 154
thymus disease associated with, 157
viscerotropic disease associated with, 154–155

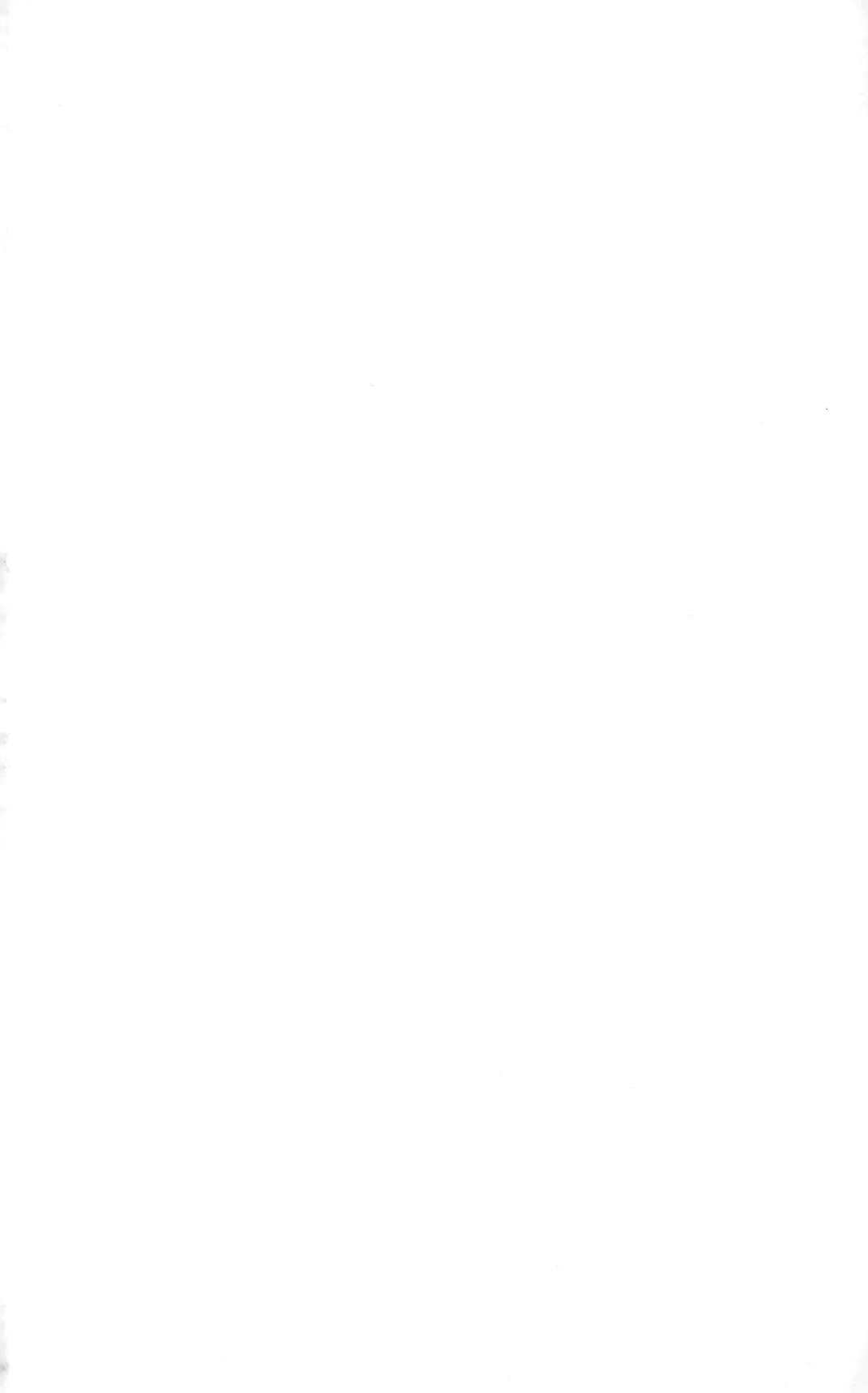

# Changing Your Address?

Make sure your subscription changes too! When you notify us of your new address, you can help make our job easier by including an exact copy of your Clinics label number with your old address (see illustration below.) This number identifies you to our computer system and will speed the processing of your address change. Please be sure this label number accompanies your old address and your corrected address—you can send an old Clinics label with your number on it or just copy it exactly and send it to the address listed below.

We appreciate your help in our attempt to give you continuous coverage. Thank you.

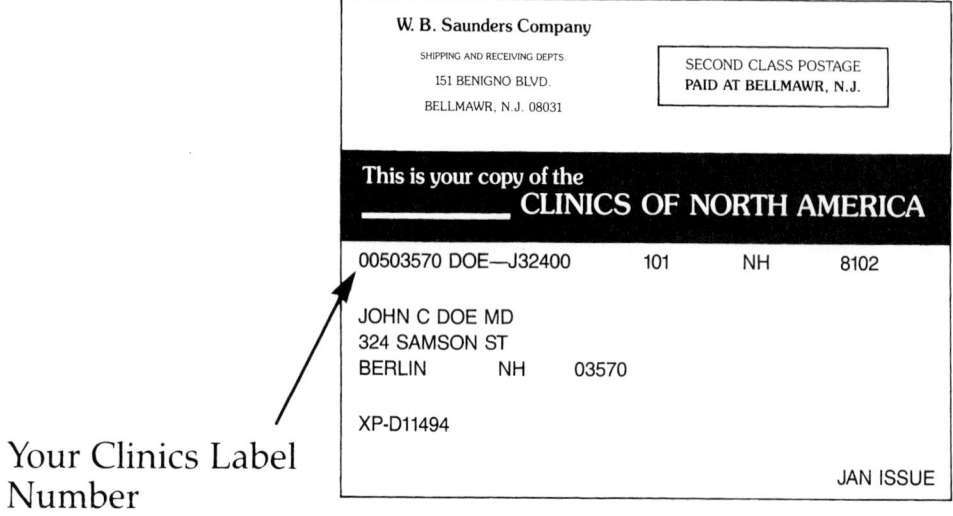

```
W. B. Saunders Company
  SHIPPING AND RECEIVING DEPTS.
       151 BENIGNO BLVD.
       BELLMAWR, N.J. 08031

           SECOND CLASS POSTAGE
           PAID AT BELLMAWR, N.J.

This is your copy of the
_____ CLINICS OF NORTH AMERICA

00503570 DOE—J32400      101      NH      8102

JOHN C DOE MD
324 SAMSON ST
BERLIN       NH      03570

XP-D11494
                                        JAN ISSUE
```

## Your Clinics Label Number
Copy it exactly or send your label along with your address to:
**W.B. Saunders Company, Customer Service**
Orlando, FL 32887-4800
Call Toll Free 1-800-654-2452

Please allow four to six weeks for delivery of new subscriptions and for processing address changes.

**YES!** Please start my subscription to the **CLINICS** checked below with the ❑ first issue of the calendar year or ❑ current issues. If not completely satisfied with my first issue, I may write "cancel" on the invoice and return it within 30 days at no further obligation.

## Please Print:

Name _____

Address _____

City _____ State _____ ZIP _____

## Method of Payment

❑ Check (payable to **Elsevier**; add the applicable sales tax for your area)

❑ VISA   ❑ MasterCard   ❑ AmEx   ❑ Bill me

Card number _____ Exp. date _____

Signature _____

Staple this to your purchase order to expedite delivery

---

❑ **Adolescent Medicine Clinics**
  ❑ Individual $95
  ❑ Institutions $133
  ❑ *In-training $48

❑ **Anesthesiology**
  ❑ Individual $175
  ❑ Institutions $270
  ❑ *In-training $88

❑ **Cardiology**
  ❑ Individual $170
  ❑ Institutions $266
  ❑ *In-training $85

❑ **Chest Medicine**
  ❑ Individual $185
  ❑ Institutions $285

❑ **Child and Adolescent Psychiatry**
  ❑ Individual $175
  ❑ Institutions $265
  ❑ *In-training $88

❑ **Critical Care**
  ❑ Individual $165
  ❑ Institutions $266
  ❑ *In-training $83

❑ **Dental**
  ❑ Individual $150
  ❑ Institutions $242

❑ **Emergency Medicine**
  ❑ Individual $170
  ❑ Institutions $263
  ❑ *In-training $85
    ❑ Send CME info

❑ **Facial Plastic Surgery**
  ❑ Individual $199
  ❑ Institutions $300

❑ **Foot and Ankle**
  Individual $160
  Institutions $232

❑ **Gastroenterology**
  ❑ Individual $190
  ❑ Institutions $276

❑ **Gastrointestinal Endoscopy**
  ❑ Individual $190
  ❑ Institutions $276

❑ **Hand**
  ❑ Individual $205
  ❑ Institutions $319

❑ **Heart Failure (NEW in 2005!)**
  ❑ Individual $99
  ❑ Institutions $149
  ❑ *In-training $49

❑ **Hematology/Oncology**
  ❑ Individual $210
  ❑ Institutions $315

❑ **Immunology & Allergy**
  ❑ Individual $165
  ❑ Institutions $266

❑ **Infectious Disease**
  ❑ Individual $165
  ❑ Institutions $272

❑ **Clinics in Liver Disease**
  ❑ Individual $165
  ❑ Institutions $234

❑ **Medical**
  ❑ Individual $140
  ❑ Institutions $244
  ❑ *In-training $70
    ❑ Send CME info

❑ **MRI**
  ❑ Individual $190
  ❑ Institutions $290
  ❑ *In-training $95
    ❑ Send CME info

❑ **Neuroimaging**
  ❑ Individual $190
  ❑ Institutions $290
  ❑ *In-training $95
    ❑ Send CME inf0

❑ **Neurologic**
  ❑ Individual $175
  ❑ Institutions $275

❑ **Obstetrics & Gynecology**
  ❑ Individual $175
  ❑ Institutions $288

❑ **Occupational and Environmental Medicine**
  ❑ Individual $120
  ❑ Institutions $166
  ❑ *In-training $60

❑ **Ophthalmology**
  ❑ Individual $190
  ❑ Institutions $325

❑ **Oral & Maxillofacial Surgery**
  ❑ Individual $180
  ❑ Institutions $280
  ❑ *In-training $90

❑ **Orthopedic**
  ❑ Individual $180
  ❑ Institutions $295
  ❑ *In-training $90

❑ **Otolaryngologic**
  ❑ Individual $199
  ❑ Institutions $350

❑ **Pediatric**
  ❑ Individual $135
  ❑ Institutions $246
  ❑ *In-training $68
    ❑ Send CME info

❑ **Perinatology**
  ❑ Individual $155
  ❑ Institutions $237
  ❑ *In-training $78
    ❑ Send CME inf0

❑ **Plastic Surgery**
  ❑ Individual $245
  ❑ Institutions $370

❑ **Podiatric Medicine & Surgery**
  ❑ Individual $170
  ❑ Institutions $266

❑ **Primary Care**
  ❑ Individual $135
  ❑ Institutions $223

❑ **Psychiatric**
  ❑ Individual $170
  ❑ Institutions $288

❑ **Radiologic**
  ❑ Individual $220
  ❑ Institutions $331
  ❑ *In-training $110
    ❑ Send CME info

❑ **Sports Medicine**
  ❑ Individual $180
  ❑ Institutions $277

❑ **Surgical**
  ❑ Individual $190
  ❑ Institutions $299
  ❑ *In-training $95

❑ **Thoracic Surgery (formerly Chest Surgery)**
  ❑ Individual $175
  ❑ Institutions $255
  ❑ *In-training $88

❑ **Urologic**
  ❑ Individual $195
  ❑ Institutions $307
  ❑ *In-training $98
    ❑ Send CME info

---

*To receive in-training rate, orders must be accompanied by the name of affiliated institution, dates of residency and signature of coordinator on institution letterhead. Orders will be billed at the individual rate until proof of resident status is received.

© Elsevier 2005. Offer valid in U.S. only. Prices subject to change without notice. MO 10808 DF4184

Order your subscription today. Simply complete and detach this card and drop it in the mail to receive the best clinical information in your field.

NO POSTAGE
NECESSARY
IF MAILED
IN THE
UNITED STATES

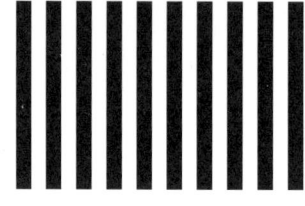

**BUSINESS REPLY MAIL**
FIRST-CLASS MAIL   PERMIT NO 7135   ORLANDO FL

POSTAGE WILL BE PAID BY ADDRESSEE

PERIODICALS ORDER FULFILLMENT DEPT
ELSEVIER
6277 SEA HARBOR DR
ORLANDO FL 32821-9816